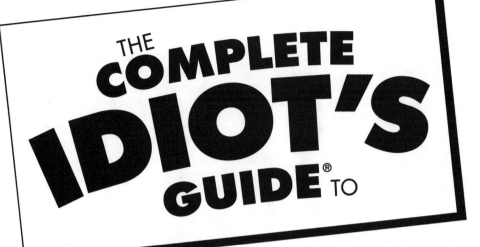

THE COMPLETE IDIOT'S GUIDE® TO

Yoga with Kids

by Jodi B. Komitor, M.A., C.Y.K.F., and Eve Adamson, M.F.A.

alpha books

Publisher
Marie Butler-Knight

Product Manager
Phil Kitchel

Managing Editor
Cari Luna

Acquisitions Editors
Mike Sanders
Susan Zingraf

Book Producer
Lee Ann Chearney/Amaranth

Development Editor
Lynn Northrup

Production Editor
Christy Wagner

Copy Editor
Susan Aufheimer

Illustrator
Jessica Wolk-Stanley

Photographer
Steven Goldberg

Cartoonist
Jody Schaeffer

Cover Designers
Mike Freeland
Kevin Spear

Book Designers
Scott Cook and Amy Adams of DesignLab

Indexer
Tonya Heard

Layout/Proofreading
Svetlana Dominguez
John Etchison
Wendy Ott
Gloria Schurick

Contents at a Glance

Part 1: Let's Get into Yoga with Kids   **1**

1   Why Yoga Is Great for Kids   3
Yoga is an ancient system of mind-body health that builds strength, flexibility, self-esteem, and imagination in contemporary kids and their families.

2   Health Benefits of Yoga for Kids   15
Yoga helps kids' bodies work at their most efficient by strengthening muscles, toning internal organs, tuning fine-motor coordination, improving posture, and helping kids sleep better, too.

3   Developmental Benefits of Yoga for Kids   29
Yoga facilitates physical, emotional, and mental development in kids from infancy through the teen years.

Part 2: Growing with the Tree of Yoga   **43**

4   Kids on the Eightfold Path   45
Yoga isn't religious, but it is spiritual. Introduce kids to yoga's Eightfold Path for better living.

5   Energized, Focused, and Carefree Kids   63
Yoga helps kids develop their emotional selves, live in the moment, focus on the task at hand, and handle problems peacefully. It also teaches parents to be good role models.

6   Kids Choose!   75
Yoga builds self-esteem in kids by fostering a noncompetitive spirit; teaching kids to respect, nurture, and love themselves and each other; and developing kids' natural creativity.

Part 3: Doing Yoga with Kids   **85**

7   Setting Up a Yoga Space   87
Help a child craft a personal yoga space.

8   Practicing Yoga with Kids   97
Find the right yoga approach for each child's unique learning style, then help each child develop a yoga routine.

9   Finding the Right Yoga Teacher or Class   111
Yoga classes can be lots of fun. Here's how to focus your yoga goals, find the right class and teacher, or start your very own yoga club!

Part 4: Yoga Songs, Play, and Postures   **125**

10 Chanting and Breathing   127
Breathing is at the heart of a successful yoga practice. Learn breathing techniques and familiarize yourself with mantras, mudras, chanting, and chakras.

11 Nature: You Be a Mountain, I'll Be a Tree   145
Yoga is designed to emulate different aspects of the natural world. Get closer to nature (and to yourself) through nature yoga poses.

12 What Animal Are You?   159
From cats and cows to flamingos and seagulls, animal play is great yoga fun.

13 Exploring the Desert   175
Desert creatures inspire the poses in this chapter—be a cobra, a camel, or a cactus!

14 Exploring the Wild   185
Kids love to get wild! Become a bucking bronco, a unicorn, a shark, a crocodile, or the formidable T. rex!

Part 5: Super Yoginis on the Move and Staying Still   **197**

15 Kids on the Move   199
Yoga for kids is full of movement, rhythm, dancing, spinning, marching, and even a little rock 'n' roll!

16 Super Yogini!   215
These super-powered poses (such as Hero Pose and the Warrior poses) increase strength and self-confidence.

17 Yoginis on Top of the World   233
Build coordination and confidence with these fun and sometimes challenging yoga poses, from Headstand to Toe-ups.

18 Yogini Fun and Games   247
Yoga games are fun with more than one! Try partner and group yoga.

19 Quiet Time   257
Stillness and deep relaxation are as much a part of yoga as action and movement.

Part 6: Especially for New Families   **267**

20 Yoga for Postpartum Moms and Brand-New Dads   269
Yoga strategies for new moms, new dads, and postpartum recovery.

21 Yoga with Infants and Toddlers   281
   Babies love yoga! Parents, soothe your infant and delight
   your toddler as you promote development.

22 Hey, Kids: Do Yoga with Your Little Brother or Sister   295
   Yoga makes for sibling fun and a strong sibling bond
   when the yoga principles for living are applied for greater
   sibling harmony.

Part 7: Yoga All Day Long!   307

23 Eating for Strong Minds and Bodies   309
   Make sure your kids and your entire family are eating for
   maximum health and enjoyment.

24 Yoga to Make Kids Feel Better   319
   Yoga is an effective natural remedy for many ailments of
   childhood, from colic to constipation to problems with
   concentration.

25 Yoga for Kids with Special Needs   329
   Yoga therapy encourages healthy development and self-
   esteem in kids with special needs, from attention deficit
   hyperactivity disorder to Down's syndrome and cerebral
   palsy.

26 Yoga for Teens   339
   As teens establish their independence, yoga provides the
   inner strength, self-esteem, and compassion required to
   help them step confidently into the adult world.

27 Surprise: A Yoga Kids Party!   347
   Everybody loves a party, especially if yoga is the theme.
   Find great party ideas and a few recipes here.

Appendixes

A Glossary   357

B Resources   363

  Index   371

Contents

Part 1: Let's Get into Yoga with Kids   **1**

1 Why Yoga Is Great for Kids   **3**

What Is Yoga? 4
   Yoga Is Union 4
   Yoga Traditions: Everything Old Is New Again 5
Working the Entire Body and Mind 6
   Building a Strong Body..7
   Building a Strong Mind 8
Yoga Is a Self-Esteem Booster! 9
Yoga for the Next Generation 11
   Kids of All Ages Love Yoga 12
   You'll Love Yoga, Too! 12
   Yoga Fun for the Whole Family 13

2 Health Benefits of Yoga for Kids   **15**

Yoga Promotes Good Internal Health for Kids 16
   Yoga Aids Kids' Digestion and Elimination...........18
   Yoga Develops Stronger Hearts and Lungs 18
   Yoga Massages Internal Organs and Glands 20
   Yoga Fine-Tunes Motor Coordination 22
Yoga Power! 23
   Muscling in on Flexibility..23
   Even More Stamina 24
   Gaining Stability and Balance 24
   All About Joints 24
Elongate for a Healthy Spine.......................................25
   Posture Perfect 26
   Energizing the Nervous System 27
Good, Restful, Refreshing Sleep for Kids......................28

3 Developmental Benefits of Yoga for Kids   **29**

From Cradle to Empty Nest...30
   Developmental Milestones for Children...................30
   Meeting Kids' Needs 34
Exploring the World with Yogini Babies........................34

Nonstop Fun with Yogini Toddlers 36
Imagine Everything with Yogini Preschoolers 38
Loving and Learning with Yogini Grade-Schoolers 38
Changing and Growing with Yogini Teens......................39

Part 2: Growing with the Tree of Yoga   43

4   Kids on the Eightfold Path   45

Introducing Yoginis to Their Spiritual Nature 46
   Can Kids Do Yoga Without Being Spiritual? 46
   Yoga Embraces All Religions 46
What Is Yoga's Eightfold Path? 47
Yamas and Niyamas for Yoginis 48
   Yama Values: Living Well in the World 49
   Niyama Do's: Learning About Yourself 53
More Adventures on the Yoga Path 57
   Control Your Body (Asanas) 57
   Breathe for Life (Pranayama) 58
   Calm Your Senses (Pratyahara).................................58
   Focus Your Mind (Dharana) 58
   Meditate (Dhyana)...59
   Touch the Divine (Samadhi) 60
Walking the Yoga Path as a Family 60

5   Energized, Focused, and Carefree Kids   63

We Live in a Hectic World....................................64
Yoga Puts Kids in Touch with Their Thoughts
  and Feelings 65
   Mindfulness: Identifying Thought and Emotion 65
   Using the Body to Calm the Mind................................67
   Using the Mind to Calm the Body................................68
   Energizing the Mind-Body......................................68
How Yoga Tames Kids' Anger 70
How Yoga Helps When Kids Feel Pressure to
  Compete..71
How Yoga Helps Kids Learn to Resolve
  Problems Peacefully 72
Walking the Yoga Walk 72

What Parents Need to Do, Too 73
Like Parent, Like Child? *73*
How Parents Handle Anger and Conflict.............*73*
Yogis and Yoginis Unite: Do Yoga with Your Kids *74*

6 Kids Choose!   **75**

Teaching Kids to Love Who They Are, Body and Soul 76
Embracing Yoga Union *76*
Learning to Trust *77*
Every Body Has Something to Learn.......................77
Helping Kids Discover How Their Bodies Work *78*
Progress Is a Relative Thing *79*
Accepting the Challenge to Grow *80*
Girls and Boys: Yogini Warriors for a Better World 80
Self-Esteem Fosters Confidence and Generosity 81
Yoga Invention: Another Chance to Shine......................82

Part 3: Doing Yoga with Kids   **85**

7 Setting Up a Yoga Space   **87**

Kids Can Do Yoga Almost Anywhere! 88
Setting Up a Yoga Space at Home 88
How Is a Yoga Space Different from a Playroom? *90*
What You'll Need....................................*91*
Room to Grow *92*
Yogini Gear: Yoga Clothes and Props 93
Honoring Your Yoga Space 94
Making Yoga a Family Routine 95

8 Practicing Yoga with Kids   **97**

The What, When, Where, Why, and How 98
Yogini Personalities 99
Selecting the Right Practice...............................106
Inside or Out? *106*
Supervised or Unsupervised? *108*
Solo, or with Others? *108*
Sticking to a Routine 109
How to Use and Where to Buy Yoga Books
and Videos 109
Encouraging a Yogini Lotus Blossom 109

9 Finding the Right Yoga Teacher or Class   111

Wanna Take a Class? 112
  Where to Look for Classes in Your Area 112
  Yoga Teachers with the Right Stuff 113
Can't Find a Class? Start Your Own Club 115
Yoga + Sports = Fun! 118
  Yoga as Part of a Balanced Exercise Program 118
  Coaxing Kids to Exercise 119
  Yogini Athletes Reach for Peak Performance 120
Yoginis with Special Needs 121
  Yoga and Children with Learning Challenges 121
  Yoga and Children with Physical Challenges.........122
Samyama: Lifelong Learning..122

Part 4: Yoga Songs, Play, and Postures   125

10 Chanting and Breathing   127

Yogini Prana Power 127
  The Breath of Life: What the Lungs Do 129
  In a Heartbeat: What the Heart Does...................130
Learning to Sit and Stand to Your Best Potential 130
Ohmmmm, My!...131
  Making Up Mantra Songs 134
  Handy Mudras 134
Breathing Through the Chakras 135
Okay, Breathe..137
  Belly Breathing..137
  Balloon Breathing 138
  Energizing Breath Exercises.................................138
  Calming Breath Exercises 140

11 Nature: You Be a Mountain, I'll Be a Tree   145

Discovering Your Yogini Nature 146
Respecting the Essence of All Things 147
Nature Play..149
  Mountain Pose (Tadasana)....................................149
  Tree Pose (Vrikshasana) 150
  Frog Pose (Malasana) 152
  Butterfly Pose (Baddha Konasana) 152
  Flower Pose 153

Star Pose *154*

Rainbow Pose (Vasisthasana) *155*

Take a Yogini Nature Walk 157

12 What Animal Are You?   159

Discovering Your Yogini Animal Nature 160

Learning from Animal Behaviors and Movements 161

Animal Play at Home and on the Farm 162

Cat Pose (Bidalasana) 162

Cow Pose 163

Downward Facing Dog Pose (Adho Mukha Shavasana) 164

Mouse Pose (Pindasana) 166

Birds of a Feather 166

Flamingo Pose 167

Eagle Pose (Garudaasana) 168

Pigeon Pose (Ekapada Rajakapotasana) 169

Swan Pose 171

Seagull Pose 172

Crow Pose (Bakasana) 173

13 Exploring the Desert   175

Destination: Desert 176

Make Like a Snake 176

Baby Snake Pose 176

Mother Snake Pose (Bhujangaasana) 177

Father Snake Pose 178

Wise and Wonderful 179

Wise Owl Pose 179

Camel Pose (Ushtraasana) 181

Desert Still Life 182

Roadrunner Pose 182

Cactus Pose 183

14 Exploring the Wild   185

Hooves and Horns 185

Bucking Bronco Pose 186

Deer Pose (Marichyasana) 187

Unicorn Pose 187

Giraffe Walk 189

Antelope Dash 190

Beware: Wild Animals Ahead! 191
  Bear Walk *191*
  Shark Pose *192*
  Crocodile Pose (Makaraasana) *193*
  Alligator Pose *194*
  T. Rex *Pose* *195*
  Tarzan Holler *195*

**Part 5: Super Yoginis on the Move and
            Staying Still   197**

15 Kids on the Move   199

Finding the Yoga Groove...199
  Who's Got Rhythm?...*200*
  The Equilibrium of Motion *200*
The Yoga Sun Dance (Surya Namaskar) 201
Go, Go, Go! 203
  Yoga Dancing..*203*
  Roller Coaster Spin..*205*
  Flopping Rag Doll *206*
  Volcano Blast...*207*
  "The Ants Go Marching" March.........................*209*
  Driving My Car *210*
  Rock and Roll...*211*
  Boat Poses *212*

16 Super Yogini!   215

Yoginis Holding Their Own...215
Yogini Strength 216
  Hero Pose (Parvatasana)..................................*216*
  Superperson Pose *217*
  Warrior I Pose (Virabhadrasana I) *218*
  Warrior II Pose (Virabhadrasana II) *220*
  Warrior III Pose (Virabhadrasana III) *221*
  Table Pose *221*
  Slide Pose (Purvottanasana) *222*
  Handstand Pose (Adho Mukha Vrikshasana) *223*
Yoga Flexibility...225
  Untying Knots *225*
  Twister Pose (Supta Parivartanasana)............*226*
  Bow Pose (Dhanurasana) *227*

Sandwich Pose (Paschima Uttanasana)............................228
Bridge Pose (Setu Bandha Sarvangaasana) 230
Wheel Pose (Urdhva Dhanurasana) 230
X Pose 231

17 Yoginis on Top of the World   233

Yoga Coordination..233
The Eyes Have It 234
Toe-Ups 235
Windmill 236
Crossovers 237
Bicycle Pose 238
Yoga Confidence..239
Pretzel Pose 239
Lotus Pose (Padmaasana)..240
Candle Pose (Sarvangaasana) 241
Plow Pose (Halaasana)..242
Fish Pose (Matsynasan) 243
Headstand 244

18 Yogini Fun and Games   247

Two Can Be as Much Fun as One! 247
Partner Straddle Stretching 248
Mirror Me 249
Assist Me 250
For the Whole Gang! 252
Whisper in My Ear..252
Yogini's Choice..252
Animal Enigma 253
Synchronized Yoga 254
Yoga Games of Your Own Design 255

19 Quiet Time   257

The Virtue of Stillness 258
Shavasana: Yoga's Peaceful Pose 258
Visual Imagery to Relax You 260
Rainbow Relaxation 260
Cloud Floating Relaxation 261
Rainforest Relaxation 262
After Visualization and Deep Relaxation 264
Moving from Shavasana into the Day 265

Part 6: Especially for New Families   267

20 Yoga for Postpartum Moms and Brand-New Dads   269

You've Got a New Baby! 270
Yoga's Postpartum Poses for New Moms........................270
   Breathing Exercises (Pranayama) 271
   Yoga Poses for Postpartum Moms (Asanas)................273
   Deep Relaxation (Shavasana) 274
When You've Had a Cesarean Delivery............................275
Hey, Dad! 277

21 Yoga with Infants and Toddlers   281

Getting to Know You..281
   Baby Breather 283
   Footsies 283
   Knees, Please! 284
   Get Hip, Baby! 284
   Yogini's Sleep Pose 285
   Up in Arms 285
   Tummy Time 286
   Upside-Down Baby! 287
   Baby Relaxation..288
Toddler Land: Learning Through Play 289
Imagine This! 291
   A Trip to the Zoo 291
   A Trip to the Park 292
   Toddler Trip 293

22 Hey, Kids: Do Yoga with Your Little Brother or Sister   295

There's a Baby in the House!..295
   How Yoga Helps When You Bring a New Baby Home 297
   Yoga Unions: Forging the Sibling Bond 298
As They Grow 298
The Yogini's Ten Steps for Sibling Synchronicity 298
   Step 1: Live in Peace..299
   Step 2: Tell the Truth 299
   Step 3: Let Go of the Toy 299

Step 4: Practice Self-Control 299
Step 5: Share and Share Alike 299
Step 6: Clean It Up 300
Step 7: Don't Worry, Be Happy! 300
Step 8: Work Together 300
Step 9: Study Together 301
Step 10: Believe in Magic 301
Loving Responsibility 301
Yoga Poses Yogini Brothers and Sisters Can
Do Together 302
Puppy Play with Downward Facing Dog 302
The Cobra Family 303
Family Picnic 303
Club Sandwich 304
Foot Massage Fun 305
It Takes a Family 306

Part 7: Yoga All Day Long! 307

23 Eating for Strong Minds and Bodies 309

Food, American-Style 310
What Do Kids in America Eat? 310
What Is Your Family Eating? 311
What Could Your Family Be Eating? 312
Food, Prepared Yoga-Style 312
Is Your Food Sattvic, Rajasic, or Tamasic? 313
Do You Have to Be Vegetarian? 314
Developing Good Eating Habits 315
Practice Mindful Eating as a Family 316
The Sacred Ritual of the Family Meal 316
*The Zen of Who You Are, What You Eat,
and What You Do* 317
Good Snacks 317

24 Yoga to Make Kids Feel Better 319

Yoga Is a Great Natural Remedy 319
Yoga, Plus Other Great Health Alternatives 320
Knowing When to Call the Doctor 321
Yoga for What Ails Kids 322
Yoga to Relieve Baby's Colic 322

Yoga for Kids' Asthma and Breathing Problems 322
Yoga for Kids' Upset Stomachs, Gas, Constipation,
    and Diarrhea 323
Yoga to Ease Kids' Aching Backs 324
    Those Backpacks Are Heavy! *324*
    Keeping the Spine Healthy *324*
Recovering from Sprains, Strains, and Breaks.................325
Yoga to Help Kids Concentrate and Increase
    Mental Alertness 326

25 Yoga for Kids with Special Needs   329

Every Kid Can Excel at Yoga 330
    Designing a Yoga Practice for Each Unique Child *330*
Yoga for Kids Who Learn Differently 332
    ADHD (Attention Deficit Hyperactivity Disorder) *333*
    Learning Disabilities *333*
Yoga for Kids Who Have Physical Challenges 335
    Too Loose: Hypermobility and Down's Syndrome *335*
    Too Tight: Stiffness and Cerebral Palsy...............................*336*
    Paralysis, Immobility, and Yoga *336*
    Too Little Tone: Hypocerebratonicity and Weak Muscles *337*
Helping Kids Believe They Can Achieve Their Goals 337

26 Yoga for Teens   339

Independence Day..340
Welcoming Teens into the Adult Community 341
What Yoga Teaches Young Men 341
    Getting Strong *342*
    Boys to Men..*342*
    Boys Growing Up Yoga Style *343*
What Yoga Teaches Young Women....................................343
    Entering the Cycle *344*
    Girls to Women *344*
    Girls Growing Up Yoga Style..*345*
Next Generation Yoginis 345

27 Surprise: A Yoga Kids Party! **347**

Yoginis Unite! 348
A Kid Party Every Parent Can Love....................................348
What Parents Need to Know About Kids' Parties 348
Keeping Kids Safe...349
What You'll Need for a Karma-Licious Yoga Party 349
Yogini Party Invitations 350
Yogini Party Decorations 350
Yogini Party Food..351
Yogini Party Favors 353
Yogini Party Fun 354

Appendixes

A Glossary **357**

B Resources **363**

Index **371**

Foreword

On Wednesday, I got the call. Jodi Komitor wanted me to write the foreword for her new book. Jodi had been a student of mine, a friend and yoga associate. We seem to always share a common view of yoga and how it applies to modern New York life. I have been teaching fitness and yoga classes for close to 20 years, and I think Jodi felt I could have some insight on her manuscript. The manuscript was overnighted to me, and of course there was the usual hate-to-rush-you-but-we-need-it-yesterday note attached. I was on my way to the West Coast to visit my daughter and to attend a yoga workshop—her idea. A family yoga weekend. With many hours of plane time ahead, I settled down to read Jodi's manuscript.

Six hours later as I landed in California, I stared out the window and thought about how lucky I was to be sharing this weekend with my daughter and doing something we both love together. I have been practicing and teaching yoga for over 10 years, and it has made a tremendous positive impact on my life and now hers as well. I felt very grateful for this ancient science's presence in my life. Wow. I had been really affected by Jodi's manuscript. I have read the ancient texts and the big, important yoga books out today, and yet Jodi's book made me think. I had learned some new lessons:

➤ *It's never too early to begin creating a positive context for life.* Yoga can help all kids and their parents practice positive ways of looking at themselves and others. That with so many negative images out there for kids to identify with, *The Complete Idiot's Guide to Yoga with Kids* offers a fun and meaningful path that helps build self-esteem during this important developmental stage.

➤ *We are all very different. Every one of us is unique, special, and whole.* Kids and adults. This book supports the notion that kids need to express themselves creatively and individually and gives you lots of great ways to do that.

➤ *Start taking care of your body when you are young.* Teaching as many adults as I do, I know how hard it is to begin a yoga program when you get older. Yoga offers a noncompetitive, physical way to exercise your body and play at the same time. Adults will find this useful, too.

➤ *Life's lessons are simple. Remembering them is complicated.* Treat yourself and your body well. Do unto others as you would have them do unto you. Play a lot. Be creative and express yourself wildly. Respect yourself and all living things, including the earth. Be true to your animal nature.

➤ *Kids learn from us and our participation in their lives.* But ultimately we learn from them. Kids of all ages will enjoy and get plenty of value from this book.

As I got up from my seat, gathered up my belongings and began to exit the plane, I thought about what an amazing world we could live in if more of us practiced yoga. What a wonderful contribution this book is—not just to parents and kids but to the whole world. Wow. This book is a simple guide to an ancient science in a complex time in history that will give kids the tools to live a positive life that contributes and gives something back. With that, I slung my yoga mat across my back, inspired to have a great weekend and feeling great about the life I had chosen. Thanks to Jodi Komitor and Eve Adamson for writing a book for all ages and giving me an opportunity to participate in it.

Molly Fox

A leader in the United States yoga community, Molly Fox has been teaching fitness and yoga for 20 years in the New York City area and currently co-owns and operates Yoga People yoga center in Brooklyn, New York, serving yoginis of all ages. Look for Molly's videos, *Yoga for Everyone, Molly Fox's Yoga Moves, Molly Fox's Yoga Sculpts,* and *Molly Fox's Yoga Stretches and Relaxes.*

Introduction

Do you remember what it was like to spend whole days just playing? If you are a child, play is probably a big part of your life. If you are a parent, you may remember when your backyard or bedroom or the long dark hallway into the den were so much more than rooms in your house—jungles, forests, forts, palaces, vast oceans, tunnels through the center of the earth.

For children, every day is an adventure because the imagination and creativity in a child is so present, accessible, and vivid. Likewise, yoga—that most ancient and most modern of physical and spiritual practices—takes on an added lightness, joy, and carefree spirit when practiced by children.

Yoga allows a child's natural creativity and imagination to flourish, aided by lots of "pretend" games, nature and animal poses, active movement, dress-up with props, and even deep relaxation. Yoga provides dramatic physical, emotional, mental, developmental, and spiritual benefits to all kids, from infants to teenagers, from the physically challenged to those challenged by learning disorders or developmental delays.

And yoga with kids can become an enlightening experience for grownups, too. Yoga can create a space for family in a way that benefits everyone, builds relationships, and forms lasting bonds and enduring memories. A treasure-trove awaits you, whether you are a child or a parent, and your family within the pages of this book. To discover it, all you need to do is keep reading.

How to Use This Book

The Complete Idiot's Guide to Yoga with Kids is divided into seven parts, each focusing on a different aspect of practicing yoga with kids:

Part 1, "Let's Get into Yoga with Kids," defines this ancient tradition and shows how yoga is as relevant today for kids of all ages as it was thousands of years ago. Yoga helps kids' bodies grow and develop to be strong, flexible, and coordinated. It promotes development in infants and toddlers, encourages imaginative play and coordination in preschoolers and grade-schoolers, and even helps teenagers with the physical and emotional challenges they face. Yoga is a great whole-family activity parents and kids will love doing together.

Part 2, "Growing with the Tree of Yoga," talks about the spiritual side of yoga. Yoga isn't a religion. It works in harmony with any spiritual belief. Yet, yoga does have something to say about how to live. Read all about yoga's Eightfold Path for better living, interpreted in ways that make practical sense for kids. Yoga's Eightfold Path helps kids to meet life mindfully, noncompetitively, compassionately, with energy and control over mind and body, and with an essential, healthy, developing love of self and others.

Part 3, "Doing Yoga with Kids," explains the nuts and bolts of a child's yoga practice. We show you how to set up a personal yoga space uniquely suited to each child's needs. We'll discuss what to wear, props, and ways to honor your yoga space. We'll also help you to determine what kind of yoga practice is uniquely suited to each child, and how to find the right yoga teacher and class.

Part 4, "Yoga Songs, Play, and Postures," is the begin-breathing, get-moving, start-pretending section of the book. You'll learn about chanting and breathing exercises, nature poses, and a whole lot of animal poses taking you all over the world, from the barnyard to the desert, from the ocean to the jungle. Get ready for some serious fun!

Part 5, "Super Yoginis on the Move and Staying Still," continues with yoga poses, movements, and games. Yoga for kids is largely centered on movement, and in this section we'll take you through lots of fun movements and dancing poses, poses to build strength, flexibility, coordination, and confidence, as well as partner and group yoga fun. Wind down with the deep relaxation called Shavasana, an essential part of any child's yoga practice.

Part 6, "Especially for New Families," is designed to help new families through the transition of a new baby with poses and techniques for relaxing or energizing new moms and dads and helping with postpartum recovery. We'll also show new parents how to do yoga with their infant and their toddler, and provide some great ideas for siblings to practice and learn about yoga together.

Part 7, "Yoga All Day Long!" talks about yoga in all the other aspects of life beyond a child's daily yoga practice. Tips and information on great nutrition for the whole family, yoga remedies for common, minor health complaints in kids, and a discussion of yoga therapy for kids with special needs are featured here. We also devote a chapter to yoga for teens and, finally, we show you how to celebrate with a super yoga kid's party for children of any age.

Yoga Bits and Bytes

Throughout this book, we'll be adding five types of boxes that offer extra information to add to your knowledge, give you tips or encouragement, and generally make yoga even more kid friendly and accessible to children (and grownups) of all ages.

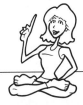

Yoga Stories

These boxes are full of trivia, factoids, or expanded background information to complete your picture of yoga, good health, and growing up.

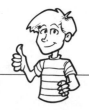

For Kids Only

These boxes are written directly to kids, interpreting yoga and related issues in ways kids can understand.

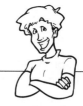

For Grownups, Too!

These boxes give grownups the knowledge, tips, and advice they need to most effectively assist kids with their yoga practice and other aspects of their lives, too.

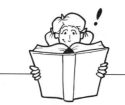

Learn About Yoga

These definition boxes clue you in on the meanings of some of the less common words in the text.

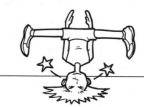

Ooops!

These boxes contain warnings and special information both kids and grownups should consider carefully.

Acknowledgments

This book could not have come about without the love and support of many people, to whom I owe my thanks.

To my Mom and Dad, who introduced me to yoga. Your love, support, guidance, and teachings have shown me the way to my spirit and led me to this path. There are no words to thank you enough for what you have given me in this lifetime. I love you, always.

To Barry, my brother, I thank you for your love, spirituality, and all that you have taught me to share with the world.

To Jaime, my brother, for your professionalism, dedication, and thirst for life, all of which have been such inspirations to me in writing this book, as well as in my career. Bless you for your guidance.

To Michael, for your love, patience, support, concerns, trust, sense of humor, and devotion. I could not have written this book without having you as the yang to my yin.

To Sonia Sumar, my first teacher who trained me to teach yoga to children. Working with you helped me to realize my desire to integrate my two passions in life: yoga and children. You are a light that continues to shine within me every day. Thank you, Renata and Jeff, for your faith in me.

To Marsha Wenig, YogaKids, your spirit and guidance hold a very special place in my heart. I am grateful for your talent, creativity, and for sharing your gift with me as well as the next generation. So glad you added your touch by tech editing this book.

To Cliff Rubin, my Webmaster, who developed my captivating Web site, which has led to many amazing opportunities, especially this book.

To Ray Evans, for your never-ending patience and "free" legal advice.

Thanks to all my friends who understood my disappearance during the months that I was writing this book.

Thank you to all the yoginis, their families, and Steven Goldberg for your patience and cooperation during the photo shoots.

To all the wonderful yoga teachers in this world, with whom I have had the honor to work, you are all so special to me and your teachings are a blessing! It is an honor to be your colleague.

Finally, thank you to all my beautiful yoginis: *William Reynolds, Sarah Gaines, Seren and Kira Helper, Sof Ciniglio, Reba Rosen, Alex Hertzfeld, Allison Martin, Sophie MacArthur, Miranda Katz, Mollie Gurian, Talia Bailey, Gabrielle LaGuerre, Hannah Sol-Morris, Cady Susswein, Stephanie Rodriguez, Ian Kinmont, Melissa Moy, Adam Eichen, David Sunshine, Michael and Emma O'Toole, Henry Millison, Robby and Gordon Menza, Claire Bentzen-Silverman, Jesse Levine-Spound, Dylan Braxton, Maxine Gunderson, David Kahn, Carrie Levine-Allman, Madelyn Widlus, Bobby Marks, Sophia Karasso, Nathaniel Bressi, Aissata Koralik-Touve, Gabrielle Levine, Leo Jagid, Alex Smith, Aziz Bowers, Isabelle Singer, Nicole Hershberg, Mary-Ann Weiss, Jessica and Grace Tregidgo, Eddie Futterman, The Borish Family, Jake Pinto-Zellner, Madelaine Lodge, Katherine Korwin, Jack Schnall, Samantha Stern, Grace MacArthur, Levi Mickelson, Samantha Goldburg, Annete Koski, CJ Junior, Logan and Madison Papp, Sofi Selig, Omar Yazbeck, Lilly Jenkins, The Students at The Manhattan New School, Nicholas Shatan, James Lipari, Ariela Roth, The Ballen Family, Ben Picariello, Michael and Emma Griffen, The Students at The Union Theological Seminary Learning Center, Antoinette and Glen Foster, Charlene De Witt, Camille Faucheux, and Alexandra Straus.* Without you this book could never have come alive. Your light, spirit, and positive energy have been an absolute delight to be surrounded by. Thank you for being your true selves and helping to make my dream come true!

—Jodi

The help, encouragement, support, and love of many helped to make the writing of this book possible. Thanks to my parents for their significant commitment to their grand yoginis, including babysitting above and beyond the call of duty. Thanks to Lee Ann for holding me up when I think I'm falling. Thanks to Joan, for auspicious beginnings. Thanks to Jodi for providing the knowledge and the sparkle that makes this book live. And thanks, most of all, to my two yoginis, Angus and Emmett, whose yogini spirits illuminate these pages and fill my life with light.

—Eve

Special Thanks to the Technical Reviewer

The Complete Idiot's Guide to Yoga with Kids was reviewed by an expert who not only checked the accuracy of what you'll learn in this book but also provided valuable insight to help ensure that this book tells you everything you need to know about doing yoga with kids. Our special thanks are extended to Marsha Wenig of YogaKids.

Marsha Wenig, C.Y.T., is a creative arts teacher, certified yoga instructor, mother, published writer, and poet. In 1996, she was a recipient of the Parents Choice Award for "her remarkable work and contribution to children" with her critically acclaimed video, *YogaKids: An Easy, Fun-filled Adventure for Children Ages 3–10.* The Coalition for Quality Children's Media (CQCM) also bestowed its Kids First! endorsement: "YogaKids models good health and heightens a child's self-awareness and esteem while encouraging them to think and experiment."

As co-founder/owner of the Dancing Feet Yoga Center, Marsha has been practicing and teaching yoga for over 16 years. With a B.A. from Rutgers University and training at UCLA, she has been teaching children in schools for the past 14 years. Her innovative programs integrate yoga, earthcare, self-expression, and creativity. Marsha's unique style combines play and warmth in ways that delight children of all ages. Check out Marsha's YogaKids Web site at www.yogakids.com.

Trademarks

All terms mentioned in this book that are known to be or are suspected of being trademarks or service marks have been appropriately capitalized. Alpha Books and Penguin Group (USA) Inc. cannot attest to the accuracy of this information. Use of a term in this book should not be regarded as affecting the validity of any trademark or service mark.

Part 1

Let's Get into Yoga with Kids

In this part, you'll get an easy introduction to an ancient and complex tradition. Yoga means union, and this tradition, which is thousands of years old, does wonders for kids who practice it today. Building strength and flexibility, concentration and focus, compassion and self-esteem, yoga is great for anybody. A child who learns yoga is developing gifts and skills that will last a lifetime.

Because yoga is a whole-body practice, it benefits both body and mind. Promoting internal health by toning organs, improving posture, and increasing strength, flexibility, and motor coordination, yoga helps kids feel great. From infancy onward, yoga promotes healthy development and fosters a creative and imaginative environment in which kids thrive.

Yoga is uniquely suited to each individual. Because it is essentially noncompetitive, each and every child can learn, grow, and succeed within his or her own personal yoga context.

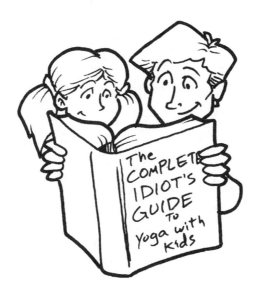

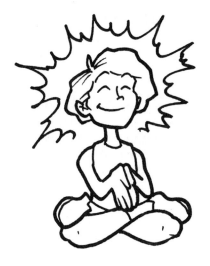

Chapter 1

Why Yoga Is Great for Kids

In This Chapter

➤ How yoga and kids are meant for each other

➤ Yoga: past, present, and future

➤ Using yoga to build a strong body and strong mind

➤ Boosting self-esteem with yoga

➤ Yoga is for everyone: babies, toddlers, grade-school kids, and teens

➤ Turning yoga into a fun family affair

Kids have strength. Kids have energy. Kids are flexible. Kids are graceful. Kids get excited. Kids calm down. Kids can move and kids can be still. Best of all, kids know how to live each moment to its fullest.

But can kids do yoga? And why should they? If you think kids don't or can't do yoga, we have a surprise for you: Kids do yoga every day!

Yoga is simply an organized system for what comes naturally to kids. It is the art of fusing body and mind for an overall sense of strength, flexibility, and well-being. Yoga moves, bends, stretches, and empowers bodies. It also moves, bends, stretches, and empowers minds. It can help kids get hold of their active lives and sometimes overactive minds. It can help kids become better athletes, better students, even better friends, siblings, and family members. Best of all, yoga can help kids to see the beauty within themselves, boosting their self-confidence, helping them feel comfortable with their bodies, and getting in touch with who they are inside.

But yoga doesn't change anything fundamental about kids. It helps kids hone, refine, and nourish what is already so beautifully present in them: the energy of life.

What Is Yoga?

Young potential yoga students often have some interesting ideas about what yoga is. When asked to describe yoga, some sit eagerly on the floor, cross their legs, hold their hands open to the sides, touch their thumbs and first fingers in a lovely but stereo-typical classic Lotus Pose, and chant the sound "Om." Others have verbal responses to the question, "What is *yoga?*" Some of the answers we've heard are …

➤ Tying yourself up in a knot!

➤ Something hippies do?

➤ Standing on your head.

➤ Just breathing.

Yoga has been stereotyped for some kids and kids may not know exactly what it is at all. Yoga isn't a demonstration of ultraflexibility. It isn't for any one group of people. It isn't a religion. It can be practiced by everyone, no matter what their beliefs. It is not just a philosophy, although it does have ideas behind it about healthy ways to live. It is, at its heart, a synchronizing of body and mind.

Some kids naturally understand the idea behind yoga, but they may have only glimpsed at what yoga has to offer. Yoga isn't just tying ourselves in knots, taking deep breaths, or sitting in a meditation position. It can involve walking like an animal, shaking your body like gelatin, reaching toward the sun, even standing on your head (when you are ready). It is also a kind of exercise, just like tae kwon do, karate, ballet or other types of dance, gymnastics, even long-distance running, baseball, or soccer.

But yoga is more than exercise and more than a sport. While any sport played well activates the mind in addition to the body, yoga is meant to bring the two together.

Yoga Is Union

Yoga is all about the connection or union between the body and the mind. The word yoga means "union," and performing different yoga postures that require mental and physical energy brings the physical body into balance with the spiritual mind.

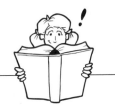

Learn About Yoga

Yoga is a system of physical and mental exercises meant to synchronize body and mind for a healthier and more aware whole self. Hatha yoga is a branch of yoga on which most modern yoga is based. *Ha* means "sun" and *tha* means "moon," together symbolizing the balancing and joining of opposites.

Yoga is essentially about balance. We don't mean the kind of balance you achieve by standing on one leg. Yes, we do such balancing, and that is a part of yoga. But to be successful at standing on one leg, your *mind* must also be balanced. Physical balance takes concentration, so in order to balance physically, you must bring your mind into balance with your body.

It may sound tricky, or strange, or not like what you are used to hearing when learning a new sport or a new skill or even a new concept in school, but that's why yoga works so well to increase your success with all those other things. Yoga helps you to move and think in a new way, a way that puts thought into movement and movement into thought.

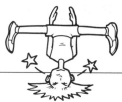

Ooops!

Some yoga poses are harder than others, and even flexible kids in good shape should start slowly, letting their bodies naturally adjust to this new "sport" or way of moving. To prevent injury and frustration, master the basic poses before attempting the difficult poses. Go slow! You'll get there.

Yoga Traditions: Everything Old Is New Again

Yet, yoga isn't such a new way after all. It is actually one of the oldest systems of physical and mental exercise ever created. Thousands of years ago, people did yoga in India. How did it start? Some people discovered that it made them feel very good, both physically and mentally, to go out into nature—into the forests and jungles, next to rivers, in view of mountains—and watch animals and nature. These people knew how to watch very closely, and found that imitating the animals and trees and mountains made them feel great, full of positive energy and good health. These people became very interested in their natural surroundings and kept inventing new poses to imitate things in their environment.

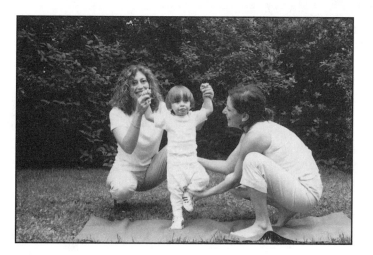

Yoga is an ancient tradition based on the observation of nature. Doing yoga is natural and fun! Jodi (at right) helps a mother and child be a tree.

Sometimes these same people wanted to communicate with nature. For example, they wanted to thank the sun for giving them warmth and light, for helping things grow, so they designed a dance for the sun. That made them feel more in harmony with the nature around them and more a part of the world.

These people in India taught what they had learned to their children, and those children passed the lessons on to the next generation, and so on and so on. Now, thousands of years later, we still do yoga for all the same reasons: to feel good, to be strong, to stay healthy, to think clearly, and to know ourselves better.

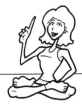

Yoga Stories

Today, doing yoga in India, where yoga originated, is a lot like doing yoga in the United States. Grownups do it, and kids do it, too, to feel better, stay healthier, and have better concentration. While yoga may not be as widespread in the United States today as it has been in India, yoga today is nothing less than a phenomenon. Yoga classes are filling up with men, women, and children. Many famous entertainers have shared their yoga experiences or are known for their devotion to a yoga practice, from Madonna to Ricky Martin. In *People* magazine's recent "Most Beautiful People" issue, the introduction just happened to mention that many Hollywood stars have abandoned sweating in gyms for the serenity of yoga.

Working the Entire Body and Mind

Yoga may look easy, or it may look impossible if you aren't particularly flexible, but yoga is neither. Adjustable for anyone of any physical ability, yoga is uniquely tailored to work your individual body and mind, and we mean your entire body and mind.

Even if you have certain physical limitations, yoga works all that is available, gently nudging your physical limits and continually challenging your mental assumptions. You thought you'd never be able to get anywhere near touching your toes? Think again. It may take a while, but if it is within your physical capability, yoga can get you there. You thought you'd never be able to concentrate in school? Think again. Yoga exercises your concentration to the point where you will be able to notice improvement. Thought you'd never find a form of exercise you could enjoy? Surprise! Yoga will change your assumptions yet again.

Building a Strong Body

Some people live for sports and other physical pursuits. Others aren't as interested in going out for the team as they are in reading a good book or hanging out with their friends. The great thing about yoga is that it can help build the physical strength, flexibility, and confidence of all kids regardless of what physical activities they prefer. Even sworn enemies of gym class can get all kinds of benefits, not to mention sincere enjoyment, from a class or personal yoga practice. Natural athletes will find their skills refined, strengthened, and more under their control.

The amazing thing about yoga is the way it works with any physical body to give it what it needs. Kids who are flexible but haven't yet developed muscle tone get stronger. Kids with strength but not much flexibility get more limber. Kids low on endurance develop greater breath capacity and staying power. Kids who are hypotonic (lacking in muscle tone) can strengthen their muscles and joints. Kids who could be athletic but may lack the confidence to go for it gain a new perspective on their abilities and can find the motivation they need to pursue the sport they've always dreamed of pursuing.

Yoga's long-term effect is greater health, confidence, and fitness, both mental and physical. Anyone can reap the benefits, anyone can participate, and anyone can enjoy yoga for a lifetime because, as your physical needs evolve and grow, so will your yoga practice.

We're not saying yoga is a miracle cure for the sedentary. It won't turn anyone into Michael Jordan or Mia Hamm, Sammy Sosa, or Rebecca Lobo (although it can certainly give a potential sports star a boost in the right direction!). But for kids looking for something different, an alternative approach to physical fitness that works every muscle, joint, and body system, or just a great new way to cross-train, yoga may be just what the gym teacher ordered.

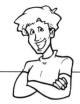

For Grownups, Too!

One reason yoga appeals to many kids who don't necessarily enjoy other sports is that yoga is noncompetitive. Everyone is a winner because each child progresses at his or her own pace, testing individual limits and achieving in unique ways. If your child has been frustrated by the fierce competition of school athletics, yoga may be exactly what he or she needs to rebuild self-esteem.

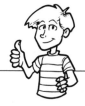

For Kids Only

Yoga is an awesome way for girls or boys to get strong. Yoga doesn't use weights, doesn't require $150 shoes, and doesn't involve any competition, but it does put you in positions where you are lifting or supporting the weight of your own body and, at the same time, stretching your muscles so they get long and lean while they get stronger. It is strength training the natural way!

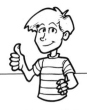

Building a Strong Mind

Now let's look at the other side of the mind-body picture. You know the kids who are in their element when it comes to working their brains. Tests? Spelling bees? Trigonometry? Haiku? No problem. For some kids, concentration is a no-brainer and the really challenging stuff is simply part of the joy of learning.

But for most kids, even the kids who get great grades or who have a reputation for being "smart," concentrating long enough to get through that medieval literature textbook chapter or all 46 math problems is a tall order. Even adults would have a hard time with some of the tasks required of school-aged kids.

Yoga's unique strength is its capacity to exercise the mind as well as the body. Although it may not make a boring lecture seem suddenly fascinating, it can help you to keep your mind on your work, and even do better on assignments and tests. A calm, serene, controlled mind that is present in the moment instead of shooting off in every direction at once will be far better prepared to figure out whether a, b, c, or d is the correct answer.

For Kids Only

Yoga is an excellent way to cross-train. For runners, yoga helps to strengthen and stretch the hips, legs, and Achilles tendons. For baseball players, yoga helps to strengthen the arms and upper body muscles. Stronger arms equal longer throws! Basketball players can benefit from increased eye-hand coordination to boost their dribbling and shooting skills, and for gymnasts, yoga helps to increase flexibility, balance, and concentration.

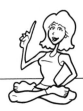

Yoga Stories

A recent Kaiser Family Foundation survey revealed that the average child in the United States spends 5½ hours *per day* watching television, listening to music, or at the computer, usually in isolation. According to author Dr. Stanley Greenspan (*Building Healthy Minds*, Perseus Books, 1999) in a recent MSNBC interview, this is far too much time learning in a passive environment. Children require active, emotional interaction with others to develop intelligence, emotional health, creativity, and other important life skills. Dr. Greenspan suggests 30 minutes is the most children should spend daily in these passive or nonemotional, interactive learning environments.

How does yoga do it? The postures and exercises of yoga aren't easy. Some require difficult balances. Some require finding and working the edge of your flexibility or strength. Some simply require lots of concentration to keep track of what arm and what leg goes where.

This kind of brain exercise coupled with physical exercise requires you to think only about what you are doing, and that means you are present in the moment. You aren't thinking about the essay due tomorrow or what you'll eat for lunch. You aren't thinking about the phone conversation from you-know-who last night or what that note said that you intercepted in study hall. Or, if you are thinking about those things, you'll realize it because you won't be able to hold that Tree Pose or that Headstand. You'll tip over. And you'll try again.

One of the original purposes of yoga was actually to help get the distracting body under control so the mind could develop its concentration and inner stillness through *meditation*. That's why yoga necessarily works both body and mind. The philosophy of yoga suggests that body and mind can't really be separated. They are both an intrinsic part of you. What affects one affects the other. Once you've tried it, you'll understand how the physical exertion of yoga becomes a mental exertion as well, and as your body becomes stronger, more flexible, and freer, so does your mind. Talk about a full contact sport!

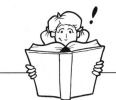

Learn About Yoga

Yoga isn't all about poses. A complete yoga practice also includes **meditation,** which is a way to train the mind by teaching it to become very still and aware of the moment, not jumping around to what happened before or what might happen next. Meditation can be practiced by sitting still, walking slowly, or even lying down. Yoga exercises help to control the body so it isn't as distracting during meditation.

Yoga Is a Self-Esteem Booster!

Adults and children both know school can be pretty hard on self-esteem. Even if kids feel great most of the time and have lots of friends, they may have a tough time in some of their classes, or maybe they don't make the team—whether volleyball or debate. Perhaps all their friends got cast in the school play but they didn't. Or maybe it seems like their French teacher really has it in for them.

Grownups sometimes forget how hard it is to be a kid. "Oh, to be young!" grownups like to say. "Life was so easy!" No, life as a kid isn't easy. It is full of intense challenges, intense friendships, intense betrayals, disappointments, and sometimes overwhelming stress. How is a kid supposed to store up any self-esteem? Sheesh!

Yoga encourages kids to feel confident and self-assured.

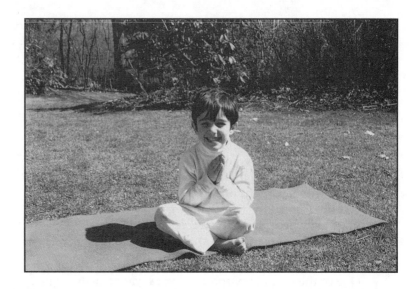

Yoga can help. Really! Kids who practice yoga have before them surmountable challenges. They learn to practice poses and do exercises they've never tried before, things they never imagined they could do. When they see they can finally stand on one leg or balance upside-down, they feel good about themselves.

Yoga can yield quick results with consistent practice. One day, you can't even touch your knees. A week later, you can reach your shins! When you maintain a personal yoga practice, you become more self-aware and you will notice your success. It is something tangible that you can see, even measure. You did it! And you can feel great about your continual successes.

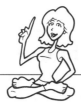

Yoga Stories

You may have heard that yoga can help you learn to do supernatural things like read minds or even levitate. Wouldn't that be fun? However, most experts agree that yoga's benefits are a little more down-to-earth. However, regular yoga practice might make you feel so good that the change will seem like magic! Runners know about a feeling called a "runner's high" that happens after running long distances. People who practice yoga often experience a similar "natural high" during and especially after practicing yoga, a feeling of lightness, easiness, joyfulness, and elation.

Another way yoga makes you feel great about yourself is in the way it taps into the power of nature. Mountain Pose is more than standing straight and still. It is learning to feel the power, majesty, and strength of a mountain. Tree Pose helps you to feel the towering height and easy movement of a great tree. In Cat Pose you are as cool as a feline and as self-assured. In Lion Pose, you really are king of the jungle. (And doesn't school sometimes seem like a jungle?)

Nature is full of indomitable creatures and impressive objects, and yoga doesn't just copy them. Through yoga, you can, in a way, become those things. And when your practice is over for the day, you can take some of that strength, confidence, power, and tranquil spirit away with you. Doesn't that feel great?

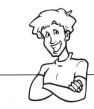

For Grownups, Too!

How do you raise kids to be ethical in this day and age? It isn't easy when so many institutions have questioned and undermined beliefs society used to hold as truth. Yoga is a ready-made, nonreligious philosophy of ethical living, as well as a system for greater physical and mental health. Yoga advocates nonviolence, truthfulness, sharing, good health, and self-respect as well as respect of others. What great lessons for kids to learn!

Yoga for the Next Generation

It's a new millennium and that's exciting for kids. This is their world, the world kids are growing into. If you're a kid, soon you and all the other kids your age will be the leaders, making decisions, shaping societies, writing laws, and raising kids of your own. How will you run things? How will you change things? How will you do things different from the way grownups are doing them now?

We find kids to be wellsprings of sparkling optimism, ready to take on the world and change it for the better. What better tool to make those dreams and visions come true then yoga?

How can such an old, old system be relevant for the next generation of kids? That's the magic of yoga. It is timeless, yet more relevant today than ever before, when kids are under so much pressure to perform, to make important decisions, and to settle ethical dilemmas.

In a world overrun by mass media, kids need somewhere to turn that doesn't involve looking passively at a screen but instead involves turning their vision inward to discover their potential power, strength, and beauty. Yoga nurtures the spirit as it hones the body, helping kids to find the path that leads to kindness, love, empathy, and service rather than to selfishness, greed, hate, and violence. Our world could use more *yoginis*.

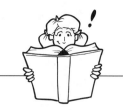

Learn About Yoga

Who is a **yogini?** A junior yogi, of course! While traditionally, a yogi was a man who practiced yoga and a yogini was a woman who practiced yoga, we find it easier and more satisfying to use the term "yogini" to refer to any child who practices yoga, regardless of gender. For our purposes, "yogi" refers to any adult who practices yoga, also regardless of gender.

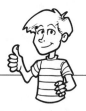

For Kids Only

Teenagers, you probably hear all the time about how many changes you are experiencing. It's true! Your body is going through immense physical and chemical changes, signaling the peak of puberty. Coping with all these changes can be ultrastressful on the mind. Yoga is a great way to help balance your emotional and spiritual self as well as your fluctuating physical self. It can make you feel a little more balanced.

Kids of All Ages Love Yoga

Once upon a time in India, yoga was practiced by grown-up men only. Today, however, yoga is for everyone, of any age. Even babies? Sure, even babies! Babies are natural yoginis and spontaneously perform many yoga poses just because it is a part of their developmental exploration of the world. Even toddlers? Why not toddlers? Toddlers think yoga is great fun. Who needs Saturday morning cartoons when you can prowl around the living room with Mommy or Daddy, being cats or tigers or lions? Slithering through the kitchen like a cobra or bouncing down the hallway on all four paws like a dog? Toddler heaven!

What about preschoolers? Preschoolers are fantastic yoginis. Their blossoming imaginations find yoga not only easy to understand but almost obvious. Of course it feels good to be a tree, to do a sun dance, to float like a boat on an imaginary ocean. Why wouldn't it?

Grade-school kids love yoga, too. Sometimes it's just plain fun to play Camel or Cobra or Cat. Grade-school kids can also appreciate their own progress when practicing yoga regularly. A newly mastered balance pose can be a triumph to a proud fourth grader. A second grader able to arch into a beautiful Wheel Pose may want to demonstrate her skill to everyone, or may keep the triumph quietly and happily to herself.

Many teens can make wonderfully astute, sensitive, and accomplished yoginis. While hormones rage and school and life seem disaster ridden, a daily yoga practice can be an oasis of tranquility and personal achievement. Even when nothing else seems to be working, teens can return to yoga and find that they can move easily and gracefully through the Sun Dance. And everything suddenly seems a little sunnier.

You'll Love Yoga, Too!

Maybe you still think yoga is too hard, or even too easy. Too boring? Too challenging? You can't do it because you just aren't that flexible?

We can almost guarantee that you will love yoga. How do we know? Because yoga isn't like a sport where you have to play it one way or no way. It is more like an art. You can do yoga your way. You can choose the poses, the movements, and the methods that speak to you, that you find fun or fascinating or relaxing or energizing. Yoga is for you. It is all about you. And it will make you feel great.

Even the least flexible among us can do a Mountain Pose (see Chapter 11). With a little practice, almost anyone can balance on one foot in a Tree Pose (see Chapter 11), even if just for a second or two. Who can't lie down and practice deep relaxation? And who wouldn't enjoy leaving the self behind for a little while to play the parts of nature?

But we don't need to convince you. All we ask is that you read this book and see what appeals to you, what compels you, and what seems like fun to you. You decide. You choose. You make your yoga practice yours and see where it takes you. You may be surprised at the person waiting inside. You are an amazing soul worthy of all the love the universe has to offer. Find that soul and nurture it through yoga. What have you got to lose?

Yoga Fun for the Whole Family

For some kids, yoga is a private affair, something to do on their own. For other kids, especially younger kids, nothing is more fun than a family affair. But can mom, dad, big sister, baby brother, even grandma and grandpa get into the act? Of course! Yoga is great fun for the entire family.

Traditionally, yoga is a system of self-examination, and practicing yoga individually is still a highly effective way to develop both physically and spiritually. Today, however, group yoga is also a perfectly wonderful way to practice yoga. Group yoga is a fun variation to an individual yoga practice that helps kids learn and grow in ways they might not if they only did yoga on their own. Group yoga helps kids pay attention to each other, helps them focus, and encourages empathy. When practiced with the whole family, it can nurture relationships and encourage self-expression and expressions of support for other family members.

Any pose can be transformed into a group pose. Don't just be a tree, be a whole forest! Don't just be a fish, be a whole school of fish swimming in tandem. A mountain range is more impressive than a single mountain, and a whole garden of flowers is more glorious than a single bloom.

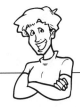

For Grownups, Too!

For adults eager to get started, sample what we mean by a family yoga practice by doing a gentle Downward Dog pose. Then encourage your young child to crawl under you and to try being a Cobra sliding under the Dog. See Chapter 12 for instructions on how to do Downward Dog Pose and Cobra Pose.

There are also plenty of poses grownups can do that kids can help with or participate in by climbing under, over, or on top. (Grownups, consider the presence of your toddler on your stomach as you rock in Boat Pose or hold a Bridge Pose an added muscle strengthener!)

Other reasons why family participation in a yoga practice is so important are that it establishes exercise, good health, and self-care as a family priority, and a fun one at that.

Families that move together and play together bond better and develop deeper, more meaningful relationships than do families that don't communicate or, at best, watch television together all night. Get up, get moving, and get together. Yoga is family bonding at its best!

The Least You Need to Know

➤ Yoga is an ancient Indian system of physical and mental exercise meant to synchronize body and mind for a stronger, healthier whole self.

➤ Yoga is great for kids, who already have a natural understanding of what it means to emulate nature, pretend, create, and move in new and different ways.

➤ Yoga helps kids of any age get stronger, more flexible, and more confident about their bodies.

➤ Yoga also helps kids learn to concentrate better and increases attention span, which helps with schoolwork as well as a personal sense of well-being.

➤ Yoga is great for self-esteem. Kids can see their progress and feel good about their accomplishments.

➤ Yoga isn't just for kids. The whole family can participate in a lively and interactive yoga practice.

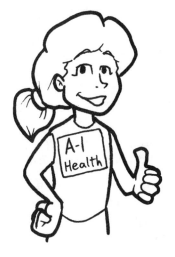

Chapter 2

Health Benefits of Yoga for Kids

In This Chapter

➤ Yoga helps kids stay healthy, inside and out

➤ Build flexibility, strength, and stamina with yoga!

➤ Yoga practice lengthens and strengthens children's spines for greater overall health

➤ Kids who do yoga may have a more restful sleep

Yoga is lots of fun and great for self-confidence, but it has excellent physical benefits, too. Learning to develop and maintain good physical health in childhood will set great patterns for later in life. A yogini today is a fit adult down the road (and, we hope, an adult who still practices yoga!).

Yoga is good for kids, physically, in many ways. It isn't just a cardiovascular exercise, although it can be vigorously cardiovascular. It isn't just strength or flexibility building, although it does those things, too. Yoga retrains the entire body to position itself in a way that allows it to function most effectively. It helps to align the spine, free and strengthen breathing, massage internal organs, and fine-tune coordination.

Just as important for health, yoga brings positive, loving energy into the body and into the self, promoting mental and spiritual health. Medical researchers are uncovering more and more ways in which mind and body are linked, and yoga improves health from both sides!

Yoga Promotes Good Internal Health for Kids

You can see the shapes of a few of your muscles and some of your bones under your skin, but a whole lot more is going on inside your body than muscle and bone. You've got all kinds of internal organs, like your stomach, colon, heart, lungs, kidneys, and liver. You've got glands, too, like your adrenal, endocrine, pituitary, and thyroid. And then there is your brain, which keeps the whole business running smoothly most of the time.

What goes on inside your body? Much more than we can list, but here are a few of the highlights of your body's internal workings—the inside story of your insides!

➤ **Circulatory system.** This is how your internal organs get nourished and stay free of waste. Blood carries oxygen and other nutrients all over your body, then picks up waste products and removes them. It all happens through the action of your heart, which is the pump that powers the whole system.

➤ **Digestive system.** This is how you make use of the food you eat. From your mouth to your stomach to your intestines and all the way through, food is chewed, digested, broken down by different glands, and the nutrients extracted, to be distributed by your circulatory system.

➤ **Endocrine system.** This is where all those hormones come in. Hormones are produced by different organs and glands in your body, and they affect your growth, metabolism, health, and eventually, reproduction.

➤ **Excretory system.** This is how you eliminate waste. You don't use every speck of the food you eat. Some of it ends up as waste and it's got to go somewhere! Some of it comes out of your skin, through sweat. Some of it is exhaled out of your lungs. Your kidneys and liver process some of it, and the rest comes out the other end of your large intestine. These waste products have to be eliminated from your body to keep them from interfering with good health and proper functioning.

➤ **Integumentary system.** This is your skin, which does more than help eliminate waste through perspiration. It also protects your body, regulates your temperature, and actually breathes. It is also the organ through which you can feel things.

➤ **Muscular system.** This is all your muscles. Some of your muscles move because you want them to move. Others move without your conscious direction, like your heart and breathing muscles. Altogether, they give your body much of its shape and allow every single movement you make, whether kicking a soccer ball or smiling. Pretty handy!

➤ **Nervous system.** This system is command central, controlling all your movements and all the activities of your organs, glands, and body chemistry. It even produces your thoughts! Your nervous system includes your brain, your spinal cord, and all the nerves that branch out from them.

16

➤ **Reproductive system.** This is the system that controls your ability to create life. It is governed by certain glands that are different in girls and boys. Girls have ovaries that produce egg cells after the beginning of menstruation. Boys have testes that make sperm cells.

➤ **Respiratory system.** This is your breathing system. Most of the time, you probably don't even notice that you are breathing, but the process is pretty complex and an important way to deliver oxygen to your body. Air comes in through your nose and/or mouth, travels down your trachea into your bronchial tubes and then into your lungs. The oxygen in the air you inhale is then absorbed by blood in the lungs. Carbon dioxide waste is released and then travels back out of the body as you exhale.

➤ **Skeletal system.** This is the system that holds you up! Your skeleton includes your bones and joints. It gives structure to your movements, and protects your internal organs, too. And, without your skeleton, you'd have no way to support all that skin and muscle.

Do you think all that stuff just works without any maintenance? Actually, you maintain your internal body all the time, even without realizing it. Everything you eat affects your internal chemistry. Breathing delivers oxygen to your body and removes carbon dioxide waste. Exercise keeps muscles and bones in shape. Sleeping helps your body to repair itself.

But you can do more to help your body stay healthy and strong. Yoga targets specific areas, massaging organs and glands, building muscle strength and flexibility, gently working joints, and helping the nervous system to work more efficiently and productively.

Let's look a little more closely at what yoga can do for kids' bodies.

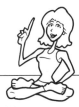

Yoga Stories

Did you know you have 206 different bones and over 600 different muscles? Among other things, your bones protect different parts of your body. For example, your ribs cover and protect your heart and lungs and your skull protects your brain. The bones of your skeleton fit together at joints. Ankles, shoulders, and elbows are joints. Without joints, your skeleton could not move or bend. Your body has more than 200 joints in your skeleton. There are 56 joints in your hands alone.

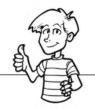

For Kids Only

To get the most from your yoga practice, or any active physical activity, don't eat for at least 90 minutes (preferably two to three hours) before you start. Your body will work best on an empty stomach. You can't expect your body to move as quickly or easily when it is busy trying to digest food, and a body in active movement may not digest food as well, causing stomachaches or other discomfort.

Yoga Aids Kids' Digestion and Elimination

Yoga has lots of bending and stretching poses that help move and stimulate the digestive system. Because yoga is cleansing, it also promotes the elimination of waste.

Some kids get constipated, especially when they don't eat enough fiber or when they get nervous about something. Yoga can help with constipation, too. Poses like the Bow Pose, especially the Rocking Bow Pose (see Chapter 16), the Cat and Cow Poses (see Chapter 12), and Breath of Fire (see Chapter 10) are especially good for facilitating healthy elimination. Also see Chapter 24 for more on how yoga can help problems related to digestion and elimination.

Yoga Develops Stronger Hearts and Lungs

Your heart has a big job. It is the powerhouse for your entire *cardiovascular* system. It beats constantly, all day and all night, moving fluids such as blood through your body, delivering nourishing oxygen and other nutrients, and picking up waste products.

The heart and lungs are a team that keeps adults and kids moving to the right rhythm.

(Drawing by Wendy Frost)

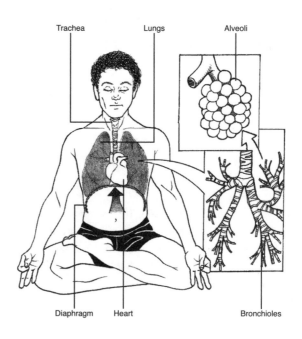

Trachea   Lungs   Alveoli

Diaphragm   Heart   Bronchioles

18

Your lungs are just as important. They help you to breathe air in and out. Your lungs and heart work together as a *cardiopulmonary* team. Your lungs bring in oxygen-rich air and pass it to your blood, which then circulates, powered by your heart pump, around your entire body, delivering oxygen and picking up carbon dioxide waste, which then gets passed back to the air in your lungs and exhaled out of your body. It's a great system.

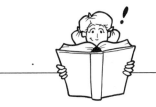

There's a difference between kids and adults in how fast their hearts pump and how many breaths per minute they take. Kids usually have a normal resting heart, or pulse, rate of 80 to 100 beats per minute; the normal resting pulse rate for adults is 60 to 80 beats per minute. Adults take 12 to 20 breaths each minute at rest, while kids normally take 20 or more, depending on their ages!

Learn About Yoga

Cardiovascular refers to your heart and blood vessels. **Cardiopulmonary** refers to the joint workings of your heart and lungs.

Time yourself. Find a watch with a second hand. Sit quietly in a chair and count how many times you breathe in one minute. Then, take two fingers and put them on your Adam's apple on your neck. Slide the fingers about an inch and a half to the side and press until you can feel the carotid artery pumping blood through your body! Using the watch's second hand again, count how many times in one minute your heart beats to push blood through the artery. Now you know your resting respiratory and heart rates!

As humans age, their heart and respiration rates tend to decrease, as shown in the following table.

Normal Vital Signs for Children at Rest

Age	Heart Rate (Beats Per Minute)	Respiration (Breaths Per Minute)
Infant*	140	40–60
1 year	130	22–30
3 years	80	20–26
10 years	75	18–22

*From birth to about six months of age, infants are nose breathers, meaning they breathe only through their noses and have not yet achieved the developmental ability to breathe through their mouths.

You may not think yoga does much for your heart and lungs because you imagine it is more about stretching. Yoga can be really good exercise, increasing your heart rate and breathing to help expand lung capacity and heart strength. A vigorous Yoga Sun Dance (see Chapter 15) can really get that heart pumping.

Yoga also includes specific exercises designed to train your breathing. You will learn to breathe more deeply and with greater control, expanding your lung capacity.

One of the breathing exercises we like to do is called Breath of Fire (see Chapter 10). This exercise is a fast breathing exercise, but between each round, we hold our breath for 15 seconds, then 30 seconds, and eventually, when we increase our lung capacity, one minute. The more you practice these exercises, the easier and more nourishing your breathing will become. You might also be able to swim underwater for a longer period of time!

Yoga does something else very important for the heart. In yoga, the heart is considered to be the physical center for love and the place from which we can emit love and positive energy. Yoga practice helps fill the heart with love, reenergizing it and renewing us so we are better able to emit that love into the world. There is no better heart medicine than love, for the self and for the world!

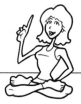

Yoga Stories

During an average lifetime, the heart beats 2.5 billion times without stopping. According to *Gray's Anatomy* (a fact-filled coloring book for children by Freddy Stark, Ph.D., adapted from the classic work by Henry Gray), during a single minute, a healthy heart can pump over 10 gallons of blood through 60,000 miles of blood vessels. One full round-trip through the entire circulatory system takes only 30 seconds. Pretty incredible!

Yoga Massages Internal Organs and Glands

You may have had a back massage before, but you've probably never had a liver massage, or a thyroid gland massage. Because of the unique way the body moves in yoga poses, all your internal organs and glands get pressed, or unpressed, massaged or released, in all kinds of ways. It's not all about muscles when it comes to yoga. Every inch of you, inside and out, gets a great workout.

For example, your thyroid gland, the gland that controls your metabolism (the rate at which you burn up the food you eat and that affects your energy level), is in your throat. It doesn't get much action when you play volleyball, but in Candle Pose the thyroid receives a gentle squeeze, helping to keep it toned and functioning.

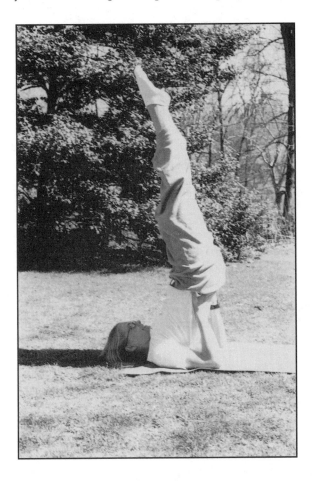

Yoga poses such as Candle Pose massage internal organs, which help keep your body happy and healthy.

Your liver is a large organ in your abdominal cavity that helps digestion and elimination by producing substances such as urea and bile that help other organs do their jobs. Gentle pressure and then release on the liver may help this important organ stay active and healthy, and what better way to massage your liver than with Twister Pose (see Chapter 16), a pose that twists your middle body, or torso?

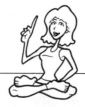

Yoga Stories

According to the American Heart Association, almost half of American kids between the ages of 12 and 21 are not vigorously active on a regular basis, and physical activity declines dramatically during adolescence. With so many opportunities for sedentary activity available to kids today (television, video games, Internet surfing, and more homework than ever before), it's no wonder kids don't move as much. Apparently, schools aren't forcing the issue, either. Daily enrollment in physical education classes has declined among high school students from 42 percent in 1991 to 27 percent in 1997.

You may wonder if anyone really needs to massage and tone his or her internal organs. Let's look at it another way. Your internal organs are part of your body, part of you. We believe that bodies—all parts of bodies—are meant to move.

Movement is life. The more television, computers, and telephones become a part of our lives, the more people are tending to become sedentary. They sit. They lie down. They watch, or type, or talk. Yoga helps to balance all that sitting around with movement of all parts of the body, to keep everything vibrant, moving, flushed with nutrients, active, and alive.

Yoga Fine-Tunes Motor Coordination

Yoga does more than physically massage your body. It also fine-tunes your nervous system by teaching the body to better coordinate all its parts. Whether large movements like Bear and Giraffe Walk (see Chapter 14) or small movements like Toe-Ups (see Chapter 17), yoga tweaks your gross and fine motor coordination. Chanting and hand-clapping exercise help eye-hand motor coordination, too.

Yoga involves paying very close attention to the movements of the body, and this trains the nervous system to pay attention to what the body is doing. Kids who are growing quickly may sometimes feel a little off-balance, even clumsy, although chances are nobody else notices.

Any body would have trouble adjusting to such rapid physical changes, but yoga helps to balance all those systems in your body that don't always feel particularly coordinated. Whether you find you are better able to keep your eye, or racquet, or foot on the ball, or simply feel more comfortable in your body as you walk down the halls or home from school, yoga helps you gain more control over your body.

Yoga Power!

Sometimes, kids feel like they have boundless energy. Toddlers are tireless until they collapse into naptime, and afterwards they are at it again, pushing their limits at every turn. Preschoolers can move nonstop from morning until bedtime and take pride in their bodies and their strengths. When kids become mature enough to notice how their bodies differ from the bodies of other kids, however, they may not feel so physically invincible.

Because yoga is noncompetitive and personally tailored to you, during your yoga practice, comparison isn't relevant. Yoga enhances your strengths and strengthens the areas where you can use more balance. It gives you power over your body without even taking into account how you compare to anyone else, and it gives you the power to feel pride in your progress and your own personal evolution, whether that involves gaining flexibility, strength, coordination, concentration, self-confidence, or all of the above.

Muscling in on Flexibility

We would like to clear up a common misconception right now: *You don't need to be naturally flexible to do yoga!* Lots of people think they can't do yoga because they aren't flexible. First of all, anyone, and we mean *anyone,* can do yoga. Yoga is meant to work with your individual abilities and within your individual limits. Yoga does increase your flexibility, no matter how flexible or inflexible you are when you begin. Just try it, and you'll see.

But yoga also increases muscle strength. Some kids *are* naturally flexible, but don't use their muscles much. Yoga helps add strength to flexibility as it adds flexibility to strength, optimizing both for a more balanced body.

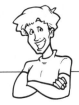

For Grownups, Too!

Here's an exercise kids can do with parents or other adults—or even with a friend! One person lies down on the floor, on his or her back, in Shavasana Pose (see Chapter 19). The other person talks the person on the floor through a gradual relaxation, working from toe to head, asking the person to consciously relax every muscle, one body part at a time. Next time, switch places.

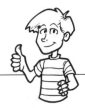

For Kids Only

Even if you are naturally flexible, you can still benefit from yoga poses that don't necessarily push the limits of your flexibility. If your knees practically rest on the ground in Butterfly Pose (see Chapter 11), you can still benefit from doing it because it will help strengthen your joints and muscles. Then you can work on lengthening your spine and deepening your breath. The benefits of yoga extend beyond flexibility.

Even More Stamina

Do kids really need more stamina? Stamina doesn't mean hyperactivity, it means physical staying power, and everyone can benefit from it. More and more young children are becoming sedentary, but yoga can get them up and moving again, developing young muscles and strengthening young bones and joints.

Older kids are more likely to feel the need of a stamina boost, especially when stress mounts and life gets difficult. Whether you find it virtually impossible to get moving in the morning, or are plagued with the mid-afternoon slump and can hardly stay awake in class, yoga can help increase your energy level.

Yoga postures and exercises help you feel invigorated and alive. When your energy level starts to drop, try a Yoga Sun Dance (see Chapter 15) or three rounds of Breath of Fire (see Chapter 10) to jump-start your engine.

The other energy-related problem kids sometimes have is sleep difficulty. Infants, toddlers, preschoolers, grade-schoolers, and teens can all have trouble winding down at night. We'll cover this in just a few moments, in the section "Good, Restful, Refreshing Sleep for Kids."

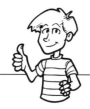

For Kids Only

Need a quick pick-me-up? Try Helicopter Pose. Here's how you do it: Stand in the middle of an open space with plenty of room. Extend your arms out to either side, and spin for as long as you feel comfortable (30 seconds is plenty of time—don't spin so long that you lose your balance and fall over!). Slow down gradually and stop slowly, then wait a minute if you are dizzy. Feel the surge of energy!

Gaining Stability and Balance

To stand on one leg, you must have a quiet, balanced mind. A balanced mind helps balance the body. To stand as stable as a mountain, you must have a mind that feels comfortable settling into a state of stability. A stable mind helps stabilize the body.

Some days, you will probably be better able to achieve physical balance than others. Begin to notice when you feel more or less balanced. If you have a cold, are menstruating, or just having a bad day, you may find your balance and stability are a little off. Yoga promotes balance all the time by working the balance-promoting aspects of the body—the muscular, circulatory, and endocrine systems—as well as the mind, which can help overcome temporary physical instabilities. The more you practice, the more balanced your life, your body, and you will be.

All About Joints

Without your joints, your bones couldn't begin to do the amazing things they can do. Your knees, hips, elbows, finger joints, ankles, and all the rest of your joints, allow your muscles to move your skeleton to perform amazing movements—drawing, playing an instrument, dancing, jumping, hugging. But joints and arches need to move to stay strong, flexible, and workable!

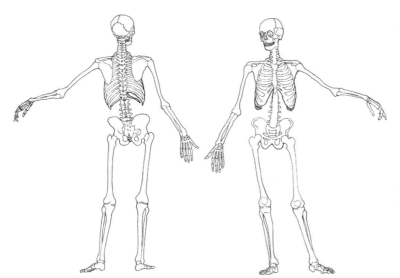

Joints and muscles make this skeleton move!

(Drawing by Wendy Frost)

Yoga helps to strengthen joints and ligaments. If you've injured a knee or a rotator cuff in the past, yoga can help to rehabilitate your joints. If you've never injured a joint in your life, yoga can strengthen the tissues that support your joints, to help prevent a future injury.

Elongate for a Healthy Spine

Spines aren't straight, exactly. They are sort of like a stretched out letter S. But just for the sake of example, imagine your spine is like a straw you would use to drink from a big cup of juice. Not the bendy straws, but a straight straw.

When the straw is straight, we have no problem sipping the juice. But as soon as the straw is bent over, the juice has trouble flowing through the straw. It might also help kids straighten their spines if they imagine a balloon gently lifting the tops of their heads upward as they walk around during the day.

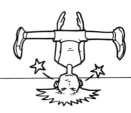

Ooops!

People often believe that if they have an injury they can't exercise. Actually, although you should use caution when moving the affected area, yoga is a great way to rehabilitate after an injury. Check with your doctor about what movements are acceptable, and ask a qualified yoga teacher for direction (see Chapter 9).

A healthy spine.

(Drawing by Wendy Frost)

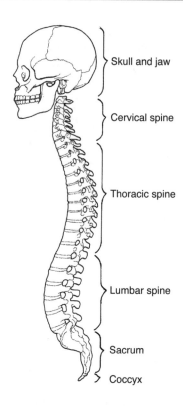

Skull and jaw

Cervical spine

Thoracic spine

Lumbar spine

Sacrum

Coccyx

So it is with your spine. It is in your best interest to keep the straw straight. A strong, straight spine allows the fluids and nutrients in our body to flow freely and easily inside us. If you slouch or bend over, your bodily fluids and your breath may become blocked.

In yoga, we also envision life energy flowing through channels in our bodies. A cramped, bent spine blocks that life energy so it can't reach every part of our bodies. Blocked energy, according to yoga, can keep the body from staying at its healthiest.

In other words, it is healthiest for our bodies to keep a straight, strong spine. An elongated spine is a tall spine and a healthy spine. Many yoga postures concentrate on elongating the spine as well as keeping it flexible and strong.

Posture Perfect

We're ready to debunk yet another myth, although this one isn't specifically about yoga: There is no such thing as "perfect." There *is*, however, an appropriate posture for your individual body—even though your body may change continually. And your posture has nothing to do with what is appropriate posture for anyone else but you!

Yoga helps us be more conscious and aware of our bodies, and consequently our posture, at all times. Yoginis who are in tune with their bodies can adjust them throughout the day to keep the spine elongated and straight.

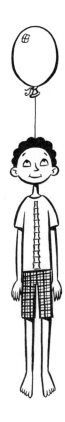

Imagine a balloon attached to a string that moves up through your spine and out the top of your head, ready to float you up to the sky. As the balloon lifts you upward, feel how your body moves to stand straight and tall.

Regular yoga practice will help you notice when you are slouching or slumping over your desk, when you are sliding back into your chair, when you are hiking up your shoulders or cramping your neck. Yoga helps you get used to the way a healthy posture feels for your body, so you can keep coming back to that posture even when you aren't practicing yoga.

Energizing the Nervous System

We've already talked about the way yoga helps balance our bodies and our nervous systems, increasing our balance, stability, and motor coordination. Yoga can also help relax and maintain the nervous system through meditation, which is another part of yoga.

Just like your muscles, which can repair themselves and get stronger during your rest periods between workouts, your nervous system needs to rest occasionally, too. Periodic meditation sessions, where you allow your mind to slow down and rest, help reenergize and rejuvenate your mental process. You'll be amazed at how refreshing it is to be quiet for a while, for both kids *and* adults!

Good, Restful, Refreshing Sleep for Kids

Bedtime can be an issue at any age. Some babies go right to sleep whenever they are put in their cribs, but many wake often or resist falling asleep even when they are tired. Toddlers and preschoolers often transform bedtime into a power struggle. Grade-schoolers and teens may find they don't get enough sleep because they stay up late studying, watching TV, or working on the computer.

Getting a good night's sleep is extremely important for kids of all ages. Kids (and adults, too) who are sleep deprived have more trouble concentrating, have less energy, and have more trouble with coordination than kids who get enough sleep.

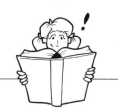

While bad sleep habits can be changed, *insomnia* is a more difficult problem for some kids. Yoga promotes sounder sleep, helping to ease insomnia and even bad dreams. Yoga relaxes us and helps manage stress, a common cause of sleep disorders.

Yoga also helps active, high-energy children relax when bedtime comes. It can be a high-energy activity, but even at its most vigorous, yoga balances the body so it is better able to make that transition into dreamland. Although other forms of exercise can make sleeping difficult, don't be afraid to practice yoga before you go to bed. Sweet dreams!

Learn About Yoga

Insomnia is the chronic inability to fall asleep or to stay asleep long enough or well enough to feel alert during the day.

The Least You Need to Know

➤ Yoga promotes healthy digestion and elimination through specific posture positions and exercises.

➤ Yoga builds heart and lung strength because it is aerobic; it also includes breathing exercises.

➤ Yoga increases flexibility and strength, balancing kids wherever they need it most.

➤ Yoga strengthens and elongates the spine to promote ideal fluid, air, and energy flow throughout the body.

➤ The vigorous yet calming effect of yoga helps kids of all ages sleep well.

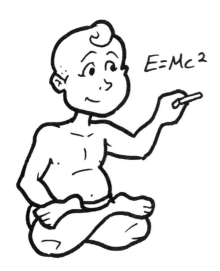

$E=Mc^2$

Chapter 3

Developmental Benefits of Yoga for Kids

In This Chapter

➤ Yoga reflects the natural patterns of child development, maximizing the body's potential

➤ For yogini babies and toddlers, parents are a key element in yoga fun

➤ Yogini preschoolers and grade-schoolers stretch and test their independence

➤ Yogini teens establish a positive sense of self

Yoga does more than help kids stay healthy and relaxed. Yoga supports and encourages the development of growing bodies, one of the primary reasons yoga is so helpful to kids.

Childhood is a period of physical change that will never be repeated in a lifetime. It offers a rare and brief opportunity to achieve body awareness and to take advantage of the developing systems of the body, as they become fully formed for the very first time.

Life in contemporary society is often less than supportive of the developmental process, but yoga, as we'll describe in more detail later, does more than support development. It is a reflection of development in its organic and ideal state.

Child development is a widely studied area with many controversial viewpoints and theories. We don't intend to debate them in this book, but we will examine the various ways in which children develop from infancy through the teen years, and show how regular yoga practice can stimulate, enhance, or as we've mentioned, reflect that development.

From Cradle to Empty Nest

If you think yoga is solely a human-made set of exercises, watch an infant for awhile. Nobody teaches a baby how to move. Nobody says, "Hey, Junior, hear that noise? Why don't you lift up your head to see what it is? Yes, very nice Cobra Pose, Junior."

While yoga was originally designed as an imitation of natural processes—whether a cat stretching or a tree swaying in the breeze—it is also based on movements the healthy human body makes naturally. This system was designed to put the body where it wants to be, moving in the directions and ways it naturally wants or needs to move, and that is why yoga helps bodies to stay healthy and keep the life energy flowing properly.

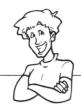

For Grownups, Too!

If you've ever sat back and watched your infant play and explore, you may be astounded at how flexible she is. How effortless it seems for her to reach up and grab her toes. What a simple matter to raise her head and legs and rock on her tummy. You may feel stiff and inflexible in comparison. Regular yoga practice can help to bring back some of that flexibility in your fully grown adult body.

Infants can do yoga in a more structured way than simply figuring it out on their own, however. Until a child is able to understand how to follow directions or play games, an adult can move an infant into developmentally appropriate yoga poses. This is nothing unnatural. The adult is simply showing the infant what its body can do, helping it to feel the potential of the human body from birth. This is how yoga supports, stimulates, and encourages development in infancy.

As children grow, yoga does the same thing. In a society where we don't always need to move very much, yoga helps remind us that our bodies were meant for moving, and moving in more ways than just walking, sitting, standing, or kicking a ball. Yoga keeps the entire body in play, working its range of motion, revealing its potential.

And just for the sake of you adults reading this book, yoga can help you reach and maintain your physical and spiritual potential throughout your entire life, even into the golden years.

Developmental Milestones for Children

Ever wonder if your child is "on track"? Parents may compare their children's development with the lists in books on the subject, and your pediatrician probably asks, during checkups, whether your child can do certain things such as crawl, wave, or eat with a spoon. Older kids soon become conscious of their own development in relation to others. "Am I normal?" a child may wonder.

We don't really like to say that children of any age should or shouldn't be able to do any specific thing. Children develop at their own rates and may develop more quickly in some areas than others. One two-month-old infant may already smile and recognize specific voices, while another may not. Both are probably "normal." Serious developmental delays should be assessed and addressed by a qualified health care professional.

Children who get involved in yoga at an early age often manage to reach developmental milestones earlier than kids who don't engage in much physical activity. Sedentary kids may lack the increased muscle tone and coordination yoga encourages. Yoga isn't about competition, of course, and we don't encourage you to compare your child to others. We do, however, wish for each child to have the opportunity to maximize his or her potential, including kids with developmental delays, who are more likely to meet milestones faster if they practice yoga regularly.

However, just to give you an idea about what level of yoga practice your child is probably capable of at what age, we include the following table. It is not meant to make anyone believe his or her children aren't progressing "normally." It is simply a guideline to help each individual parent and/or child assess general capabilities at different ages.

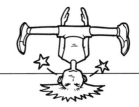

Ooops!

There exists quite a wide range of normal when it comes to child development. What is normal, anyway, besides a setting on your washing machine? Only your child's pediatrician or other qualified health care professional can assess appropriate development in your child. If you have a concern about your child's development, talk to your health care professional.

Stage	Age	Developmental Milestones
Infant	1 month	Can respond to sound by blinking, crying, or quieting, becoming startled, or changing respiration rate. Is already moving, stretching, flexing, and wiggling, testing the limits and capabilities of the body.
Infant	3 months	Begins to reciprocate to voices and faces, and begins to lift head, neck, and chest off the ground. A three-month-old can follow objects with his or her eyes, smile responsively, and can hold things like rattles or blankets. Baby knows you are there!
Infant	6 months	Begins to imitate, babble, grasp small objects, and play with his or her own hands. Can control head welland raise body on hands. Many can sit with support, roll over onto their backs, and creep or scoot. Infants six months and older can easily do the Yogini Sleep Pose (see Chapter 21), lying on their backs and bringing both feet over their heads with the help of their hands.

continues

continued

Stage	Age	Developmental Milestones
Infant	9 months	Can gesture, begin to crawl, pull to a standing position, cruise by walking and holding on to furniture, or even walk alone. Can poke with fingers and shake, throw, and drop objects. Loves to imitate and play interactive games like peek-a-boo. Nine-month-old babies can perform a nice Snake (Cobra) Pose (see Chapter 13), lifting their heads and chests off the ground from a stomach-lying position.
Infant	12 months	Cruises or walks, can follow a rapidly moving object with eyes, understands simple verbal commands, begins to imitate sounds, and may say a few words. By the first birthday, many kids enjoy Downward Facing Dog Pose (see Chapter 12), with the body in an inverted V, feet and hands on the ground.
Infant	15 months	Stands and walks without help, shows interest in pictures, makes requests by pointing, physically expresses emotion (affection by hugging, anger by throwing a tantrum), and imitates more complex activities.
Infant	18 months	Walks up stairs with help, throws a ball, jumps in place, pulls and pushes toys, and may be able to remove some clothing.
Toddler	24 months	Runs, kicks a ball, goes up and down stairs with two feet on a step, turns doorknobs and unscrews lids, can pick up objects from the floor without falling over, talks a lot, can put on clothing, refers to self by first name, and pulls people to show them something.
Toddler	30 months	Can stand on one foot momentarily, can jump a short distance with both feet, can move fingers independently.
Toddler	36 months	Can pedal a tricycle, climb stairs with alternating feet, can dress self almost completely, can feed self, and can begin to learn games with simple rules.
Preschooler	4 years	Can speak intelligibly, can tell the difference between fantasy and reality, can climb well, can follow two- or three-step instructions, can sing a song, and can hop on one foot.
Preschooler	5 years	Can skip, listen to stories, and engage in elaborate fantasy play, and can follow more complex rules for games. Loves to role-play.

Stage	Age	Developmental Milestones
Grade-schooler	6 years	Climbs well, tests limits of body (speed, throwing distance), becomes more self-reliant. By age six, many yoginis can do the Rock-n-Roll Pose (see Chapter 15), curling into a ball with knees pulled into the chest and rocking on their backs.
Grade-schooler	8 years	Can perform many chores for him- or herself, develops a sense of personal competence, can use logic to solve problems, and is interested in how things work. May begin to acknowledge alternative viewpoints. Peers become increasingly important.
Grade-schooler	10 years	Establishes peer group leaders, friends become even more important as does independence from family, accepting of increased responsibility, and especially needs family support for self-esteem and self-confidence.
Adolescent	11–14	Puberty usually hits during this time. Girls and boys both experience a growth spurt and develop secondary sexual characteristics, although these changes usually happen to girls about two years earlier than they do to boys. Feelings of vulnerability and sensitivity about appearance are common at this age. Privacy and peer conformity become extremely important, and physical activity patterns are established that often last for a lifetime.
Adolescent	15–17	Puberty is usually fully established in girls by this age, and boys are on the way, having gained muscle mass in addition to secondary sexual characteristics. Questions about values, beliefs, and identity are common, and a tendency toward future-oriented thinking begins (how current actions will affect a future outcome). This is the age to test rules, and family support is crucial. Depression due to circumstances such as relationship problems or losses is common.
Adolescent	18–21	Puberty in boys and girls is over and done with by this age, and "children" are busy achieving their adult selves, making career decisions, and often moving out of the family home. Older adolescents are more self-confident and comfortable with who they are, although high-risk behaviors may peak at this stage.

Meeting Kids' Needs

Whether a child is progressing according to the preceding table or not, yoga enhances and encourages natural development. We are all very different, physically, emotionally, and spiritually, but yoga is right for anyone. Whether a parent helps to move a baby's ankle in circles or a teenager hones his or her sense of balance, yoga gives kids what they need in terms of shaping and facilitating their own development.

Cognitive and emotional development are also enhanced by yoga. Preschoolers striving for more independence can find it by accomplishing Candle Pose (see Chapter 17) all by themselves. Teens in need of increased body confidence can find it not only through an increase in muscle tone and flexibility but also by practicing and instituting yoga principles of internal strength and flexibility, love, acceptance, and noncompetitiveness.

Yoga is also a wonderful endeavor for kids who are experiencing developmental delays and have special needs, which we'll discuss in detail in Chapter 25. Yoga may actually improve the rate and quality of development, helping kids to meet those developmental milestones at an age-appropriate rate (as assessed by your health care professional).

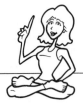

Yoga Stories

According to Sonia Sumar, internationally renowned yoga therapist and author of *Yoga for the Special Child* (Special Yoga Publications, 1996), children with Down's syndrome, cerebral palsy, attention deficit disorder (ADD), and learning disabilities can benefit immensely from the developmental stimulation of yoga. Many of her students with special needs have caught up to their peers and are now developing at an age-appropriate rate, or have made other remarkable strides in all facets of development from physical to behavioral.

Exploring the World with Yogini Babies

Now let's take a look at how yoga is specifically suited to kids of different ages, and what better place to begin than the beginning of life, in infancy?

Babies obviously aren't capable of following the instructions or getting into some of the poses accomplished by older kids, but that doesn't mean they can't do yoga!

Apart from the natural yoga positions babies tend to put themselves into as they explore the world and test their physical limits, an adult can help an infant into different yoga poses by gently manipulating the baby's arms, legs, and torsos.

The feet are a great place to start. Gentle massages on the feet, foot rotations, and ankle flexion and rotation will prepare a baby for future yoga poses, as well as send relaxation signals.

Our feet are our foundation, so even before your infant can walk, foot exercises can help to promote strength and flexibility in the ankles and aid in the formation of the arches.

Babies can also do knee bends and hip rotations with help from an adult; these are great for babies with colic, gas, or constipation. A gentle spinal twist is extremely beneficial for a baby, working the entire spine to help keep it flexible and healthy. The spinal twist also stimulates the central nervous system.

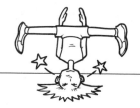

Ooops!

Moving an infant's body into yoga postures must be done with extreme caution, and adults should first learn the proper way to do this under the guidance of a certified children's yoga instructor (see guidelines on how to find one in Chapter 9). Babies are surprisingly flexible and strong, but adults must nevertheless be gentle and never push an arm, leg, or spine further than it naturally wants to go.

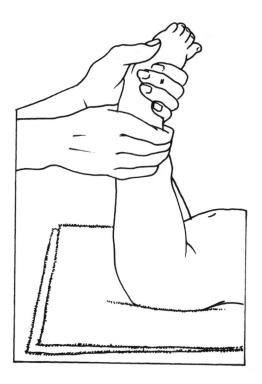

Gently massage baby's leg and foot, smoothing up the leg to the tips of the toes. (See Chapter 21 for details.)

(Drawing by Wendy Frost)

Lateral and parallel arm raises strengthen arm muscles and allow for flexibility in the shoulders, which will help an infant prepare for crawling.

Exercises for babies lying on their tummies include leg lifts and knee bends to help strengthen the lower back muscles as well as the legs. Infants can even do a version of the headstand, where an adult inverts the child to a 45-degree angle. The baby rests on mom's or dad's legs, which are straight out in front. The adult then bends his or knees, inverting the baby. This pose is beneficial in many ways. It reverses the flow of internal fluids, massages internal organs, and stimulates the central nervous system.

Gently invert baby for a few seconds and then return baby to a prone or upright position.

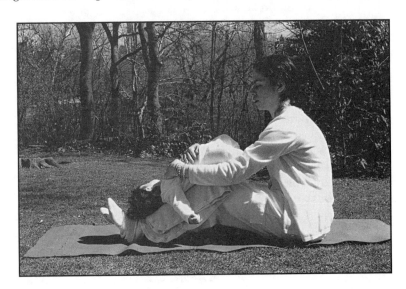

Finally, finish an infant yoga session with a rest and deep relaxation. Play soft music, give your baby a massage, and dim the lights or get a softly colored light bulb for your baby's room.

Nonstop Fun with Yogini Toddlers

Toddlers can do many of the same poses infants can do. Toddlers love to do yoga with an adult, and they can contribute more than an infant can, getting into and out of poses by themselves with just a little guidance and support from the participating parent or older sibling.

Toddlers can, of course, do more poses than infants can, too. For example, toddlers enjoy touching nose to knees, because the toddler can hold her own knees and lift up her head to reach them, with adult assistance. This is a great pose for relieving gas and colic and for stretching and elongating the muscles of the back and neck.

Toddlers (and preschoolers, too) tend to have relatively underdeveloped abdominal muscles, and knee bends work to strengthen these muscles, as well.

The Yogini's Sleep Pose (see more toddler poses in Chapter 21) is also a fun toddler pose. This is a pose children do all the time without realizing it is yoga! The child lies on his or her back and brings both feet over toward his or her head. An adult can help to lift up the head to meet the feet. This pose is actually a forward bend in a prone position, elongating the spine and creating flexibility in the hips and knees.

Gentle backbends are appropriately introduced during the toddler stage. Snake Pose (also called Cobra Pose, see Chapter 13) and Half Bow Pose (see Chapter 16) are achievable. For Snake Pose, rest the toddler on his or her belly, then scoop your arms under the toddler's arms and gently lift the toddler's upper body (not to the point of discomfort). For Half Bow Pose, the adult can bend the toddler's knees and raise the lower body, including the legs, hips, and lower back. Both of these backbending poses elongate the spine and strengthen the back muscles, help to keep the spine in alignment, and help to relieve constipation and gas. Follow with a forward bend to counter the backbend by doing Mouse Pose, which we sometimes call Child's Pose (see Chapter 12).

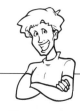

For Grownups, Too!

Toddlers are such natural yoginis that they will often discover yoga poses during their own play before you get a chance to show them! Give your toddler the space and opportunity for creative physical play and you might just end up witnessing the invention of several new yoga poses your family can include in its practice.

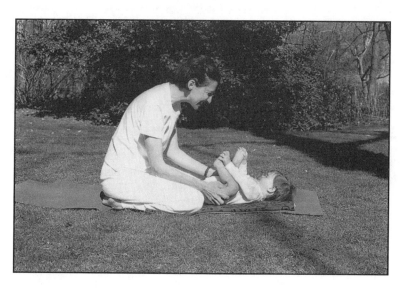

Toddlers are natural yoginis who love physical play as they discover what their bodies can do. This mom and toddler practice the Yogini's Sleep Pose.

Imagine Everything with Yogini Preschoolers

Preschoolers are even more independent in their yoga practice. They may not even want any help—they can do it *themselves!* This is the chance for the parent to step back and play the role of a facilitator. Parents no longer need to put the child into the poses.

Preschoolers are pretty much ready to do most yoga poses. They can fly like a butterfly, stand tall like a tree, and explode like a volcano. Accuracy and form are less important at this stage than are having fun and capturing the spirit of the pose. Safety is important; however, we would advise not correcting a preschooler's form unless safety is at stake.

For example, in a classic Snake Pose, the legs are together. If your preschooler's Snake Pose has a split tail (legs not together), that's fine. Let it be. However, if your child is doing Candle Pose (see Chapter 17) and turns his or her head from side to side, a parent should encourage the child to "Look at the flame on your feet!" because too much neck movement in this position, where weight is settled into the neck, might cause an injury.

Yoga with preschoolers is a blast! Meow and stretch like a cat, fly like a butterfly, be still like a mountain, swim like a fish. It's preschooler heaven! This is the stage where children—and their game parents—can really get into the feel of being one with nature. Forget about grown-up worries and take a cue from your preschooler yogini—be carefree during your yoga session and have fun!

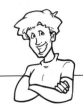

For Grownups, Too!

Preschoolers enjoy Downward Facing Dog Pose (see Chapter 12), but enjoy it even more when they can "walk" each other or be "walked" by a parent. One person pretends to hold a leash, and "walks" the other, who moves around the room in Downward Facing Dog Pose. Barking adds to the fun, and for a real burst of giggles, let preschoolers lift their legs for a pretend doggy bathroom break.

Loving and Learning with Yogini Grade-Schoolers

Yoga for grade-schoolers is similar to yoga for preschoolers, except that as grade-schoolers continue to grow, they will notice increased capability to perform certain poses. Parents can still refrain from form corrections at this stage. The key again is to have fun!

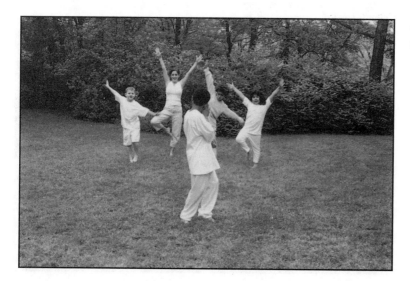

Grade-schoolers love playing yoga games.

Grade-schoolers are increasingly interested in other people, both parents and peers. This is the age to do lots of partner poses and big group poses. Play yoga games and really stretch and strengthen that imagination!

Grade-schoolers gain a lot of physical benefits from a regular yoga practice, but they also gain an important sense of their own being, getting in touch with who they are as they increasingly understand that they are an individual with unique qualities and a singular place in the world. Yoga can help grade-schoolers get in touch with their emotions, feelings, and moods, and may even help them to learn control over their behavior—a great big step for a grade-school child, and one that may help the child to feel he or she is truly no longer a "baby."

Changing and Growing with Yogini Teens

Teenagers are fully capable of practicing yoga all by themselves. Some prefer independent practice, others prefer to practice yoga with friends, a teacher, a parent, or all of the above.

Physical activity patterns set in the teen years are often an indicator of future activity patterns. Sedentary teens often become sedentary adults, and physically active teens often stay that way into adulthood. Regular yoga practice for teens can help establish healthy fitness habits for life.

Through yoga, teens learn healthy, lifelong fitness habits. This pair practices Warrior III.

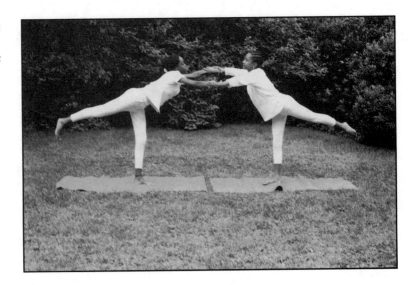

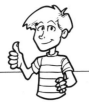

For Kids Only

Yogini teens, try Group Flower Pose, a challenging group yoga pose, with your friends. Sit in a circle with at least five other yoginis. Each person assumes Flower Pose (see Chapter 11), bending knees and bringing arms under each knee. Sit close enough and bring your arms under far enough that you can hold your neighbor's hand, causing knees to lift. Keep your feet together and balance. This is very tricky but lots of fun.

Parents should refrain from correcting inexact form in their teen yoginis. Reminding children about what goes where is fine, but yoga shouldn't become an arena for family discord. Parental correction may sound like a criticism, even if it wasn't intended to be.

Parents should keep yoga a positive experience for their teenagers, who will benefit from the physical exercise, the stress-relieving aspect of yoga, and the increased self-confidence and body acceptance yoga promotes.

Teens are also increasingly interested in values—which to choose, which to reject—and may be especially interested in yoga's Eightfold Path, which offers (non-religious) guidelines for living a productive, spiritually fulfilling, and healthy life. Continue on to the next chapter for a more complete discussion of yoga's Eightfold Path.

The Least You Need to Know

➤ Yoga can promote and enhance the natural process of child development by engaging the body in its full range of motion.

➤ Adults can move an infant into certain simple yoga postures to relieve physical discomfort, mobilize the growing infant body, and help the infant to relax and sleep well.

➤ Adults can help the increasingly independent toddler to achieve a variety of yoga postures to increase strength, flexibility, and burgeoning physical development.

➤ Yoga for preschoolers is a treasure trove of imaginative play. Yoga for grade-schoolers helps to increase the ability to achieve different postures, sometimes through partner and group yoga poses and yoga games.

➤ Teens can practice yoga independently or with an instructor, helping to set good fitness patterns for life, increase self-esteem and body confidence, and establish other habits and even values for living.

Part 2

Growing with the Tree of Yoga

This part describes yoga's spiritual side. Yoga respects and can enhance any spiritual belief, encouraging kids to think and act compassionately and with respect to themselves and others.

Yoga has a specific system to accomplish these goals. Thousands of years ago, an Indian sage named Patanjali developed a systematic description of yoga in his Yoga Sutras, in which he described yoga's Eightfold Path. This path delineates the steps to whole-body health and personal fulfillment in the form of compassionate values, healthy and productive habits, exercise, breathing techniques for better health, sensory control, greater focus, meditation, and a personal communion with divinity, whatever that means for the individual.

In this part, we interpret the Eightfold Path in a child-friendly way, helping kids to use it for their benefit, to live mindfully, calmly, with self-control and dignity, empathy and love.

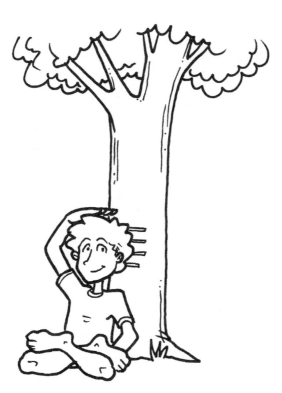

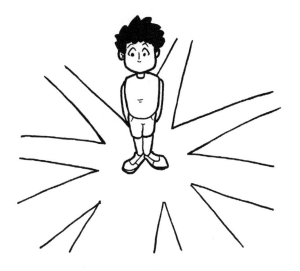

Chapter 4

Kids on the Eightfold Path

In This Chapter

➤ Walking yoga's Eightfold Path

➤ Spirituality for kids

➤ Yoga values and good habits

➤ Yoga exercises for the body and breath

➤ Calming the senses, focusing the mind, and learning to meditate

➤ Getting in touch with the divinity within

Yoga is great exercise, but it isn't just about doing yoga poses. It is a way of life! Yoga is a system of living that includes exercises for the body and for breathing, guidelines for how to live with productive, love-based values and habits that encourage self-respect and respect of others, and a number of different, progressively advanced techniques for centering the mind, increasing concentration, and exploring spirituality.

While some kids might be interested in only the fun yoga exercises, kids of any age may find the other aspects of yoga helpful, interesting, and a great road to self-improvement and confidence, as well as a tool for exploring the more spiritual aspects of life.

Introducing Yoginis to Their Spiritual Nature

Kids have a natural affinity for the spiritual, and no matter what spiritual path parents prefer to model for their kids (if any), parents may find that kids tend to find the idea of reality beyond the physical an easy concept to grasp. Kids also appreciate guidelines (even if they don't always act like they do). They want to know what will produce positive consequences for their lives, and what will produce negative consequences.

Rather than enforcing a doctrine, yoga instead gives kids a tool for spiritual exploration. Kids may have big questions and yoga doesn't seek to answer those questions. That is the parents' job, or the job of your religion. Yoga simply encourages kids to find their own spiritual identity. What a wonderful gift for a child!

Can Kids Do Yoga Without Being Spiritual?

Of course, not all families are spiritually oriented and some may not find this aspect of yoga compelling. Some kids are uncomfortable with the more spiritual-seeming parts of a yoga practice, like singing chants or saying the word *Om*. That's fine!

Even without its spiritual aspect, yoga can be a fine tool for physical and mental growth, teaching physical control, mental tranquility, and self-confidence. It can even be instructive in what values are most beneficial to the individual and the society as a whole. When a student is ready, he or she may decide to explore some of the more spiritual and/or lifestyle-oriented aspects of yoga.

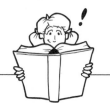

Learn About Yoga

The word **Om** is meant to imitate the original sound of the universe at creation and is the vibration that connects all beings in the world. It is often repeated to help focus the mind during meditation, symbolizing unity with all things. It also makes a great vibration when spoken by a group, connecting everyone together.

But remember, above all, yoga should stay fun. If yoga doesn't stay fun, challenging, and evocative to kids, if they don't love it, they won't keep doing it and its many physical and emotional benefits will go untapped.

In other words, if a child is interested in the tools for spiritual growth yoga offers, great! If not, fine. This is exactly what we mean when we say yoga meets the needs of the individual. It gives a child what he or she needs at this moment in life.

Yoga Embraces All Religions

Some parents may worry that yoga might contradict or be at odds with the spiritual guidance they choose to offer their children. But yoga isn't a religion or even a belief system. It is a method that can be applied to any belief system, Christian or Jewish, Buddhist or Muslim or Hindu, even atheist. It is also appropriate for spiritual seekers without any religious affiliation.

At its heart, yoga embraces all religions and respects any search for spiritual truth. While it does contain guidelines for living (see the sections on Yamas and Niyamas coming up a little later), the principles these guidelines espouse, such as nonviolence, truthfulness, and an avoidance of excess, make universal sense. Any young person can be a yogini, no matter what else he or she believes.

What Is Yoga's Eightfold Path?

Sometime way back around the second century C.E. (Common Era), in India there lived a man named Patanjali. While we know virtually nothing about him, he was responsible for organizing centuries of yoga thought, practice, and philosophy into a concrete system, explained in a large text called the Yoga Sutras. This work explains yoga—what it means, how to practice it, how to benefit from it, and how to live it. It is sort of the bible of yoga.

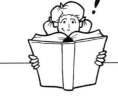

While many kids may not necessarily be interested in reading the Yoga Sutras (they are a collection of aphorisms, succinct but often enigmatic), they might be very interested in the ideas contained in them. One of the books of the Yoga Sutras goes into specific detail about living your life the yoga way. Patanjali divides the practice of yoga into eight parts, which he calls the *Eightfold Path*. This path consists of eight different aspects of living yoga, from physical exercises to breathing techniques to meditation to healthy values.

The point of the Eightfold Path is to incorporate yoga into life. It encompasses the whole of yoga, revealing yoga's true purpose: to maximize the potential of the self through the recognition of one's own inner goodness and the inner goodness in all others. Sounds pretty lofty, doesn't it? And not too child friendly? On the contrary.

> **Learn About Yoga**
>
> Yoga's **Eightfold Path** consists of a list of five values or universal guidelines for living called **yamas,** a list of five habits of expressions of values called **niyamas,** and discussions of the importance of yoga exercises (**asanas**), breathing techniques (**pranayama**), sense withdrawal (**pratyahara**), concentration (**dharana**), meditation (**dhyana**), and interaction with divinity (**samadhi**).

Patanjali's Eightfold Path consists of eight different aspects of yoga practice. They are ...

> ➤ A list of values, or personal attitudes to cultivate, called *yamas.*

> ➤ A list of healthy and productive habits to develop, called *niyamas.*

> ➤ Yoga exercises for the body, called *asanas.*

> ➤ Breathing exercises to energize and calm the body, called *pranayama.*

> ➤ The practice of calming and stilling the senses, called *pratyahara.*

➤ Focusing techniques to increase concentration, called *dharana*.

➤ Meditation, or *dhyana*.

➤ Spiritual communion, called *samadhi*.

Kids and adults can grow together with yoga's Eightfold Path.

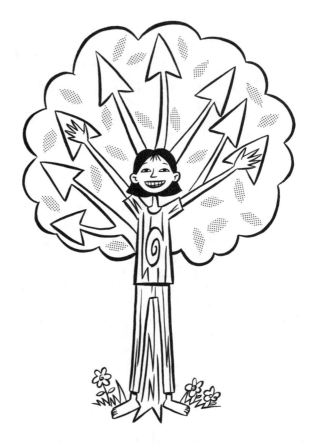

This may all seem a little confusing, so let's break down the Eightfold Path and talk about it piece by piece. You'll see that not only is it kid friendly, it makes a lot of sense for the whole family, too.

Yamas and Niyamas for Yoginis

How do we know what is right? How do we know what is good for us? How do we make decisions about dilemmas in our lives? Yoga philosophy has a few opinions on the subject that may help yoginis and their yogi parents live well and productively, in harmony with those around them.

You've probably heard of the Golden Rule. Maybe you even recite it to your kids: Do unto others as you would have others do unto you. That is at the heart of the yamas and niyamas.

These guidelines for living, divided into two groups—attitudes or values, called *yamas,* and healthy habits, called *niyamas*—are not meant to be religious in any way. They are simply physically and spiritually healthy, love-based attitudes and habits that lay the groundwork for a fulfilling and productive life.

Yama Values: Living Well in the World

The first group of guidelines are the yamas, or attitudes. Yamas are guidelines for personal attitudes about life and how to live it, teaching a productive and respectful way to react to one's environment and to other people. Let's look at each of them, and some of the ways kids can cultivate these values:

1. Live in peace.

The first yama, called *ahimsa,* is about cultivating a nonviolent attitude in every aspect of your life. That means refraining from harming anyone or anything. This yama can be as simple as vowing not to be mean to your little brother, or as complex as deciding to become a vegetarian so you don't support violence to animals. The idea is to get rid of malicious thought, mean words, and violent actions, surrounding yourself with an aura of peace, kindness, and love.

Parents can promote nonviolence at home in many ways. Limit viewing of violent television shows and movies, discourage violent games or ban toy weapons from the house, and most importantly, model nonviolent behavior for your children. Help your children to deal with conflicts and anger in a productive, nonviolent way, by using words instead of physical aggression, by working for creative solutions, and by putting love first.

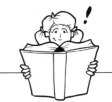

Learn About Yoga

Patanjali's Eightfold Path is sometimes described as a tree with eight limbs. Two limbs of Patanjali's Eightfold Path consist of **yamas,** or values, and **niyamas,** or good habits. Yamas are guidelines for personal thought, behavior, and reaction to one's environment and other people. Niyamas are productive habits to cultivate that will help the yogini honor his or her own spirit by maximizing physical, emotional, and spiritual potential.

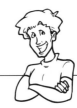

For Grownups, Too!

Although the different steps in the Eightfold Path don't necessarily have to be a part of a yoga practice, nor do they need to be accomplished in order, the order is designed to be progressive. In other words, first work on living well according to yoga guidelines, then get the body under control with exercise, then develop breathing control, etc.

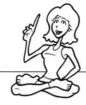

Yoga Stories

In India, where yoga first started thousands of years ago, many people are vegetarian, eating no meat, poultry, or even fish. In the United States, many people who practice yoga don't choose to be vegetarian, although many do, and some even choose to be vegan, eating no animal products at all, including dairy products and eggs. Vegetarian diets can be healthy for kids, especially if they include dairy products and eggs, and plenty of fresh, natural, preferably organic fruits, vegetables, and grains at every meal.

2. Tell the truth.

The second yama, called *satya,* is about deciding to tell the truth and act according to the truth, rather than lying or trying to deceive people, even yourself. People sometimes think lying can get them out of trouble, or at best, keep someone from getting their feelings hurt. Maybe they even lie to themselves, sometimes. They might believe a little lie won't hurt anyone. However, lies hurt the soul of the person telling them, and truth, even if it stings at first, is always the most straightforward way to deal with things. People trust those who tell the truth, and truthfulness leads to personal integrity.

Parents should help their kids with truthfulness, because this is a tough one. Always encourage kids to be open to you, and don't immediately punish them when they are honest, even if it is about a broken rule or an undesirable behavior. Talk about how much you value and respect the fact that they told you the truth, and recognize how difficult it must have been. And, of course, once again, model truthfulness for your children. If your kids catch you lying to get yourself out of trouble whenever it is convenient, they can hardly be expected to internalize truthfulness as a value.

3. Don't take what isn't yours.

The third yama, called *asteya,* is about refusing to steal. We don't just mean shoplifting or bank robbery, although we certainly would discourage such practices! We also mean stealing the ideas of someone else, like copying a school paper, or taking the credit for something that should go to someone else. Refusing to steal could include stopping yourself from stealing the attention away from someone who is getting it all. A kid who acts up because she thinks her friend is having a better birthday party than she had is stealing attention; a kid who keeps interrupting his little sister when she tries to talk is stealing, too.

Parents can encourage the refusal to steal by reinforcing the value of their children's own ideas. Why would your child need to plagiarize if your child knows his or her own ideas are worthwhile? And as far as shoplifting goes, let your child understand that this serious crime has grave consequences, and is also a betrayal and deeply disrespectful to a fellow human being who doesn't deserve to have his or her possessions taken away. Even a store is run by people, and yoga recognizes the value and goodness inherent in all people.

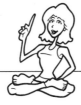

Yoga Stories

One of the principles in yogic thought is that of karma. Simplified, karma means that everything you do puts out a certain energy into the universe that will return to you. For example, if you make an effort to be honest and truthful, it will come back to you in some way, such as the return of a lost wallet. If you are open, caring, and loving to others, you will receive openness, care, and love. We like to call the awareness of or adherence to this principle karma yoga.

4. Master your urges.

This yama is most relevant for kids in the throes of puberty. Called *brahmacarya,* which is sometimes translated as chastity, this yama is about controlling the sexual urge so it doesn't control you. The intense hormonal changes associated with puberty are often accompanied by strong sexual desire (although not always). Brahmacarya is about refusing to let this desire cause you to diminish or disrespect anyone, including yourself. It doesn't necessarily require sexual abstinence, although some yoginis choose to practice abstinence. It really involves the control and proper expression of sexual energy, however parents care to interpret that for their children.

Regular yoga practice can help teens and preteens to channel sexual energy into a physical pursuit not fraught with the many consequences of teenage sexual activity. It reminds kids how valuable and worthwhile they are, so they may be less willing to give in to situations or pressures with which they aren't comfortable.

Discussing sexuality is, of course, of the utmost importance. Who knows what children will imagine if parents don't explain why control of the sexual impulse is so very important, especially in contemporary society where sexually transmitted diseases are rampant, sexual activity among teens is high, and sexual violence is so common.

51

Kids prepared for what puberty has in store will be better able to maintain their self-control and make smart decisions when confronted with challenging circumstances related to sexuality.

5. Do you really need it?

The last yama is about refusing to indulge in greediness. Called *aparigraha,* this yama has to do with distinguishing want from need, and living on what you need rather than expending energy on collecting more and more possessions. Possessions are seductive. Kids can easily fall prey to this mentality, especially when they get competitive and overly concerned with what or how much their friends have.

Kids who get possession-obsessed, always wanting more toys or better clothes or nicer electronic equipment, can benefit from this yama, which encourages the yogini to examine the effect of excess possessions. Possessions distract the yogini from more worthwhile endeavors, like exercise, meditation, schoolwork, and social relationships. When valuable possessions are lost, broken, or stolen, the possessor suffers. Plus, owning lots of stuff means you've got lots more stuff to keep, maintain, clean, and worry about. Is it really worth it? The pleasure you get from obtaining possessions is pretty short-lived. You might get a rush buying something and using it a time or two, but then it just becomes just one more thing to be responsible for.

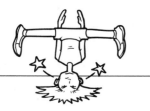

Ooops!

Conspicuous consumption of food is one thing, but eating disorders, including bulimia or binge eating, are quite another. Kids who suffer from these disorders can't just decide to stop bingeing; they need medical assistance. If parents suspect their child has an eating disorder, they should talk to a qualified health care professional immediately. Eating disorders can be treated successfully, but if left untreated, can result in serious physical consequences.

Aparigraha can also refer to greediness in other areas besides possessions, such as food. Greed when it comes to food (also known as gluttony) is unhealthy for the body, wasteful, and expensive. Does a child really need the whole pizza, or will two slices fill him or her up? Greed can also refer to someone's time (does a child spend four hours every night on the phone so that no one else can call?), or even attention (does a child answer every question in class and dominate all discussions so no one else has a chance to get a word in?). Aparigraha goes hand in hand with asteya, refusing to steal. People without lots of possessions, who don't demand more than their fair share of attention, are less likely to be the victims of theft.

Parents should help their kids evaluate how much their kids really need in terms of clothes, personal possessions, and even attention. Gently remind them of the value of simple living when you catch them getting possession-obsessed. And yet again, model simplicity in your home and in your own behavior, encouraging an environment of sensible consumption.

Niyama Do's: Learning About Yourself

Niyamas are habits and they are an outgrowth of the yamas. Once you have established healthy, loving attitudes and values, you can express them through healthy habits that are both self-honoring and respectful of others.

1. Keep it clean.

The first niyama, called *saucha,* is about cleanliness and purity. This refers to several things. Good hygiene is one. Parents should encourage their kids to keep their bodies, hair, nails, teeth, and so on clean. Good hygiene is more than healthy—it encourages self-respect. *Saucha* also means dressing in clean clothes, and living in a clean environment. A lot of kids have a hard time keeping their rooms clean, but this is just one more healthy habit to develop that encourages personal discipline. Plus, a clean, uncluttered living environment helps unclutter the mind.

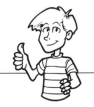

For Kids Only

Some of the reasons for avoiding greediness are obvious, but indulging in greed has a subtle negative effect on the entire psyche. If you are always focused on what you don't have and how to get more, you don't have room in your consciousness to appreciate and cherish what you *do* have. You will become less happy, less content, because you are always looking for something bigger and better.

The food kids eat should also be pure. Fresh, healthy food is best. The less processed and chemical laden, the better. The closer the food looks to the way it came out of the earth, the better. And no less important, acting, speaking, and thinking purely is a part of saucha. We won't try to dictate for you what pure actions, words, and thoughts are, except to say that they should be an outgrowth of the internalized values listed earlier in the section on yamas.

And of course, parents who set a good example by practicing good hygiene, keeping the living space as clean as possible (we know, we know, it isn't always possible), eating healthy natural food, and acting in a way that embodies the five yamas, will have kids who, at least eventually, will probably come back to those habits.

2. Chill out.

The second niyama is called *santosha,* and that means contentment. This habit has to do with putting the nongreed yama into practice. Living simply and frugally, cultivating a calm attitude, and learning to accept what you have as enough is the practice of *santosha.*

Some people wonder if *santosha* means you should never strive to get ahead in life or to achieve something better. Not at all! Yoga advocates evolving to become a happier, more fulfilled, more loving, more fully realized human being. But we all know that won't happen by getting more *stuff.* It happens by working on *you* and by learning to

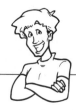

For Grownups, Too!

One great way for a family to cultivate contentment together is to make it a point to get together each day (dinner is often a good time) and have each family member share the best thing and the worst thing that happened to them that day (or the high and low point). Everyone stays in closer touch and parents may never again hear the response "nothing" when they ask their kids what they did today.

be kind, loving, and of service to others. Those aren't easy tasks if you are too busy being upset or discontent or frustrated about who you are or how much stuff you don't have.

Parents should help kids cultivate contentment by cultivating it themselves. As a parent, do you complain a lot in front of the kids about needing more clothes or a bigger house or more free time? Do you often act frustrated, irritable, or dissatisfied? Think about that. Parenting is a tough job and sometimes it is impossible to get through the day without getting frustrated or irritable, but if you can cultivate contentment by allowing time for yourself to relax and reenergize, by respecting your own needs as well as the needs of your family and co-workers, and by consciously trying to reorient your thinking away from the accumulation of possessions, you'll be setting a super example for your kids.

3. Cultivate self-discipline.

The third niyama is called *tapas,* which means concerned effort or serious trying. We think of this niyama as self-discipline. Self-discipline can be difficult at first, but it is an amazingly powerful skill for kids. Some kids might think they just aren't disciplined, but self-discipline is largely a matter of habit. The more you practice it, the better you get.

Traditionally, yogis practiced self-discipline by doing things like standing for a long time without moving, fasting (not eating for a period of time), or observing long periods of silence. We don't suggest kids engage in such extreme measures, but they can practice self-discipline all the same. Working on homework every night at the same time for a certain length of time is a good discipline. Practicing yoga exercises every day is another. Kids can learn self-discipline playing in organized sports, practicing music lessons, adhering to a natural diet and foregoing the soda and candy bars, or by committing to regular volunteer work. Almost anything we do can become a practice of self-discipline if we commit to it and stick to it.

Parents should help their kids acknowledge and work on their self-discipline skills by assisting them in finding opportunities to practice and reinforce their successes. And don't do it for them, or remind them so constantly that they couldn't possibly do anything. The point is *self*-discipline, remember?

Self-disciplined parents are, yet again, a great example for their children. If kids can watch firsthand how self-discipline happens, they will be better able to find and encourage that quality in themselves.

4. Be studious.

The fourth niyama, called *svadhyaya*, means study, but it doesn't necessarily refer to homework or reading spiritual texts, although that may be a part of *svadhyaya* for some yoginis. This niyama is really about self-study, or contemplation of the individual. Kids who spend time each day really considering who they are and actively investigating the question "Who am I?" will find all the other yamas and niyamas easier to achieve.

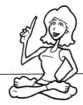

Yoga Stories

For kids interested in exploring the spiritual traditions and philosophies of the world, here is a brief reading list to get you started. Reading these works with your parents can engender some interesting discussions:

➤ Bhagavad-Gita

➤ Yoga Sutras of Patanjali

➤ *Siddhartha* (by Herman Hesse)

➤ Tao Te Ching

➤ The Bible

➤ The Torah

➤ The poetry of Rumi

➤ The Way of a Pilgrim

➤ The Kabbalah (excerpted versions are available)

➤ Writings by the Dalai Lama

➤ Writings by Thich Nat Hahn

How do kids learn to study on their own? Parents can engage kids in conversation that guides them. Encourage them to read beyond what is assigned for school, specifically books or articles that might address areas of interest for them or areas of questioning. (We know it can be difficult to push kids to read, and we don't want kids to develop negative attitudes toward reading, but finding what interests your kids and encouraging reading in those areas can make reading a positive experience.)

Following are some questions parents might ask their kids to get them thinking about themselves and their purpose and place in the world. Kids can certainly ask themselves these questions, too, even writing the answers in a journal. In addition to encouraging self-study, such questioning can bolster kids' self-esteem. And remember, keep the arena open, loving, and supportive, never accusatory or prying. If a child doesn't want to talk, don't push it:

How would you describe your personality?

What are your strengths?

What are your goals for this year? or, if that is too big, What are your goals for today?

Are there areas in your life you would like to improve?

What is your plan for improving them?

What do you like best about yourself?

What do you think your friends like about you?

Have you ever thought about the purpose of your life?

How do you see your role in the family?

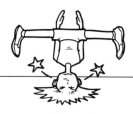

Ooops!

As a parent, when talking to your child about himself or herself, listen for negative talk or comments that truly seem at odds with your perception of your child. Are you missing something, or might your child be suffering from depression? If you think your child has a problem, keep the lines of communication open and seek counseling from a professional.

What might you like to be when you grow up?

In what ways do you think your friends and family need you?

In what ways do you feel supported and helped by your friends or family?

What do you think is important in life?

Do you think you usually act according to what you believe is right?

Parents can also make it clear to their children that whenever they feel like talking, parents are available. This reminds kids that what they have to say, and by extension, who they are, is valuable and worthy of contemplation and cultivation.

5. Consider divinity.

The final niyama, *ishvar-pranidhana*, has to do with thinking about and even committing to a higher power. This could be anything, depending on who you are and what you believe—God, Goddess, the universal power of love, positive energy—whatever divinity or a higher power means to you. This niyama involves focusing on and aspiring to that ideal, committing yourself to the love and energy, and accepting the aid that may come from that higher source.

If your family has never been involved in a particular religion, you might consider going to different places of worship together to see what different traditions have to say on the subject of divinity. If you aren't interested in religion per se, you might talk about what goodness is, what love means, or how one can harness positive energy in life. Whatever your individual focus, this final niyama can give kids a sense that their values and actions have a focus, a purpose, and are even powered by something beyond themselves and their own best interest.

More Adventures on the Yoga Path

Wow, all those yamas and niyamas, and those were just the first two limbs on Patanjali's Eightfold Path! Remember, even though traditionally the yamas and niyamas are meant to be dealt with before proceeding along the Eightfold Path, you don't need to master them before attempting the yoga exercises. We like to approach the whole Eightfold Path as one, spending some time here, some time there, until the whole thing eventually becomes part of everyday life.

The other limbs on the Eightfold Path are the subject of most of the rest of this book, so we will handle them only briefly here.

Control Your Body (Asanas)

The third limb consists of the asanas, or yoga exercises, and comprise the major portion of this book. The yoga exercises are what many consider to be the fun part, but they also have a very serious purpose.

Engaging in true spiritual contemplation isn't easy. Have you ever tried meditating? Your nose itches, you get restless, your mind races. It's hard to settle down, living in this fast-paced world of ours.

Thousands of years ago, yogis had the same problem. They wanted to spend time nurturing inner contentment, studying themselves, and contemplating divinity, but their bodies kept distracting them! Bodies like to move, and so the yoga asanas were created to keep the body in optimum health and allow the mind to remain alert and at ease.

Asanas have plenty more benefits for kids today besides helping to get the body under control so it isn't as distracting to the mind. Asanas give kids an outlet for excess energy and help to generate energy when needed, too. They allow kids to express their creativity and keep their bodies healthy. They help kids gain control over their growing and changing bodies. They promote inner contemplation and give kids the opportunity for social interaction when practiced in groups. See Chapter 11 to begin your practice of yoga asanas.

Breathe for Life (Pranayama)

Pranayama is the breathing part of yoga. Of course everyone knows how to breathe, but not everyone knows how to breathe really well, to get the full benefit of every inhale and exhale.

Pranayama teaches the yogini how to increase lung capacity, nourish the body with breath, and generate internal heat energy or a cooling relaxation response. See Chapter 10 to begin your practice of pranayama.

Calm Your Senses (Pratyahara)

Pratyahara is the part of yoga that works on calming the senses. Thank goodness for our senses, which help us to get the most possible enjoyment out of life. We can look at a sunset, smell bread baking in the oven, taste a fresh crisp apple, hear the waves breaking on the beach, feel the soft grass under our feet. Our senses also protect us. If we hear a car coming, we know to get out of the way. If we smell rotten food, we know not to eat it. If we accidentally touch a hot stove, we automatically withdraw our hand without even having to think about it.

Although our senses are vital for providing us with information, enhancing our enjoyment of life and protecting us against danger, sometimes too much information coming in can also be distracting. You may have experienced trouble falling asleep at night because of a bright moon outside or the sound of a dripping faucet.

Because children rely so much on sensory experiences to learn about the world around them, they often have more difficulty tuning out those experiences enough to concentrate on a particular task. Your kids might know what it's like to be so distracted by a ticking clock or the sight of other children playing that they can't concentrate on the test they're trying to take.

Learning to control the senses is as helpful as learning to control the body through asanas. Controlling and resting your senses allows your mind to work without these distractions. Old Hindu texts equate this process to a turtle withdrawing into its shell. Special yoga techniques exist for controlling or filtering the amount of information entering through the sensory channels. One technique is to sit very still and center the mind on a single point until you don't notice the distracting sensory information around you.

Focus Your Mind (Dharana)

The sixth limb of the Eightfold Path, dharana, involves learning to focus the mind, or concentrate. Yoga philosophy talks about how people tend to concentrate on outward things. Of course we do! Our senses perceive so much in the world that what we're sensing naturally becomes the focus of our attention most of the time. Concentration techniques involve concentrating on a single point, such as a light or a sound, long enough to internalize it or become one with it.

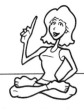

Yoga Stories

When Jodi (children's yoga teacher extraordinaire and co-author of this book) taught first grade, she implemented a program called "How Does Your Engine Run?" based on principles developed by occupational therapists Mary Sue Williams and Sherry Shellenberger. Their structured curriculum guides children through a series of activities designed to teach them how to use self-awareness, sensory experiences, and environmental modification to help them change their energy and concentration levels. Many of Jodi's students had a poor ability to regulate their energy level and their behavioral state. For example, when children were unable to settle down for a quiet activity, Jodi might dim the lights and put on soft music. For lethargic children, Jodi had frequent stretch breaks to get them moving.

While many kids may not be interested in protracted periods of concentration on a single point, they can practice this limb of the Eightfold Path in other ways. Generating the self-discipline to study, read, practice a sport, or continue to play an instrument even when they are tempted to quit will help to hone concentration skills. Even informal meditation sessions practiced regularly where the child concentrates on one thing—a favorite color, perhaps, or a few words to a favorite song—will help to exercise and increase the child's ability to concentrate.

Meditate (Dhyana)

Both calming one's senses and focusing one's mind, the fifth and sixth limbs, sound like meditation, and they are indeed meditation techniques. This seventh limb, however, is what happens when the last two limbs have been successful. Dhyana is the practice of meditation where the senses no longer infringe on concentration and concentration on a single point is so complete that the meditator feels at one with the focus of the meditation.

These last three limbs may sound esoteric, and we will have plenty of accessible techniques to help kids develop their concentration and ability to relax and do visualization techniques that lead to a productive meditation practice (see Chapter 19). But for now, just remember that a good chunk of the Eightfold Path of yoga involves development and discipline of the mind, which is just as important as development and discipline of the body.

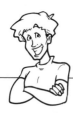

Touch the Divine (Samadhi)

The last limb of the Eightfold Path, samadhi, is really what happens when the rest of the path has been traveled. When the yogini's values and actions are founded in love, and when control over the body, breath, senses, and mind has been mastered, the result is not only a fully realized human being but a sense of overwhelming joy at the realization that every person is part of the divine force of love.

Again, this limb can mean different things for different people and isn't meant to convey any religion or doctrine. Achieving samadhi may not even be a goal. It is, however, considered the culmination of a traditional yoga practice—the end result, or goal. We feel that it can mean something different for every child or adult who practices yoga.

For Grownups, Too!

While Chapter 19 will teach you and your child some great ways to relax and meditate, one easy meditation technique (some would call it meditation training rather than real meditation) is to sit comfortably and count your breaths. Inhale: one. Exhale: two. Count to 10, then start back at one. Keep your mind focused on the counting and push other thoughts away gently. This technique is great for calming and centering both kids and adults.

Walking the Yoga Path as a Family

Living the yoga way is a great way to help kids establish the good health habits, personal discipline, self-control, spiritual fulfillment, and sense of self-worth they need to make the most of their lives. Yoga really is a complete program for life, one that can begin at any age.

It is also the perfect family activity everyone can enjoy together at times, separately at other times. A family walking the yoga path together shares a bond with a strong moral center based in love and mutual respect.

Families that do yoga together form lasting memories, common ground, and a closeness they might not otherwise achieve. As a parent, let yoga become a path for your family, and keep in close touch with your kids all the way through their own adulthood.

The Least You Need to Know

➤ Yoga is more than exercises; it is an Eightfold Path consisting of a list of helpful values, a list of good habits, exercises, breathing techniques, sense withdrawal techniques, concentration-enhancing techniques, meditation, and spirituality.

➤ Kids are interested in spirituality and can benefit from spiritual exploration.

➤ Yoga values include nonviolence, truthfulness, not stealing, sexual control, and not being greedy.

➤ Good yoga habits include cleanliness in hygiene, environment, and thoughts; contentment; self-discipline; self-study; and interaction with whatever the individual feels constitutes divinity, a higher power, or spirituality.

➤ Kids practicing the Eightfold Path with their families may establish a closer connection and better communication with parents throughout childhood and into adulthood.

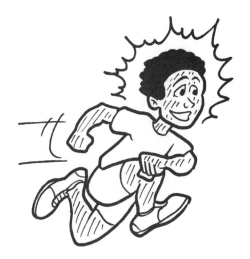

Chapter 5

Energized, Focused, and Carefree Kids

In This Chapter

➤ Yoga—the ultimate stress management tool for kids

➤ Teaching mindfulness and maintenance of the mind-body

➤ How yoga helps kids deal with anger, the pressure to compete, and conflict resolution

➤ Why parental modeling is essential for healthy child development

Life in the modern world gets pretty stressful. Adults know what it is like to feel fragmented, exhausted, forgetful, and burdened with worries. But kids aren't immune, either.

Lots of kids today report high levels of stress. What do kids have to be worried about? Plenty. Homework, friends, romantic relationships, money, jobs, their parents, their siblings, their futures—the same stuff grownups worry about. Kids may worry more today than ever before, and they are certainly under lots of stress. But that isn't all bad.

Kids learn from stress. They learn responsibility, self-discipline, organization, money management, and strategies for building and maintaining relationships. But too much stress for too long has the opposite effect. Stress is supposed to be a short-term thing, not something to endure for weeks and months at a time. Our bodies aren't made for it, and kids who suffer from chronic stress can find coping with daily life extremely difficult.

Yoga is the ultimate coping strategy. It teaches kids how to maintain high energy, stay focused, and prioritize their stressors for more effective stress management.

We Live in a Hectic World

Many of the undesirable qualities in the world today are things under our control. We can make a conscious effort to simplify our lives, be less materialistic, be more caring and giving, and be a better family member and friend.

However, there is much about the world today we can't change. The behavior of other people is a big one. The divorce of parents, the betrayal of a friend, the chronic illness or death of a loved one, even random violence are all realities in the lives of lots of kids, and these are things kids can't control.

Environmental stresses are also often beyond the control of kids. School can be extremely difficult, both in its academic and social aspects. Sometimes life at home isn't a picnic, either. Changing environments with a move is difficult, too, even if the move is to a more desirable location.

And then there are the internal stressors. Sometimes kids feel insecure or negative about themselves. They may take on too much, requiring perfect grades and participation in lots of extracurricular activities, or they may feel unable to take on much at all.

What's a kid to do? Stress management is an important skill for kids, and regular yoga practice is a great place to start.

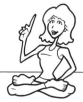

Yoga Stories

Kids may not be able to control all the stresses in their lives, but they can affect their body's ability to handle them. While regular yoga practice is an excellent technique for stress reduction, lifestyle changes can reduce the effects of stress too. Positive steps kids can make in their own lives include ...

➤ Eating healthy food at regular times each day.

➤ Getting regular exercise.

➤ Avoiding excess caffeine.

➤ Avoiding alcohol, tobacco, and illegal drugs.

➤ Practicing self-affirmation. ("I can do this." "I am worth the effort." "I can feel good about this." "I'm doing a good job.")

➤ Noticing and consciously ceasing negative self-talk. ("I can't do it." "My life will always be miserable." "Nobody likes me.")

➤ Making an effort to build a network of supportive friends.

Yoga Puts Kids in Touch with Their Thoughts and Feelings

Yoga may look like exercise for the body, but it can also have a surprising effect on the mind and emotions. Yoga can make kids feel surprisingly emotional. When we practice yoga, blocked emotions and feelings can be released and different energy centers may be stimulated.

Sometimes in yoga classes, students will even cry, or behave inappropriately at the end of class. This can be confusing for the students, who wonder where their outbursts came from. Part of practicing yoga is recognizing and honoring those emotions as they are released. It's okay to feel suddenly angry or sad or frustrated, or on the flip side, to feel sudden joy or excitement. Kids might even find they travel the entire range of emotions during a class.

One important way to manage stress is to get emotions out in the open. Having friends and family members to talk with about feelings is important, but sometimes kids may not even realize they are holding their feelings inside. It may not make sense to some people that physical exercise can release emotional feelings, but we believe the mind and the body are so inextricably linked that they have a constant and pervasive influence on each other. Work one, and you work the other. Exercise the body, and the mind will begin to clear itself of the things that are keeping it from doing its best work.

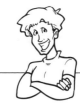

For Grownups, Too!

Yoga breathing techniques are a powerful way to cleanse the body and release negative emotions. When practicing yoga breathing, concentrate on inhaling love, joy, and positive energy, and exhaling self-doubt, sadness, and negative energy.

Mindfulness: Identifying Thought and Emotion

Practicing *mindfulness* means being acutely aware of and present in each moment. Have you ever gone through the whole day on "automatic pilot," going through the motions but never really paying attention to how you feel or what you are doing? Life may be easier on automatic pilot, but it is much less satisfying and productive.

Yoga cultivates mindfulness. During yoga, we constantly scan our physical and emotional bodies, moving slowly and really tuning in to each movement and position. How does this pose feel?

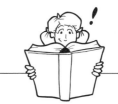

Learn About Yoga

Mindfulness is a state of awareness in which a person is consciously present in each moment as it happens rather than dwelling in the past or the future, or automatically performing behaviors.

What are you thinking as you do this movement? What sense impressions do you have during this series? What does your body feel like now? We don't encourage the use of mirrors when practicing yoga with kids. Instead, we look within ourselves. Mindfulness is keeping your senses open and looking within.

Jodi and her yogini assistant help the group practice mindfulness during deep relaxation.

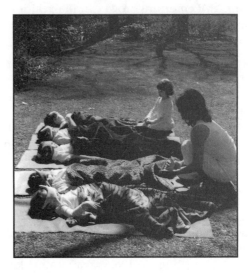

The perfect time to begin practicing mindfulness is during deep relaxation (called *Shavasana* in yoga; see Chapter 19). Eventually, mindfulness can extend beyond the yoga practice to enhance everyday life. Being truly present and aware while doing homework, eating dinner, or spending time with the family can make each day a special gift—because each day is a special gift. Sometimes we just forget to notice!

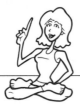

Yoga Stories

Sometimes we escape stress via chemical means. People may think caffeine will help them stay awake or energized, alcohol will help them relax or feel less inhibited, illegal drugs will help them escape problems or keep friends, or aspirin or ibuprofen will cure chronic headaches. While some medications are necessary to correct certain problems, excessive use of chemicals to modify the body's stress response can actually make matters worse by causing a physical or emotional dependency, by suppressing the immune system, and by increasing the chance of accidents. Natural stress-reduction techniques like yoga are healthier, safer, and create a more balanced state.

Using the Body to Calm the Mind

The Chinese call it "monkey mind," that feeling when your mind is racing out of control, flitting here and there, thinking about everything you have to do but unable to concentrate on actually doing any of it. Most grownups know how it is to feel overextended and disorganized, but kids know the feeling, too. Imagine monkey mind for a teenager:

> I can't believe I haven't even started that English paper. And I have to read a whole history chapter, and do 45 math problems by tomorrow. I'm really hungry! And what did Jennifer mean when she said my hair looked different? And I wonder if I'll get invited to that party. I hardly got any sleep last night but I've got so much homework! And what will my mom say when she sees I haven't cleaned up my room yet? And what if I don't get to play in the game this week? Does the coach think I'm not good enough? And what if I do get to play? What if I screw it up? I'm so restless, I can't sit still. What if I let everybody down? And if my little brother comes into my room one more time I'm going to scream!

Or, imagine monkey mind for a grade-schooler:

> Oh no, nobody else is wearing jeans today. We all said we'd wear jeans today. If I don't get this multiplication thing soon, everyone will laugh at me. Why are those people looking at me? Do I look funny? Is something wrong with me? I have no idea what the teacher is talking about. I'm really hungry. I can't believe my parents are making me go to Aunt Sarah's house after school. How boring. What if I hate the lunch today? Why didn't I bring my lunch? I wish I could be playing outside. School makes me miss all the good weather. Maybe I could go home for lunch and change out of these jeans before anyone notices. I'm so restless, I can't sit still. If the bell doesn't ring soon I'm going to scream!

These are just examples, of course. Even very young children can experience monkey mind and other effects of stress. A child's stress may be expressed in a completely different way, but if a parent asks a child if he or she ever has racing thoughts, we bet the answer is "Yes."

One of the amazing things about the link between the body and the mind is that moving the body actually helps to release mental energy, too, helping the mind to slow down, cease its chatter, and relax.

Yoga exercises are particularly suited for helping to calm and quiet the mind. Yoga exercises take concentration, and the mind can't scatter every which way if it is busy focusing on balance or the movements of a Yoga Sun Dance. At the end of a yoga workout, the body feels pleasantly energized, and the mind wonderfully serene, as if you've given your mind a mini vacation or internal massage.

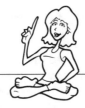

Yoga Stories

Here's a little test to show you how your mind can affect your body, and vice versa. Find a friend, sibling, or parent to help you, then stand tall and raise one arm out to the side. Hold it strongly, then think about something positive: someone you love, something you love to do, etc. Have your partner try to press your arm down and feel how hard it is to press down. Now, try it again. Think of something negative: something you don't like to do, something you dread, something that makes you nervous. Have your partner press your arm down again. It will be much easier! End with a third try, thinking about something positive again. *Voilà*, your arm is strong again!

Using the Mind to Calm the Body

Of course, the mind-body interchange goes both ways. Just as physical movements help calm the mind, the mental exertions of yoga help calm the body.

The physical signs of stress are more obvious in some kids than others. While some might display hunched posture, irritability, and low energy, others might be hyperactive with irregular eating and sleeping habits, while others act fine but seem to get every cold and flu virus that comes along. What can the mind do about that?

Much of the effort of yoga postures is a mental effort. When the mind learns to focus and concentrate, the body becomes more centered and organized. Energy flows more freely. The immune system works more effectively. Posture straightens. Anything that gets the mind under control will help to get the body under control.

The Body Scan is a good example. The Body Scan is a technique that involves lying relaxed and still. The body doesn't *do* anything. The mind does all the work. Working from toes to head, the mind concentrates on relaxing each body part, one at a time. The effect of this mental exercise on the physical body is amazing. It is one of the most physically relaxing of relaxation techniques, the classic example of the interrelationship between the body and the mind.

Energizing the Mind-Body

People tend to think that things like the Body Scan or meditation in the Lotus Position represent the extent of yoga's physical challenges, and that the point of yoga is relaxation. As we've already mentioned, yoga can be physically strenuous, and it can also be exceptionally relaxing. At the same time, however—and this is one of the paradoxes of yoga—it is incredibly energizing, for both the body and mind.

There we go again, lumping the body and the mind together. It might be easier to just call the whole package the "mind-body," because really, that's what we are. (While it might be even more yoga-accurate to say "mind-body-spirit," that's getting unwieldy.) Because yoga moves and relaxes the body, and quiets and relaxes the mind, the overall effect is one of increased energy, ready and waiting with mindfulness and a positive spirit, to live each moment to its fullest.

Yoga is about balance. If you feel sluggish and lethargic one day, doing yoga will bring you increased energy and momentum. Yoga is great for kids with low energy. One of Jodi's students has autism and a very low energy level. At times, doing even a simple yoga pose can be challenging for him. But he does it, and his yoga practice benefits him in many ways. He enjoys Yoga Dancing, Lion's Breath, and Mother Snake Pose, during which he likes to shake, roar, and hiss!

When kids are feeling overly stimulated yoga also works its magic, balancing the other way to bring renewed relaxation and ease. Another student of Jodi's often enters yoga class feeling disorganized and overstimulated. He displays difficulty focusing on the task at hand and his attention span is limited. However, after an entire yoga class, and especially after a deep relaxation or meditation, he is noticeably more focused, organized, and steady. Beginning this student's classes with a deep relaxation before moving into other poses has made a world of difference. This student and other kids who tend toward overstimulation also benefit from doing poses that involve gross motor movements, like Bear Walk (see Chapter 14), Crossovers (see Chapter 17), and the Yoga Sun Dance (see Chapter 15).

The point is that healthy bodies and focused minds feel energized but not overactive, serene but not lethargic, and that's where yoga brings us, to that lovely and ultimately centered middle ground where our bodies and minds can work the best.

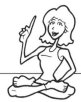

Yoga Stories

The philosophy of yoga and many other Asian philosophies include the notion of yin and yang. Yin and yang are two opposing forces that make up all things in the universe. Yin refers to the moon, darkness, and female forces, and yang refers to the sun, light, and male forces. Neither yin nor yang is superior or inferior. They complement each other and balance each other. This is also the goal of yoga. Each person has both yin and yang forces within, but individuals tend to have more of one or the other. Both girls and boys can tend to be more yin or more yang in nature. Yoga helps bring the yin and yang of the mind and body into balance.

*The ancient symbol for
yin and yang, the balance
of opposing energy states.
Yoga brings kids' minds
and bodies into balance.*

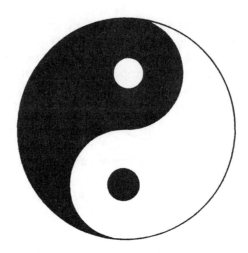

How Yoga Tames Kids' Anger

Whether the child is a frustrated toddler who can't make someone understand what he or she wants, or a frustrated teen who doesn't agree with a particular opinion or rule expressed or enforced, parents probably know what it is like to see their kids angry.

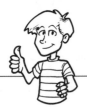

For Kids Only

Yoga poses can help release angry emotions, but you can help yourself, too. While it doesn't apply to all situations, remember that you have the power to let things go. Sometimes it helps to remember the big picture instead of focusing on the little things. This is a complicated concept, but it might be something for you to consider the next time you feel angry.

Anger is a difficult emotion for kids. They feel it strongly, but they have learned, or are in the process of learning, that there are acceptable and unacceptable ways to express it. But express it they must. Repressing anger can lead to future problems. The challenge is learning to express anger in an appropriate and productive way.

But all those anger-management solutions are sometimes hard for children to reach. How do you talk out your problems when you are so mad that all you want to do is yell or punch a pillow? Yoga can help kids handle anger, letting it out in a nonviolent but effective way until they are able to address the problem in a more rational manner.

Lion's Breath (see Chapter 10) and Volcano Blast (see Chapter 15) are two effective poses for the release of angry emotions. Kids can think specifically about what is making them angry as they do these poses. It really works!

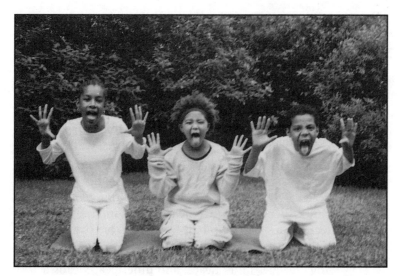

Lion's Breath is a great yoga pose for releasing angry emotions or helping transform bad moods into good moods!

How Yoga Helps When Kids Feel Pressure to Compete

A big source of stress for a lot of kids today is the pressure to compete. Whether the child is on the football team or in the chess club, is a swimmer or a singer, is trying for an academic scholarship or the title of "most rowdy in school," competition is part of life, especially for teens. Not that younger kids are immune, either! We've witnessed a pretty fierce argument between a four-year-old and a five-year-old over which one was "cooler."

Yoga can be an oasis for kids caught in a competitive world. Yoga is noncompetitive to the core. No mirrors, no contests, no losers, no trophies, no titles. In yoga, the student examines the self. Yoga builds self-esteem so that kids won't feel the need to compete. Even in yoga games, there are no winners and no losers. Kids love the feeling that they don't have to compare themselves to anyone else. They don't have to measure up to anyone, and there is no need to be "the best one," except to be the best possible individual they can be. Kids, in turn, feel safe and confident!

For some kids, allowing yoga to be noncompetitive may be difficult. They may begin by comparing their progress to the progress of others, and this can be a difficult transition to make, into the realm of noncompetitiveness. This is where parents can really help. Kids receive so much of their self-image from their parents, and parents should make a conscious effort to do things with their children that teach kids to love themselves. A child who has that inner confidence won't feel so pressured to compare him- or herself with others.

How Yoga Helps Kids Learn to Resolve Problems Peacefully

One of the skills kids must learn to become successful adults is conflict resolution. Toddlers are clearly unable to negotiate a settlement when it comes to who gets the toy train. They will either persist or give up. Preschoolers are already learning to work out conflicts—"I'll play with the train first and then I'll give it to you." Grade-schoolers and teens have even more advanced conflict resolution skills.

But sometimes, even for adults, conflict resolution can be tough. Some situations are simply unfair. In others, anger or other emotions may cloud the issue. But the regular practice of yoga in all its manifestations, from the yamas and niyamas to the exercises and breathing techniques, can help kids learn effective conflict resolution at an early age.

Yoga teaches inner peace, and inner peace leads to peaceful relations with others. Yoga teaches the student to focus on what is really important, to let go of the little things, to give to others, and to be selfless. The practicing yogini may be quicker to grasp the concept of peaceful communication.

That doesn't mean yoginis should be doormats. Yoga wasn't created so people could get walked over. Instead, yoga helps put problems in perspective. The child who walks away from an argument because it is unimportant radiates a much different energy than the child who backs down in an argument because he or she is full of fear or lacks self-confidence. The child who walks away is unconcerned about the reactions of others and chooses to spend his or her energy in more fruitful ways. That child has set an example that will help to promote peace in the immediate environment and ultimately, in the world environment.

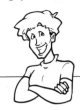

For Grownups, Too!

The next time you and your child have a disagreement, get out a tape recorder and record your conversation. Sometimes, just the action of getting the tape player can dissolve the tension. If not, play the tape back later, after you have both cooled off. You may both learn something about the way you sound to each other when you are angry. Perhaps everyone involved will find a way to modify his or her approach next time around.

Walking the Yoga Walk

We've talked a lot about what yoga *can* do for a child, but will the child actually reap the benefits? Going to yoga class then forgetting about yoga the rest of the time may not have much of an effect, but the child who decides to walk the yoga walk can be positively transformed, not into a different person but into the whole person he or she has the potential to be.

Children who have already taken the step toward reading this book, or who have accepted the opportunity to do yoga, either in a class or on their own, are already open to yoga and have already begun to walk the yoga walk. They are already open to new ways of being, and that in itself is a giant leap for humankind.

What Parents Need to Do, Too

Of course, you parents reading this book have taken a big step, too. Perhaps you suspect yoga can be beneficial to your child, and you are eager to help your child fulfill his or her potential in whatever way you can. Great!

But as we're sure you know, your job doesn't end with the purchase of a book. Your job every single day is to model the behavior you would like to see in your children.

Like Parent, Like Child?

Today, your child may do everything he or she can do to act like the opposite of you. You like baseball? She leaves the room at the mention of the game. You love reading? He would rather watch TV? You say tomato? She says—you get the picture.

But here's the thing about kids. As they attempt to establish their independence from you, they are constantly testing to find out who they are as individuals, different from you. Yet, it's a big, scary world out there and kids need to know they are anchored somewhere. When they are unsure (even if they don't look or act unsure), they are looking to you for an example of how to act, what values to have, even what to think. They may ultimately decide to disagree with you, but they are watching you, and your behavior will influence theirs, like it or not.

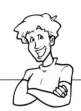

For Grownups, Too!

The best way to help your children commit to a regular yoga practice is to practice yoga yourself. Yoga has incredible benefits for parents—stress reduction, relaxation, body confidence, increase in focus and concentration (helpful when you can't remember where you put those car keys!), and a place for spiritual exploration. Set a great example for your kids while you help yourself!

That's a pretty big responsibility, one of the most awesome responsibilities of parenting. You can talk yourself blue in the face, but kids notice if you don't do what you say. Yet, modeling represents parenting's most rich opportunity. The public service announcements speak the truth: Your kids *do* listen to you, and they watch you, too. They may be good at disguising their listening some of the time, and it may sometimes take them awhile to respond to what you say and do. But your behavior matters.

How Parents Handle Anger and Conflict

One of the most important ways your behavior affects your kids is in the way you handle anger and conflict. A violent or explosive response to conflict can affect your kids in a lot of ways, none of them very positive. Everyone loses his or her temper

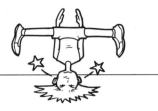

Ooops!

Adults, if you believe you have a problem dealing with conflict or anger, please seek help. A counselor can help with anger management. Your regular yoga practice, including meditation, can also help overstressed parents deal with anger. Yoga's message of nonviolence, inner peace, self-love, and honoring the divinity in others can have a powerful diminishing effect on angry emotions. That's great modeling!

once in a while, but as an adult and a parent, you have a responsibility to your child.

When conflict arises, we urge you to remember that your children will internalize your responses in one way or another. How do you want them to be able to handle conflict in their own lives, as adults? Act as you would have them act.

Yogis and Yoginis Unite: Do Yoga with Your Kids

Whether you think you "need" yoga or not (we believe it is highly beneficial for everyone!), practicing yoga with your kids is an indescribable bonding experience. Yoga brings young children together with their busy parents, and older kids can find something in common with parents on a physical and an intellectual level.

As the traditional family dinner fades into distant memory, a family yoga practice can take its place. For families who manage both, all the better! Families who spend time together in love and growth maintain an indestructible bond that will last a lifetime and serve as a foundation on which kids can build a life, healthy relationships, and families of their own.

The Least You Need to Know

➤ Modern life is hectic and stressful for kids, but yoga can give kids a healthy and productive tool for stress management.

➤ Mindfulness means being present in each moment, totally focused on what you are doing and feeling.

➤ Working the body can calm the mind, and working the mind can calm the body. The two are so interrelated that we like to refer to the mind-body as a single entity.

➤ Yoga can help kids deal with anger, modify the urge to compete, and deal more peacefully and productively with conflict.

➤ Parents need to model behavior for their kids because kids are paying attention to how parents act.

➤ Doing yoga together is a great family bonding experience.

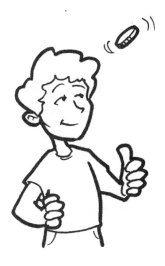

Chapter 6

Kids Choose!

In This Chapter

➤ Yoga and the whole child

➤ Fostering self-love through yoga

➤ Learning has many faces

➤ Yogini girls, yogini boys

➤ The benefits of fostering self-esteem

➤ Sparking creativity by inventing new and unique yoga poses

How often do kids get to make decisions for themselves? How often do they feel like they have power over their own lives? Coaches, teachers, parents, and counselors set rules, guide kids, and try to help them become adults. We try to let kids make their own decisions and exercise control, but for whatever reason, it doesn't always turn out as such. Yoga can be a refreshing change for kids in a world where adults make the rules. Even in a yoga class with a teacher, the emphasis isn't on following rules or doing things in exactly the right way. The only rule is that kids cherish themselves and work at an individual pace toward physical, mental, and spiritual fulfillment. That's a rule that gives kids power over their own lives.

Teaching Kids to Love Who They Are, Body and Soul

If a child is to love her body, she must know her body. If a child is to love his soul, he must know his soul. Kids are incredibly sensitive when it comes to what they can and can't do, how they look, how other people perceive them, how they compare to others, even to what they might be able to do *too* well. Yet, most of this awareness has to do with the external, and kids tend to internalize those external judgments: *If I look like this, I must not be worthwhile*, or, *If my friend said that about me, it must be the way I really am.*

Yoga flips this way of perceiving, helping the child to see his or her internal worth first, so that the child's inner light can radiate outward, transforming the external from the inside out. If kids love their inner selves, their souls, they can also learn to cherish and nurture their bodies.

Kids practicing yoga learn to appreciate their inner light, to nurture it, and to share that glow with friends—proud, happy, confident yoginis!

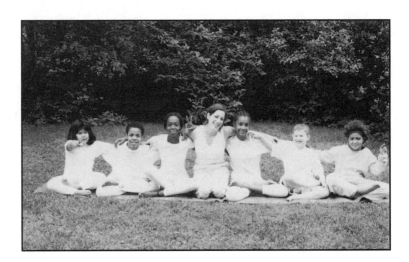

Embracing Yoga Union

The word yoga means union, from the root *yuj,* "to yoke." One of the most important ways yoga teaches kids to love themselves is by joining or yoking the body with the mind, and the mind-body with the soul. The body is integral to the self, of course, but kids who embrace yoga union begin to understand that body is only a part of the self. The mind, the emotions, the body's energy, breath, thoughts, feelings, and soul—all these things are part of the self, and just as essential as the body.

Embracing yoga union also means using this knowledge to maximize the potential of the self. Yoga makes the body stronger, more flexible, and freer, and does all these same things to the mind, the emotions, the body's energy, the breath, thoughts, feelings, and the soul. Kids who learn to see themselves as a united whole, rather than a collection of body parts, will be getting the most possible benefit from a yoga practice. They also tend to bloom like flowers.

Learning to Trust

Of course, a parent telling a child, "You are more than your body—you are also your mind, feelings, soul ..." isn't likely to mean much to him or her. First, the child must trust his or her parents and must also trust the process of yoga. This isn't always easy. Children learn at an early age that they can't always trust everyone and everything.

Parents can begin to build trust by treating their children with respect. Children treated with respect learn to trust. If a child opens up or shares something important with a parent, or asks something of a parent that is of great importance, the parent should really listen, respond, and address the child's needs in a caring and respectful way. Parents can also help their children to trust the yoga process by being supportive, encouraging, and never critical.

Every Body Has Something to Learn

Nobody knows everything. Not parents, not teachers, not kids. Everyone has something to learn. If you are naturally flexible, yoga can teach you about strengthening your body. If you are naturally strong, yoga can teach you about flexibility. Yoga can open up new worlds, of emotional expression, physical confidence, spiritual questing, and self-esteem.

And, no matter who you are and what you can or can't do, yoga can teach you about yourself. Nobody can know you like *you,* and nobody can know a child like the *child him- or herself.* A child is an endlessly unfolding person. Yoga can set a child upon the journey of the self, a journey full of wonder, mystery, surprise, and joy.

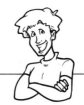

For Grownups, Too!

One of the jobs of a good yoga teacher, and any adult involved with a child, is to help kids love themselves by acknowledging that each student is unique and special. Everything a child does and says is important! Listen while making eye contact. Ask questions to show you are listening. Adults can play an incredibly important role in helping kids feel important and worthwhile.

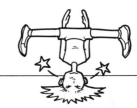

Ooops!

We don't believe in correcting yoga poses kids do, unless they are in an unsafe position that could potentially strain or injure a part of the body. If their form isn't exactly like the teacher's or the picture in the book, that's fine. Insisting on perfection for children can make them feel inadequate and turn them into perfectionists, and being a perfectionist is a very stressful existence.

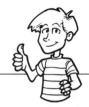

Helping Kids Discover How Their Bodies Work

Although yoga is about more than the body, it uses the body to tap the other realms of the self. The body is yoga's tool, and when kids understand how their bodies work, they will be better able to use their bodies. They will also be more comfortable with their bodies.

Knowledge of basic anatomy is important for yoginis, and kids think body knowledge is fun, too. Kids love to sing the "head bone connected to the neck bone" song, or "dance" with different body parts doing the "Hokey Pokey." Lots of books out there teach children about their bodies, and kids can extend that knowledge by drawing skeletons or making skeletons out of Silly Putty, clay, or Play-Doh (kids love skeletons!), by talking about how their muscles look and where they attach, and by moving individual muscles and watching how their shapes change under the skin. For example, ask the child to flex and extend his or her arm to see how the arm's shape changes. Families might also enjoy the fun book *Dem Bones,* by Bob Parner (Chronicle Books, 1996).

Help kids learn about how their bodies move with muscles on a skeleton.

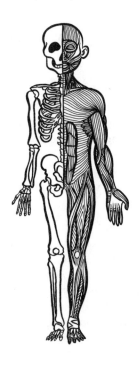

Parents should try to answer their children's questions about anatomy as openly as possible, and if they don't know the answer, find out! Open and frank discussion about anatomy, from head to toe, is an important step toward helping kids to nurture and cherish their bodies.

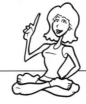

Yoga Stories

Most people probably take their internal organs for granted. They are inside you, working full-time to keep your body functioning, but do you know what they look like? Your insides are actually a rainbow of colors. Most of the internal organs come in different shades of tan or pink. Your liver and spleen are a purplish-brown. Your adrenal glands are bright yellow; the fat in your body is slightly less yellow; the outside of your brain is light gray and the inside is almost white; and your blood, of course, is red.

Progress Is a Relative Thing

A source of frustration for many kids is slow progress, especially when compared to other kids. We've said many times already that yoga is noncompetitive, but that doesn't mean kids won't compare their relative progress.

But that's just it: Progress is relative. Yoga is an opportunity for kids to learn how to gauge their own progress without comparing it to others.

Children may also get frustrated when they don't feel they are progressing fast enough. Kids love immediate gratification. What's the reward if you can't touch your toes after your second yoga practice? This is the perfect opportunity to teach patience and persistence. Practicing yoga for a short time each day will allow kids to reach their goals. Maybe not tomorrow, but eventually.

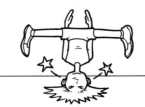

Ooops!

Patience in a yoga practice is important to prevent injury. Children must remember to treat their bodies with care. Pushing themselves beyond their limits could cause an injury.

The best way to see progress with yoga is to practice it often. One long, weekly session will be slower to yield results than shorter daily sessions. The more frequently a child practices, the faster he or she will see results.

Accepting the Challenge to Grow

Children grow, physically, whether they want to or not. But growing in maturity, growing emotionally, and growing spiritually are challenges yoga can help kids to accept and relish. Each individual grows and changes constantly in so many different ways. From babies to teens, puberty to menopause, size 2T to 14, growing is an essential and exciting part of life.

Yoga helps the mind and spirit grow along with the body, giving kids the confidence they need. Whether yoga helps kids to take on responsibility and become more disciplined, or gives them the inner strength and courage to ask questions about meaning and goodness, truth and spirituality, yoga is as much a tool for growth as it is for health. It can lead kids toward adulthood with a flourish.

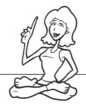

Yoga Stories

Puberty marks the onset of adolescence, the period during which children gradually become adults. Puberty hits teens and preteens anywhere between the ages of 9 and 12 (earlier or later in some cases) and is marked by an increase in hormone production to adult levels. This increase precipitates rapid growth and the development of the sex organs and secondary sexual characteristics such as pubic hair, breasts on girls, and lower voices in boys. This rapid increase in hormone production can also contribute to elevated emotions.

Girls and Boys: Yogini Warriors for a Better World

It is tempting to offer separate sections for the ways in which yoga can help girls and boys grow and mature and become fully realized individuals. We might say things like, yoga helps girls with moodiness, jealousy, or body image, and yoga helps boys with aggression, competition, and respect for others. But as soon as we say these things, we realize how wrong we are.

Sure, boys and girls have distinct differences. Everyone knows that. The differences are physical, chemical, emotional, all of that. Yet, even more distinct than the differences between genders are the differences among individuals. Whether the child is a boy or a girl, he or she might be equally likely to deal with moodiness, jealousy, a poor body image, aggression, an overly competitive spirit, or a lack of respect for others. Either gender may often feel depressed, suffer from eating disorders, have problems with social interaction, feel angry, or become antisocial.

On the more positive side, girls and boys can both have self-confidence, a healthy body image, pride in their accomplishments, empathy with others, generosity, kindness, and the ability to form healthy relationships with others. We are all people, and much the same in what we need to thrive.

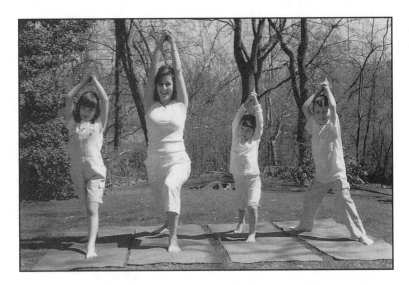

Jodi with yogini warriors for a better world!

The point is that boys and girls practicing yoga become warriors of a sort—warriors for peace, goodness, truth, generosity, kindness, and love. Yoga teaches kids to "fight" for goodness and love in the world. It gives them a purpose and a vision. With kids like that suiting up for battle, we'd have to say the future looks pretty bright.

Self-Esteem Fosters Confidence and Generosity

We probably don't have to tell you the benefits of self-esteem, but we would like to suggest that kids can experience a power and pride they may not find elsewhere when they realize they can do yoga postures and movements they never dreamed they would be able to do. When a child accomplishes something beyond his or her expectations, the child grows. The child will want to share his or her pride and power with the world.

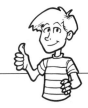

For Kids Only

For a great boost of self-confidence, try doing the three Warrior Poses (see Chapter 16). Warrior Poses are based on movements and positions of ancient warriors, and in yoga, they aren't meant to be aggressive or violent. Instead, they help the yogini feel a sense of power and force. Stand strong and feel that nothing and no one can bring you down!

Parents can boost the experience for their children by reinforcing their accomplishments. Parents should express interest and happiness at their children's progress, no matter what it involves. Children who know their parents are proud, too, will feel like they can accomplish anything. And they can!

Self-esteem does more than help a child. It helps the world. A confident child who believes in him- or herself will have the inner resources to help others in many ways. In the words of Marianne Williamson (from her book *A Return to Love,* HarperCollins, reissued 1996): "... As we let our own light shine, we unconsciously give other people permission to do the same." Yoga's gift to a child becomes a child's gift to the world.

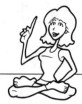

Yoga Stories

We quote here a larger excerpt from Marianne Williamson's book *A Return to Love,* which speaks for itself:

"Our deepest fear is not that we are inadequate. Our deepest fear is that we are powerful beyond measure. It is our light, not our darkness that most frightens us. We ask ourselves, who am I to be brilliant, gorgeous, talented, and fabulous? Actually, who are you not to be? ... Your playing small doesn't serve the world. There is nothing enlightened about shrinking so that other people won't feel insecure around you. We were born to make manifest the glory ... that is within us. It is not just in some of us; it is in everyone."

Yoga Invention: Another Chance to Shine

One of the things kids seem to enjoy the most is inventing their own yoga poses. Kids love to let their creative sense run wild during a yoga practice, and parents can encourage a child's imagination to bloom during yoga time by supporting the creation of new yoga poses. Parents should let their child's creativity and sense of invention shine, and let his or her enthusiasm radiate throughout the entire household. Every one will feel the positive energy generated by the creative process, and the child may come up with some poses that will become family favorites for generations!

Even very young children can make up yoga poses. If they are old enough to do yoga poses, they are old enough to invent a yoga pose. Kids may also enjoy renaming old standards to fit their own personalities. Downward Dog Pose may become Cocker Spaniel Pose if your family pet is a Cocker Spaniel, or Sally Pose if that is the name of your dog. Snake Pose may become Python Pose if your child has a pet python. Tree Pose might become Pineapple Tree Pose. Rag Doll Pose may become The Raggedy Ann Pose. Lion's Breath may become Wild Thing's Breath. Some kids like to rename poses in ways that don't make much sense to adults but are spirited, fun, and unique. Why not?

Infusing your family yoga practice with this kind of creative spirit is what makes yoga not just fun but unforgettably fun. Laugh, learn, and create together as you get stronger and more flexible. You are making memories and cultivating a child with vision.

The Least You Need to Know

➤ Yoga teaches kids to love their whole selves, body, mind, and spirit.

➤ Yoga fosters trust, body confidence, and self-esteem.

➤ Yoga helps kids accept the challenge of physical, emotional, and spiritual growth.

➤ Both boys and girls can benefit from taking on the discipline and vision of a yoga practice.

➤ Kids with nurtured self-esteem can change the world!

➤ Kids love to invent their own yoga poses, and the entire family can share in the spirit of creativity during yoga time.

Part 3

Doing Yoga with Kids

This section shows you exactly how parents and kids can start practicing yoga. We'll talk you through the creation of a unique and personalized yoga space and show you how to maintain and honor that space. We'll also help you define your yoga goals and craft a practice specifically suited to a child's individual needs and learning style, and tell you how parents can encourage children in ways that make yoga nothing but a positive experience.

For those interested in taking a yoga-for-kids class, we'll offer advice on finding the appropriate class for your child and the right teacher. Yoga is a great way for young athletes to cross-train and balance their athletic abilities and physical development. It is an excellent therapy for kids with physical or learning challenges, and a way of life children can embrace in whatever way is appropriate, fun, and rewarding for them.

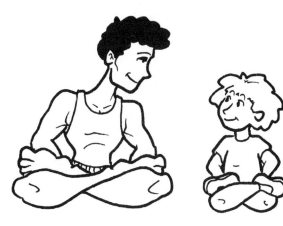

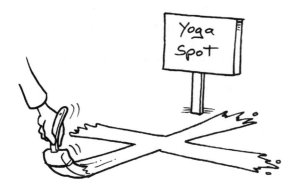

Chapter 7

Setting Up a Yoga Space

In This Chapter

➤ Yoga, the portable sport

➤ Where to practice yoga at home

➤ Setting up and honoring your yoga space

➤ What to wear and what props to use

➤ Incorporating yoga into your family routine

Perhaps you have decided to give yoga a try. Great! Now what? Do you practice in your living room? On the bed? In the playroom? In the backyard? How do you know what to do?

Perhaps you will find a great yoga class for kids (see Chapter 9 for more on the subject of choosing a yoga class), or perhaps you will decide to practice yoga on your own. Either way, a child will need a space at home to practice, and that space should have certain qualities that will make the most of each yoga session.

Creating a yoga space needn't be complicated or expensive. It simply requires some attention.

Kids Can Do Yoga Almost Anywhere!

Yoga is a flexible activity. Kids can practice it here and there, almost anywhere! Kids might find that Alternate Nostril Breathing is useful to relax during a test. They might enjoy sitting in Butterfly Pose while watching television, or engaging in some spirited Yoga Dancing to let off steam after school. Tree Pose can help kids get focused before a study session, and Breath of Fire in the morning before breakfast is a great way to get energized. We really mean it when we say that yoga is a way of life—it is portable and can serve you well wherever you go.

But even yoginis who practice yoga throughout the day need a yoga space to practice at home. Let's look at how to create such a place.

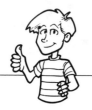

For Kids Only

Yoga in school? Sure! Yoga can help you get through the day relaxed, poised, and feeling great. Yoga breathing exercises can energize or calm you all day long, and some poses like Balloon Breathing (see Chapter 10) can be practiced right at your desk without anyone even knowing it, to help keep you concentrating in class.

Setting Up a Yoga Space at Home

Look around your house for open spaces. If you have a playroom, it might have a nice open floor space (when it isn't covered in toys!). What about the living room? Can a coffee table or a chair be moved back for a yoga session, and then replaced? Does the child have a spacious bedroom? What about a den or family room? And don't forget the outdoor spaces. A large, sturdy deck, a patio, or even a nice, open, flat space on the grass are all potential yoga spaces.

Make a list of the potential yoga spaces inside and outside your home (you'll want at least one space inside for yoga practice in inclement weather). Then, survey each item on your list for the following qualities:

➤ **Can the space be private?** Can doors be shut or can family members understand not to enter during a yoga session?

➤ **Is the space quiet?** Television noise, loud talking, constantly ringing phones, and other reminders of the chaotic outside world aren't helpful to a yoga practice. Perhaps phones, televisions, and talking can be curbed during yoga practice. Otherwise, you need to find a space that is separate from these noise sources.

➤ **Can the temperature be regulated?** Outside spaces are wonderful for yoga practice, but when the weather is chilly or sweltering, yoga is best practiced inside where the thermostat can be adjusted for comfort. When children's bodies are cold or overheated, they don't respond well to yoga poses.

➤ **Can breakables be stowed?** A wide-open living room containing shelves with china figurines, glass coffee tables, or other breakable objects can be a precarious place to practice yoga. Some yoga movements are quite active, and some balance poses take some practice. Kids need to be able to concentrate on yoga, not on avoiding that shelf of framed pictures or that curio cabinet of Fabergé eggs.

➤ **Is the floor nonskid?** Slick linoleum floors can be too slippery for yoga, but wood is good, as long as you use a towel or mat for floor poses (not for standing poses, unless the mat is nonskid, and don't forget to take off your socks to keep from slipping!). A clean, soft carpet without too deep a pile is also great for yoga.

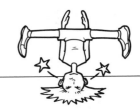

Ooops!

A nice big bed or a plushy couch may look like an inviting place to practice yoga, but mattresses don't provide the support necessary to perform yoga poses effectively. You'll get more out of yoga if you practice it on the floor on a carpet, rug, or yoga mat.

➤ **Is the room filled with distractions?** A television sitting in the room can be a distraction even if it's not turned on. Can it be covered with a scarf or an afghan? A desk piled with homework can be a constant reminder of work that remains undone—not conducive to relaxation and concentration on yoga.

➤ **Is the room easily de-cluttered?** Piles of junk, toys, laundry, and other clutter can work against the goals of yoga. Remember, a cluttered room makes for a cluttered mind, and a clean, neat room helps the mind to stay clear and focused. Practicing yoga in a clean, clear, uncluttered space is remarkably different from practicing yoga amongst clutter.

Lots of families already have a "kid room" such as a family room or playroom that is probably ideal because it may already be "child-proofed," free of breakables, with wearable, playable surfaces and lots of room to play. When clutter-free, your family room or playroom can be the perfect yoga space.

On the other hand, if your playroom is terminally cluttered but your living room stays picked up and clean, you may find that the living room makes a better yoga space. Playrooms are, after all, for playing. Before a playroom becomes a yoga space, it may need a little transformation, as we'll discuss in the next section.

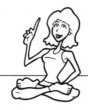

Yoga Stories

Practicing yoga outside is traditional. Thousands of years ago, people in India designed yoga poses to imitate features of the natural world, and practiced these poses in their environments. Long before air conditioning, heating, and other indoor comforts, outside was often the most pleasant, well-ventilated, well-lit place to practice yoga. Practicing yoga in a backyard or on a deck, on the beach or in a park, the yoginis today can get a taste of what the yogis of ancient times experienced during their yoga practice. While ancient yogis didn't hear the noise of traffic, they may have heard birds singing, rustling trees, wind in grass, wind chimes. They certainly felt the sun on their bodies, the breeze on their faces, and the solid earth under their feet. You can, too.

How Is a Yoga Space Different from a Playroom?

Playrooms are places to romp around, get messy, and have fun. Consequently, they are often cluttered. Playrooms also tend to have a kind of high, excited energy about them. This is where kids get to cut loose and really be kids!

But if your playroom doubles as a yoga space, it is important to distinguish the two uses of that same space. Even when yoga is full of boisterous movement, it encourages focus, concentration, and an inner state of tranquility. That can be hard to achieve in the room where a toddler dumps all the books out of the bookshelf looking for *Goodnight Moon*, where a second-grader sets up his train set, where a fifth-grader paints his masterpieces, where every kid in the neighborhood camps out to watch the cartoon channel and have popcorn fights.

A good way to make duel use of a play space is to have a transformation ritual. Before each yoga practice, parents should help their children switch gears

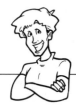

For Grownups, Too!

Clutter control is a real challenge for some kids, but many adults may find it equally challenging. The best way to teach your kids about managing clutter is by setting a good example. Get in the habit of keeping your *own* things picked up (not your child's) and expecting others to do the same. This sends a powerful message that respecting the house and keeping it clean is the responsibility of all family members.

by transforming the playroom into a yoga space. After yoga practice, the room can be transformed again into a playroom.

What You'll Need

The first step in transforming a room into a yoga space is to de-clutter. As we've mentioned, a yoga space should be uncluttered because an uncluttered environment contributes to tranquility and concentration. Pick up toys, put away books, and remove other clutter. Vacuum or sweep the floor, and open a window (weather permitting) to let fresh air in. A yoga space should be well-ventilated, but not drafty.

Some playrooms have areas that can't be de-cluttered in a hurry. Shelving units stacked with toys can be distracting. Televisions seem to have a presence in a room even when they are turned off. A stack of toy boxes suggests what is inside.

But such distractions can be quickly put out of view by draping them with sheets, afghans, and blankets. The effect of a room draped in fabric is surprisingly relaxing and transformative.

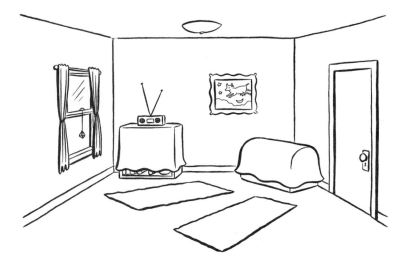

Transforming your playroom into a yoga space for kids.

Don't forget to turn off televisions, radios, and other noise sources. Turn off the ringer on the phone and let the answering machine pick it up.

Music can also do wonders to transform a room into a yoga space (although some people prefer to practice without music). A portable tape or CD player can be used to help switch the energy of the room to make it more suitable for yoga, whether relaxing or upbeat music is appropriate for your particular practice. Relaxing music is appropriate to add serenity to a yoga space, while upbeat music might be best for certain group poses or yoga games (see Appendix B for some musical suggestions).

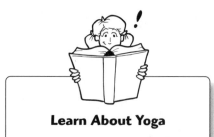

Learn About Yoga

An **ashram** is a spiritual retreat, originally associated with Hinduism but now commonly used to describe a place where yoga is taught and/or practiced.

Hang a crystal or a wind chime in the window, dim the lights or switch the light bulb to a soft color such as rose or blue, and set out your yoga gear—mats, source of music, and so on. *Voilà!* That rough-and-tumble playroom, bedroom, or living room has become an *ashram.*

Room to Grow

As a child grows and as his or her yoga commitment increases, parents might consider transforming an entire room into a permanent yoga space. Do you ever really use that sewing room? How often do guests stay in your guest room? Could you have a garage sale to clear out that junk room?

Providing a child with a permanent yoga space is a wonderful gift that will help the child nurture his or her own yoga practice and spirituality. A wide open space with appropriate flooring, furnished with nothing more than a music source, light source, any personally cherished objects hanging from the ceiling or the walls to promote serenity, and perhaps a personal altar, are all you need. An altar is a small space—a table, dresser top, shelf—where the yogini can keep things that hold special meaning. Parents should let the child choose what goes on the altar rather than trying to direct. Some possibilities: rocks, feathers, seashells, a pictured religious figure, personal artwork, photos of loved ones. An altar is a tribute to the child's selfhood, and a meaningful addition to any yoga space.

Special things are kept on a yogini's altar.

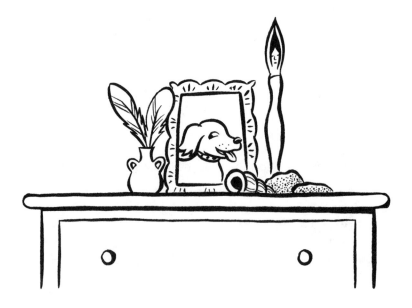

A dedicated yoga space is a nice luxury to have, but don't worry if you simply don't have square footage. The most important gift parents can give their children is love, support, and the willingness to be involved in their yoga efforts. Parental support is what really gives yoginis room to grow.

Yogini Gear: Yoga Clothes and Props

Yoga is one of those great activities that doesn't cost anything. Every child probably has clothes that are well suited to a yoga practice. Anything comfortable that allows for full movement but isn't too baggy or floppy is perfect. Large shirts can get in the way of certain poses, and can flop over a child's face during inverted poses. Too-tight clothing is also restrictive. Shorts or sweatpants and tucked-in T-shirts or tank tops are appropriate, and a leotard or leggings that fit comfortably are ideal because they are flexible but stay close to the body and out of the way.

Yoga props are entirely optional, but some of the yoga poses and games in this book do suggest the use of props. Many of these props are things you may already have at home, and keeping a basket full of yoga props nearby can inspire kids toward further invention of yoga poses.

One item you may not have is a yoga mat, also called a sticky mat. Even in carpeted rooms, yoga mats can make poses easier to achieve and can guard against slipping. Yoga mats are specifically designed for yoga and are not the same as all exercise mats. They are not thick and cushiony, but thin and skid-free. Look for them at yoga schools where adult classes are taught, in holistic or yoga-oriented catalogs, or advertised in *Yoga Journal* (see Appendix B). Some health food stores might also carry them.

If you don't have a yoga mat, keep a towel handy to use in poses where you find yourself slipping or sliding out of a pose.

We mention many other props throughout this book, which we will talk about when they are relevant to specific poses. More general props, although not necessary, can add to the ambience of your yoga space, including:

➤ An aquarium or indoor fountain with running water.

➤ Chimes.

➤ A Tibetan singing bowl (these traditional bowls make a "singing" sound when their rims are rubbed or struck with a wooden stick).

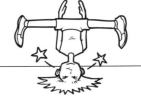

Ooops!

Yoga is best practiced barefoot, so no expensive athletic shoes are required—however, barefoot yoginis can get cold feet! Because we also don't recommend socks, which don't allow the foot a good grip on the ground, we encourage you to keep the yoga space warm. For chilly yoginis, blankets are appropriate for meditation positions.

➤ A Buddha or other spiritually meaningful figurine.

➤ Incense.

➤ Candles (but note: Kids should never use candles unsupervised).

Honoring Your Yoga Space

The last thing we would like to stress about the creation of a yoga space is that it is a place of spiritual renewal, designed to foster and encourage respect for the body, the mind, the soul, the whole self. In that spirit, we encourage parents and kids to honor the yoga space.

Make the transformation of "regular room" to yoga space a ritual. Parents should encourage their children to assemble the yoga space with reverence and mindfulness. Parents should pay attention to what they are doing as they assist their children. This will also help both to get into the right frame of mind for a yoga practice.

Also, especially if you have a dedicated yoga space, treat the room with respect. Don't pile it with junk or allow it to get really dirty. We would even suggest that all family members, keep from both thinking negative or violent thoughts and using negative or violent words when in the yoga space. Of course, ideally this would be a goal at all times, in the true spirit of the yamas and niyamas.

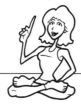

Yoga Stories

Several ancient philosophies from India and Asia describe how all space is filled with flows of energy. A recently popular ancient Chinese art of placement called feng shui has to do with arranging spaces and environments to best promote the concentration and flow of positive energy. People in the twenty-first-century America might not think that paying respect to a room will make any difference. Maybe not. However, we believe that people generate good or bad energy according to how they speak, think, and act. The space where a child practices yoga should be a space overflowing with positive energy, where he or she can feel safe, comfortable, and loved. Parents should help generate that energy by keeping the yoga space clean and serene, a sacred place of beauty, clarity, and focus.

Making Yoga a Family Routine

The last thing we would like parents to consider in this chapter is how to fit yoga into their child's busy schedule. It is amazing how busy kids are. School, homework, extracurricular activities such as sports practice and music lessons, concerts and games, family activities, religious activities—the list goes on and on. How are you ever going to find time for yoga?

First, yoga is one of those things that seems to magically *expand* your time. It gives kids more energy and focus so they can use their time more efficiently. Second, most things that result in positive long-term benefits require a commitment, and yoga is no exception.

A good way to help kids make the commitment to a regular yoga practice is to incorporate yoga into the family routine. Don't just pencil it in—yoga deserves a permanent marker! Every family has a routine they go through at least some of the time. Maybe yours has a morning routine—get up at 6:30, eat breakfast, feed the dog, take a shower, brush your teeth, get dressed, go to school, and so on. Right before breakfast might be the perfect place to add 20 minutes of yoga, and a morning yoga routine might just make the rest of the morning go so smoothly that no one will have to get up any earlier.

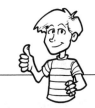

For Kids Only

Feeling grumpy early in the morning? Greet the day with a Sun Dance in your bedroom before you interact with the world, and you may find the day ahead looks a little more pleasant and full of sun. See Chapter 15 for a step-by-step explanation of how to do a Yoga Sun Dance.

Other options are to make a commitment to a family yoga session each afternoon after school or each evening before bed, whichever suits your family best. On some days, a child may decide to practice yoga alone. That's fine. Parents can practice alone, too, and may welcome this short period of solitude. On other afternoons or evenings, kids may be excited to show their parents a new pose, further progress in flexibility, or simply be eager to play some fun yoga games with their parents.

The point is to make yoga a part of your family life. Let the family's daily yoga practice be an open invitation to everyone, parents and kids, for communication on a physical and spiritual level. Parents should honor their commitment and encourage their kids to do the same. Yet, parents shouldn't let it become a chore or something they force their kids to do.

If children see their parents practicing yoga, they'll be more likely to understand what commitment is all about than if their parents immediately relent and join them in front of the television. We can't say it enough: Family time is precious, and the family that practices yoga together builds a strong and lasting relationship.

The Least You Need to Know

➤ Kids can incorporate yoga into their entire day: when they first awake to energize before school, at their desks in school to aid concentration, between classes for relaxation, and after school to wind down or regroup.

➤ Create a yoga space at home where kids can practice each day in a safe and tranquil environment.

➤ Even a hectic, messy playroom can be simply transformed into a yoga space with draped sheets, music, soft lighting, and the right props, including a yoga mat.

➤ Honor your yoga space to keep it filled with positive energy.

➤ Parents can demonstrate to their kids what it means to make a commitment to a yoga practice.

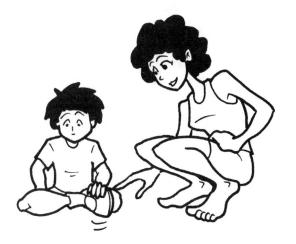

Chapter 8

Practicing Yoga with Kids

In This Chapter

➤ What, when, where, why, and how to practice yoga

➤ What yogini personality is your child?

➤ Find out which your child prefers: in or out, supervised or not, solo or with friends?

➤ The importance of committing to a routine

➤ Books and videos as yoga resources

➤ Your role as cheerleader

You've got the space, you've got the clothes, you've got your yoga mat, you've got the motivation, and you want to get started. Of course! If you're a parent wondering how to begin, this chapter is just for you. If you're a child reading this book on your own and are looking for ideas and inspiration, this chapter is also for you (although we generally address this chapter to parents, we hope kids won't be deterred from reading it). But before you and your child jump right into the poses, let's iron out a few details. How should you start? When should you practice? What kind of practice is best for your child?

Because yoga is so individualized, each practice will be different, but we can offer some guidelines and general structure to help your child get the most from his or her yoga practice.

The What, When, Where, Why, and How

What kind of practice would best suit your child? You might consider taking a class, practicing from a book, working one-on-one with a certified yoga teacher, following a yoga routine from a video, or just letting your child go at it alone. Take the quiz in the following section to determine your child's individual learning style to help you further define what kind of yoga practice would be ideal.

When should you practice yoga? Any time! Morning, midday, afternoon, and evening are all great times to practice yoga. However, yoga works best on an empty stomach, so wait until at least two hours after a meal before practicing, to give your body a chance to finish digesting. Poses such as a vigorous Yoga Sun Dance or inversions are particularly difficult on a full stomach.

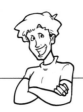

For Grownups, Too!

Appreciating and cherishing the natural world is consistent with yogic principles. Beyond practicing yoga outside, encourage your yogini to interact with the natural environment whenever possible. Go on family field trips to natural areas, make observations about plants and animals you see, and talk as a family about ways to help preserve the environment, like recycling, not littering, and practicing other ways to conserve natural resources.

Where should you practice yoga? We've talked about creating a yoga space in the last chapter. Consider your yoga practice mobile, however. Outside, inside, at a friend's house, in a park, wherever the yoga spirit moves you!

Why should you map out a practice and stick to a routine? Yoga may be fun to practice here and there, whenever the mood strikes. However, to reap the maximum benefit, it should be practiced on a regular basis, preferably at approximately the same time each day. Your daily routine can vary, but having a plan is often the best way to stick with something.

How should you practice? We'll go into more detail as we get into the poses, but in general, we recommend a routine something like the following:

➤ Chanting

➤ Eye exercises

➤ Breathing exercises

➤ Yoga poses including balancing, backbending, forward bending, and inversions, including yoga games, partner poses, and other yoga fun

➤ Deep relaxation

This order can be varied somewhat, and some items can be omitted. For example, you can skip the chanting, the inversions, or whatever may not feel right on a certain day. Overall, however, this routine makes a nice, complete, and thorough workout that is both energizing and relaxing for body and mind. A typical yoga class lasts about 45 minutes. Your child's home practice session might last about that long, shorter, or longer, depending on your child's age, interest, and attention span.

Yogini Personalities

Your child is an individual. He or she might not necessarily enjoy what a friend, neighbor, or parent enjoys. Your child has individual needs and preferences, strengths and interest. Every child has a unique spirit, his or her own personal strengths and challenges, and a personal way of taking in knowledge and understanding the world.

While children understand, comprehend, and learn in a range of ways, different learning styles or what Harvard Professor Howard Gardner calls "intelligences" exist, and each child is dominant in one or more intelligences over others. Take the following quiz about your child, or if possible or appropriate, allow your child to take the quiz to determine which types of intelligences are dominant in your child, and what approach to yoga might best suit your child considering his or her unique way or relating to the world. (The concept of using Gardner's multiple intelligences theory in conjunction with yoga for children is the signature work of Marsha Wenig and the YogaKids program.)

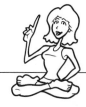

Yoga Stories

The following quote is by Harvard Professor Howard Gardner from his book *Frames of the Mind* (Basic Books, 1993), in which he maps out seven types of intelligence and explains how each individual tends to be a combination of various types, more dominant in some, less dominant in others. We believe the following commentary is great advice for parents of the developing yogini:

> "It is of the utmost importance that we recognize and nurture all of the varied human intelligences, and all of the combinations of intelligences. We are so different largely because we all have different combinations of intelligences. If we recognize this, I think we will have at least a better chance of dealing appropriately with the many problems that we face in the world."

The following quiz is loosely based on the multiple intelligences theory of Professor Howard Gardner, but we won't give away the different learning styles until after you've taken the quiz.

Yogini Personality Quiz

Consider carefully each of the following questions and answers, then circle the answer that seems most like your child (or, if you are the child taking the test, the answer that seems most like you). If two or more answers seem equally right, you may circle more than one.

1. How does your child most like to spend free time?

    a. Reading or writing

    b. Doing puzzles, figuring out problems

    c. Drawing, sculpting, building things, or otherwise working with his or her hands

    d. Playing or listening to music

    e. Playing sports, dancing, dramatics

    f. Talking or spending time with friends

    g. Spending time alone on individual, self-directed projects, or just thinking

2. What kind of books does your child most like to read, or have read to him or her?

    a. Books with an interesting or complex story

    b. Mysteries, books with puzzles or codes, anything he or she can try to decipher, solve, or uncover

    c. Books with interesting, colorful pictures

    d. Books with rhymes and/or incorporated songs

    e. Books with different textures and materials to touch, pop-up books, books about hands-on activities

    f. Books about people, books with games or activities for groups of kids, books read in a group, such as at library story hour or to a group of friends and siblings

    g. Books about self-exploration and ideas; likes to read alone and seems to think deeply about content but not necessarily discuss it with others

3. In which area does your child most excel at school?

    a. English

    b. Math

    c. Art

    d. Music

    e. Physical education

    f. Interacting with friends

    g. Working alone, being an individual

4. What kind of music does your child enjoy?

    a. Music with interesting, complex, or amusing lyrics or a strong story line

    b. Music with complicated rhythmic patterns

    c. Music that describes a scene or picture; particularly enjoys drawing or painting to music

    d. Any and all music; loves music and listens to it frequently

    e. Expressive music appropriate for dancing; loves to dance and move to music

    f. Music with lots of voices, music that his or her friends like; particularly enjoys listening to music in a group

    g. Relaxing, meditative music

5. What kind of physical activity does your child most enjoy?

    a. Acting out stories and performing

    b. Playing games involving complex rules or problem solving

    c. Imaginative play, creating active physical expressions of ideas

    d. Dancing or exercising to music

    e. Expressive dancing, sports, or martial arts

    f. Anything in a group—team sports, tag, romping around with the kids in a playgroup

    g. Solitary activities such as long-distance running, riding a bicycle alone, or taking walks

6. How does your child tend to solve problems?

    a. By talking about the problem and listening to others

    b. By trying to figure out a logical or clever solution

    c. By creating a visual map or chart of possible solutions or testing solutions by drawing pictures

    d. By thinking while listening to music, by creating silly songs about the problem, by dancing to music

    e. By role playing or acting out possible solutions, by making a game out of a problem, by engaging in physical activity to clear the mind so a solution comes

    f. By asking lots of people what they think, arriving at a solution through group consensus

    g. By withdrawing and considering the problem independently, meditating, thinking

7. What would best describe your child's group of friends?

   a. Your child and his or her friends generally have great verbal and listening skills, many friends with good communication who love to talk.

   b. Your child and his or her friends enjoy mental challenges—chess, solving mysteries, doing puzzles, and other pursuits related to logic and reasoning.

   c. Your child and his or her friends are an imaginative group, always creating visual representations of their dreams—forts, sidewalk art, snow sculptures, scrapbooks.

   d. Your child and his or her friends spend a lot of time listening to music, making music, possibly forming a band, going dancing, or being members of a singing group or orchestra.

   e. Your child and his or her friends are always on the move, playing sports, exploring, running. They often express themselves with dramatic gestures and movements.

   f. Your child and his or her friends love to be together all the time. They get along well, cooperate, and really seem to need each other. They would rather be together than apart.

   g. Your child has a few very close friends but also is comfortable spending time alone and appreciates friends who allow your child his or her privacy.

8. How does your child feel about yoga?

   a. He or she is interested in reading and talking about yoga in preparation for practicing.

   b. He or she is interested in the specific physical and mental benefits and in the process itself. What makes a balance pose work? Why are forward bends followed by backbends? How will yoga help concentration?

   c. He or she likes to look at pictures of people doing yoga poses rather than read about how to do yoga poses.

   d. He or she is interested in the yoga dances, yoga games, and rhythmic movements.

   e. He or she keeps trying out poses in preparation for class and relates the positions to other physical activities he or she has experienced.

   f. He or she can't wait to take a yoga class with old friends, or to meet new friends.

   g. He or she is interested in the meditative and self-exploration aspect of yoga.

Tally your child's score by counting how many times each letter was chosen. Each letter represents a different type of intelligence or learning style. You may have a larger number of more than one letter—for example, more a's and d's than the other letters. That's fine. Most people have several dominant learning styles, and the following descriptions for each will be relevant to your child. These descriptions of each learning style include some yoga-specific suggestions for tailoring a practice to your child.

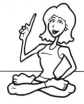

Yoga Stories

The brain is a two-sided, symmetrical structure and each side is responsible for different aspects of thought. Your left brain controls the right side of your body, and the right brain controls the left side of your body. In addition, the left brain is thought to be primarily responsible for language and words, logic, and mathematical skill, while the right brain is thought to be primarily responsible for concepts such as rhyming, music and rhythm, pictures, symbolic representations, spatial understanding, and the imagination. However, if part of the brain is injured, other parts sometimes compensate, taking over some of the functions from the injured area. Some people believe individuals tend to be stronger in either left-brain thinking or right-brain thinking.

Please remember that no one style of learning is any better than any other style. Each type is simply different. Learning your child's learning style or way of thinking will help you to help your child learn in the most effective way possible. Not only will you and your child better understand how to approach and structure an individualized yoga practice, but you may gain insight into what strategies and tactics will work best for your child in academic situations, too.

If you chose mostly a's, you have a communicator. Your child has strong linguistic intelligence and excels at reading, writing, speaking, and listening. He or she may be interested in reading about yoga and talking about it with you. Encourage this linguistically expressed curiosity! Your child is probably eloquent and creative, and may particularly enjoy keeping a yoga journal, using yoga poses to tell stories, and having discussions about yoga class with parents and friends. Linguistically oriented learners tend to do well in group situations and would probably enjoy a yoga class, either formal or informal. Before you know it, your little communicator may be running the show!

You also might steer your communicator in the direction of some reading on the subject of yoga, spirituality, and other topics sure to spark scintillating discussion.

If you chose mostly b's, you have a master of logic. Your child has strong mathematical and logical intelligence. He or she is good with numbers, abstractions, and reasoning. Don't try to get too philosophical with this child unless you are willing to back up your statements with logical proofs! The master of logic enjoys understanding the structure of yoga, wants to know the proven benefits, and may be interested in group poses that form patterns, individual poses that have a pleasing symmetry, and breathing and chanting exercises with specific sequences. Your child may also be intrigued by the idea of balance in yoga, and how to best achieve physical and mental balance through balancing different types of yoga poses. Present it as a challenge, asking your child to figure out what kind of pose would balance the pose you are doing.

Your master of logic might be interested in finding out more about *mantra yoga* and *mandala meditation*, which both focus on patterns and a systematic path that may appeal to the more logical spiritual seeker. Kids might enjoy making up their own mantras or creating their own mandala artwork.

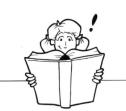

Learn About Yoga

Mantra yoga is a form of yoga that uses the chanting of mantras, which are words or groups of words meant to invoke certain beneficial vibrations when chanted. **Mandala meditation** is a form of meditation in which the meditator gazes at a mandala, which is a picture of a circular pattern that draws the eye to its center, to help the mind focus on a single point.

If you chose mostly c's, you have a see-er. Your child has strong visual intelligence. He or she is spatially oriented and likes to work with images, drawings, sculpting, and building. Your child understands things best when he or she can look at them rather than hear about them. Your child has an active imagination full of vivid pictures, colors, textures, patterns, and pretending. See-ers enjoy the guided imagery parts of a yoga practice, poses that are meant to look like specific things in nature, and any chance to draw, paint, sculpt, or create in order to understand or interpret something learned.

Encourage your see-er to keep a yoga drawing journal, drawing poses or ideas for invented poses. Your child might also enjoy doing yoga with a video or colorful picture book. Although not appropriate for all kids, some visually oriented kids might benefit from practicing some yoga poses at home in front of a mirror, so they can better see the pose. (We discourage the use of mirrors in a yoga class setting, however, as it can make many kids self-conscious.) See-ers can also be productively encouraged to look within themselves as opposed to remaining focused on external appearances.

If you chose mostly d's, you have a music lover. Your child has a strong musical intelligence. He or she is oriented toward rhythm, melody, sound patterns, dancing to music, singing, and rhythmic chanting. Music lovers thrive on practicing yoga to music and particularly enjoy yoga movements such as Yoga Dance. Encourage your music lover to practice yoga to music. Family freestyle dancing sessions can be a lot of fun, too! Your music lover might also enjoy vocalizing during certain (appropriate) yoga movements, such as howling or barking like a dog during Downward Facing Dog Pose. Music lovers often enjoy singing while dancing, chanting, and making up songs and dances related to the yoga practice. You might even add some musical instruments to your yoga practice. Your music lover may also enjoy performing his or her musical yoga for an appreciative audience.

Music lovers may also be particularly interested in mantra yoga and other forms of chanting, as well as meditation techniques that involve rhythm and/or vocalization.

If you chose mostly e's, you have a toucher. Your child has a strong kinesthetic intelligence. He or she is oriented toward touch and understands things best in a hands-on environment. Touchers love dance, sports, drama, martial arts, and inventing yoga poses by moving and working out the poses with their bodies (as opposed to thinking about the pose and then trying it). They also love yoga games that feel like sports or martial arts, the physical power of warrior poses, gymnastic-type yoga poses, and group poses in which the yoginis can be sculpted into a physical expression of an idea.

Touchers really enjoy yoga group poses and family yoga activities where everyone stays literally in touch, creating flower gardens, groups of animals, forests of trees, schools of fish, bridges, even imaginary machines or complex, multilimbed, friendly monsters.

Keep in touch with older kids, too. Besides doing yoga together, offer your stressed-out teen a shoulder rub or do something together that involves working with your hands, like cooking or working on the car. Older kids can sometimes go for long periods without physical contact from family members. Everyone gets so busy, but maintaining actual, physical contact with your kids can help them to feel more closely connected to family. And don't forget to give lots of hugs (something from which any yogini can benefit)!

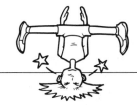

Ooops!

The quiz and other information in this chapter about learning styles are meant to help kids get more out of an individual yoga practice, not to label kids. Be careful not to assign a label to your child at the expense of noticing other strengths and tendencies.

If you chose mostly f's, you have a socializer. Your child has strong interpersonal intelligence. He or she is a people person! Socializers are good at relating to others, sharing, compromising, cooperating, and forming relationships. Socializers love group yoga in any form. They are good communicators and are empathetic. They are tuned in to friends and family members in a way that makes them wonderful to be around.

Don't forget that your socializer has needs, too. He or she may be so good at understanding, listening to, and caring for others that others take advantage. A family yoga practice is important to keep socializers grounded and feeling loved. Don't be upset by how important your socializer's friends seem to be to him or her. These relationships are teaching your child how to be a caring, giving friend and member of the community. Your socializer may enjoy starting his or her own yoga club (see Chapter 9). Kids who do yoga together strengthen their bodies as well as their friendships!

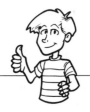

For Kids Only

It's summer, it's hot, and all you want to do is go to the swimming pool or the beach. That doesn't mean you can't practice yoga! Water yoga is fantastic, and much different from yoga on land. The difference in body weight and the way the body moves makes it a whole new experience.

If you chose mostly g's, you have a thinker. Your child has strong intrapersonal intelligence. He or she is introspective, self-directed, and likes to think before acting. The thinker may be particularly interested in meditation techniques, keeping a yoga journal, and pondering poses rather than jumping in and trying them right away. Give your thinker time to stand back and watch, taking it all in before giving it a try. The thinker has a surprising understanding of his or her own needs and interests. Focusing and concentrating comes naturally, and your thinker may resist group yoga in favor of a solitary spiritual exploration. Yoga has traditionally been a solitary activity, so let your child know you accept and support his or her individualized efforts.

Your thinker might also be interested in reading more about mindfulness, advanced meditation techniques, and the historical quests for self-knowledge of others throughout history. Take a trip to the library.

Selecting the Right Practice

With a defined idea of your child's learning style in mind, consider what type or types of practice your child will probably find most productive. Communicators get along well in groups, but your communicator might also have a strong intrapersonal intelligence and prefer to read about yoga, talk about it with a few close friends, and practice it alone. Touchers may love to practice yoga barefoot on the lawn with friends, or all alone in a perfectly tailored yoga room. Your socializer may want to take a yoga class but may prefer a teacher who lets him or her take the lead.

Now let's take a look at several choices you will have to make when putting together the right kind of practice for your yogini.

Inside or Out?

Some climates are more conducive to regular outdoor yoga practice. Others, obviously, aren't. If you have the space and the weather is nice, your yogini may still prefer to practice indoors.

While an outdoor practice can be spiritually uplifting, it can also be distracting. Wind, traffic noise, onlookers, or barking dogs can all keep the yogini from sustaining a rhythm and concentration. A stuffy living room when the sun is shining may seem a poor substitute for the park to other yoginis. If your child knows the options, he or she can decide.

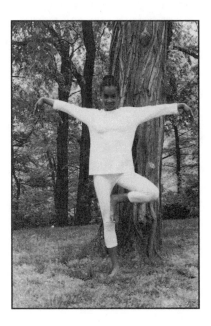

A yogini enjoys outdoor yoga practice. Be a tree!

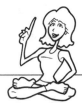

Yoga Stories

Practicing yoga outside when it's hot is better than practicing outside when it's cold. Muscles respond better when they are warm. Cold muscles can tense up and become more easily injured. In fact, there is even a form of yoga called Bikram Yoga where people practice in a room with the heat turned up very high to induce a heavy, purifying sweat and a heightened consciousness. While we don't recommend you crank the thermostat to 90 degrees while practicing yoga, we do think that yoga outside in the summer heat is lovely, as long as you keep well hydrated with plenty of fresh water and seek shelter if you start to feel dizzy, extremely tired, or experience any kind of pain. And don't forget the sunblock!

Supervised or Unsupervised?

Some kids do best with direction, under the guidance of an attentive teacher or parent. Younger kids require it. Other, older kids would much rather research the subject and pursue it on their own. Whether or not your child tends to be a thinker, a see-er, a toucher, a music lover, or a combination, he or she may or may not prefer supervision. Again, let your child decide.

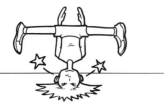

Ooops!

Although all the poses in this book are safe for kids to practice with friends, parents, teachers, siblings, or alone, some yoga poses that appear to be more challenging or advanced are best done with someone else around to help.

However, if your child commits to a yoga class with a teacher, we would also suggest you encourage your child to continue attending rather than attending only when the mood strikes. Choosing a class and committing to regular attendance will help build self-discipline, one of the good habits yoga encourages.

Solo, or with Others?

Just as some kids may prefer a teacher to self-instruction, others may prefer to practice with friends or family rather than alone. If your child likes to go at it alone, we would suggest you continue to make a family yoga time available on a regular basis, for your child to join if he or she would like. Don't force it, but keep it an option.

Practicing yoga together.

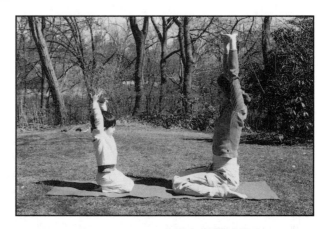

For kids who love to practice with friends, you might also encourage occasional solo practices, to remind your child that yoga is about inner exploration. Group poses can be great fun and yoga is an excellent way to spend time with friends. Solo yoga is relaxing and meditative in a completely different way, and both can help the yogini grow. It's all about balance.

Sticking to a Routine

Practicing yoga at the same time each day, for about the same length of time, is a great way to practice self-discipline, stick with your yoga, and maintain a sense of regularity in your life. Some kids today have so many activities and so much going on that having one, consistent relaxation activity each day can be comforting and energizing. Other kids who aren't involved in many activities can make yoga their extracurricular effort and feel a sense of accomplishment and involvement, even if they practice alone in their bedrooms.

Practices don't need to be completely rigid. Varying the routine from day to day according to your child's mood, energy level, and inclination at the moment can keep yoga interesting and challenging. But encourage your child (without making it an obligation) to hold the commitment to yoga sacred. If your child can stick to a daily yoga practice, he or she can soon feel able to accomplish just about anything.

How to Use and Where to Buy Yoga Books and Videos

Maybe your child isn't inclined to attend a class or practice yoga with friends. How will he or she know what to do? Fortunately, there are a number of excellent yoga books and videos available. Although many of them are for adults, older kids can still use them and benefit from them. Parents can also view these resources and adapt poses for younger kids.

A video expressly for children 3 to 10 years old is called *YogaKids*. Thousands of children have been introduced to the joys of yoga through this Parent's Choice Award–winning video. Since Jodi is a certified YogaKids facilitator, many of the techniques in this book are similar to those in the *YogaKids* video.

Books are great for communicators and thinkers. Videos are great for see-ers, touchers, and when they are set to music, music lovers. Even kids who take a class or practice with friends can use books and videos on solo practice days.

Read books (like this one!) or watch videos with your child at first. Practice together, working out the poses. When your child is ready, he or she can take it from there. See Appendix B for a list of resources for purchasing books and videos about yoga, and some titles we particularly enjoy.

Encouraging a Yogini Lotus Blossom

You can read about child development, contemplate your child's unique personality, and talk to your child about yoga until you are blue in the face, but nothing will have as strong an effect as simply supporting your little yogini. Help your child set up a yoga space. Together, gather books, videos, and appropriate yoga clothes. Present

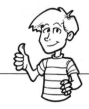

For Kids Only

Affirmations are things you say to yourself to feel great. The following affirmation is from a book called *Just Because I Am: A Child's Book of Affirmation*, by Lauren Murphy Payne, M.S.W. (Free Spirit Publishing, 1994). Try repeating it to yourself and see how it makes you feel: *I am a person. I am special. I am important. Not because of things I do, not because of what I look like, not because of what I have … just because I am.*

your child with a small gift for his or her yoga space, such as a crystal or a CD of relaxing music. And be sure to tell your child how much you love him or her and how much you respect your child's commitment to yoga.

Even younger kids can understand your emotional support. If they ask to "play yoga," jump right in, if you can. Tell them how proud you are of the way they work on their yoga poses. Applaud their accomplishments, help them explore the areas they find challenging, be an optimistic voice in the face of discouragement, and don't forget about being a good example. The parent who expresses love and emotional support will raise children who are able to express love and emotional support to others.

The Least You Need to Know

➤ Before your child begins a yoga practice, map out what kind of yoga practice he or she will benefit from most, where to practice, why a schedule and a commitment will help, and how your child will arrange his or her routines.

➤ According to Harvard Professor Howard Gardner, children have different types of intelligences or learning styles. Knowing your child's combination of dominant intelligences will help you craft a yoga program individually suited to your child.

➤ Some children prefer practicing outside or inside, supervised or unsupervised, alone or with friends, or a combination.

➤ A regular routine will help your child to get the maximum benefit from his or her yoga practice.

➤ Yoga books and videos can be a great resource to enhance a yoga practice.

➤ Support from parents is the key to yogini success!

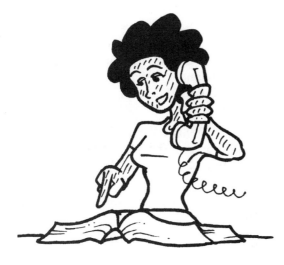

Chapter 9

Finding the Right Yoga Teacher or Class

In This Chapter

➤ How to find the right yoga class or teacher for your child

➤ No classes to be found? Start a yoga club!

➤ Yoga—a fun way to increase athletic ability

➤ How yoga helps kids with special needs master their goals

➤ The yoga concept of samyama and what it can do for your kids

After reading through and working with this book for awhile, kids might become interested in taking a yoga class. That's great! Practicing yoga in a class involves a much different energy than doing yoga solo. In a class, a yogini will be exposed to the energies of the other children, the teacher, even the energy of the room. Yoga classes can be highly motivating and fun, and can provide an arena in which a child can forge new friendships.

However, depending on the class structure, the teacher, the other students, and each child's approach and personality, a yoga class might also produce difficulties for some children. How can you pick the best teacher and class environment for your little yogini? Keep reading! We'll suggest what to consider.

Wanna Take a Class?

The first item parents should discuss with their children is whether they really want to take a class. Was it the parent's or the child's idea? If a child is happy and satisfied with a personal yoga practice and hesitates about taking a class, there is no harm in holding off. Parents might love the idea of their children taking a yoga class, but if a child doesn't love the idea, it probably won't work out.

If a child is genuinely interested in taking a class, parents should, by all means, be encouraging. A parent can be a child's best advocate and most powerful resource when it comes to finding the perfect yoga class environment.

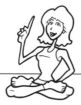

Yoga Stories

The inspiration for Jodi's studio, Next Generation Yoga in New York City, came from Jodi's first teacher, Sonia Sumar, the author of *Yoga for the Special Child*. After learning from Sonia about how to respect and love every child for his or her unique qualities, Jodi created a studio for children that was peaceful and serene, a place children would love to be. Kids feel safe and confident here, and they love to bring their friends and parents to watch. When looking for the right yoga class for a child, consider the environment and the way the child feels in the space. When Jodi's students tell her they wish their homes were more like her studio, she knows she's doing something right!

Where to Look for Classes in Your Area

The next step is to determine what yoga classes, if any, are offered in your area. Just because you can't find anything in the phone book under "Y" doesn't mean there aren't yoga classes in town, and just because you see classes only for adults doesn't mean there aren't classes for kids, either. Some of the following places might be sources of information about local classes and instructors:

➤ A nearby yoga center for adults, which might offer unadvertised children's classes, or might be willing to begin offering children's classes if the center perceives enough local interest.

➤ Magazines such as *Yoga Journal* and *Yoga International* publish a yearly issue with listings of classes, teachers, and studios around the country and throughout the world.

➤ The Internet for local and national resources and lists (see Appendix B for some helpful Web sites, including several that list certified children's yoga instructors by city and state).

➤ Health food stores.

➤ Progressive bookstores.

➤ The local library.

➤ Local holistic health practitioners such as massage therapists, chiropractors, acupuncturists, homeopaths, or herbalists.

➤ Pediatricians or their nurse practitioners (also check the bulletin board at the doctor's office for notices).

➤ Daycare centers and preschools (teachers might have heard of something, and might even be trained in teaching yoga themselves!).

➤ Elementary, middle school, junior high, or high school teachers.

➤ Physical education teachers.

Parents—and teens who are old enough to research on their own—should make a list of the classes available. Many teens do well in adult yoga classes. Now you can begin the screening process.

If you can't find anything at all (quite possible if you live in a small town or rural area), all is not lost. See the section later in this chapter on starting your own yoga club.

Yoga Teachers with the Right Stuff

A teacher can make all the difference between yoga success and yoga frustration. Some yoga teachers are brimming with positive energy as well as expertise. Others have one or the other. A few have neither. The only way to tell whether a yoga teacher is a good match for a yogini is to meet the teacher. Call and ask if you can attend a sample class. Most teachers will be happy to let a child have a risk-free trial class trial classesbefore signing up for an entire session, and a sample class will give a child a better idea of whether or not he or she will enjoy the experience.

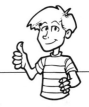

For Kids Only

Teens, if you can't find a yoga class for kids your age in your area, consider a yoga class for adults. You are practically an adult yourself, right? Talk to yoga teachers in your area and ask how they feel about teenagers in class, and about their philosophy of yoga. If you like what you hear, give it a try. Most yoga teachers will probably be happy to have you.

Yoga teachers with positive energy radiate a sense of joy and fun to share with yoginis and parents.

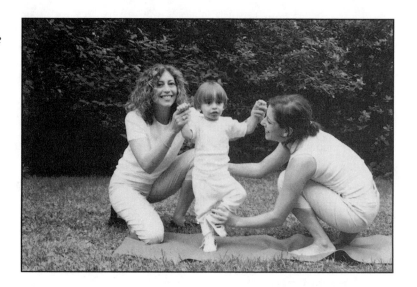

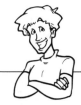

For Grownups, Too!

Wondering what to ask a potential yoga teacher to determine qualifications? Here are a few suggestions: Are you certified? What kind of training have you had? How much training have you had? Are you insured? How much experience do you have with children? What ages? What are your priorities in teaching yoga to children? What keeps you motivated? What do you enjoy about teaching yoga?

If this isn't possible, ask if you can meet the yoga teacher for an informal "interview." Good yoga teachers shouldn't object, as long as you are polite and friendly about it. And parents, take your child with you. Yoga teachers should be glad you care so deeply about the welfare and success of your child.

Once you meet the teacher, you can determine whether he or she is qualified in whatever way is important to you. First on our list would be a well-trained instructor who is experienced with children and who makes the child feel at ease.

After meeting the teacher, you should have a better sense of the teacher's philosophy and qualifications, but nothing is more telling than taking a class. Whether the parent and child take the class together or the child takes it alone, look for the following additional qualities in the teacher:

➤ Knowledge in yoga asanas and techniques

➤ Energy and enthusiasm

➤ Empathy and a sense that the teacher is "tuned-in" to the students

➤ A feeling that the teacher really likes, enjoys, and appreciates children

➤ Open and nonjudgmental

➤ Creative, inspirational, playful, and fun!

➤ Friendly and personable

You get the idea. If you are convinced the instructor is well trained and competent, and you get a good feeling about the instructor's approach and personality, you've got a winner!

Most important, no matter how a parent feels about the personality of the instructor, how the child feels is what really matters. If a parent thinks the instructor is great but the child balks, a parent should trust his or her child's instinct. If a child doesn't feel good about the instructor, chances are the experience of the yoga class won't be a positive one.

On the other hand, if a parent isn't comfortable with a teacher but the child is, a parent should try to figure out why he or she feels that way. If a parent suspects the teacher isn't sufficiently qualified or is untrustworthy, discuss those feelings with the child. If a parent is uncomfortable for some personal reason that doesn't affect the welfare of the child, let the child's judgment be the deciding factor. For younger children, parents must make the decisions, and their judgment as parents is probably on target.

In general, most yoga teachers mean well and many are wonderful, supportive, enthusiastic, caring people who can offer children a positive and fun yoga experience. It is, of course, the parent's job to feel confident that this is the case.

Can't Find a Class? Start Your Own Club

Yoga classes aren't available everywhere, and yoga classes for kids are even scarcer. So, parents, if you don't live anywhere near a yoga class but your kid is ready for some yoga interaction, consider starting your own yoga club! And teens can start one on their own, too.

Yoga clubs can be lots of fun, and as structured or unstructured as you care to make them. They can be as local as a group of siblings or as expansive as an entire neighborhood, school district, or even a town. Whether your yoga club is highly structured or highly informal, organized by you or somebody else, the best way to get things off the ground is to have a plan. That's where we come in!

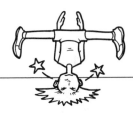

Ooops!

Even if a potential yoga instructor is qualified, if a parent or child feels uncomfortable for any reason (even if you aren't sure why), don't be afraid to walk away. Not all combinations of people work, and you don't owe anyone an explanation.

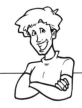

For Grownups, Too!

Some yoga classes for young kids (toddlers, preschoolers) are taught by people with very few qualifications specific to yoga, such as gymnastics teachers, aerobics instructors, preschool teachers, or others who work with kids but aren't certified to teach yoga. That doesn't mean the class won't be safe and fun. If your child has disabilities or health challenges, however, consider more seriously the specific training of the teacher.

The following steps for organizing a yoga club needn't be followed exactly or in order, but they will give you a general idea of how to go about the process:

1. **Appoint someone to be in charge.** This can be a temporary, rotating, or permanent position, but unless someone is organizing, chances are nothing will get accomplished. If you are the type who likes to organize and make things happen, go for it! If you aren't comfortable in this role, seek out a neighbor or adult friend with great organizational skills and enthusiasm to take on the project. Kids can be great motivators, and surprising in their ability to mobilize a group to action. A yogini teen might have fun gathering friends together for a yoga club, or a teen experienced at babysitting who enjoys small children might be the perfect candidate to organize a yoga club for toddlers or preschoolers.

2. **Determine interest.** Ask around school, preschool, or the daycare center. Talk to parents, teachers, and the kids themselves. Who would attend such a club? How often would they attend? Do people seem excited or are they unsure about what yoga is? (Show them this book!)

3. **Give your club a name.** The name should be something kids love, but if you can't think of one right away, assign your club a temporary name. How about "Yoga Club"? Direct and to the point. A few other possibilities we like: Yoga Tots, Yoga Babies, Yoginis United, Who Wants to be a Yogini?, Nirvana Network, Samadhi Society.

4. **Draw up a plan.** Decide on a location for meetings, a time, how long meetings will last, and set a trial period, such as a month or two, during which you vow to keep up the club so it has a chance to become established. Your plan might include a weekly meeting at a local recreation center for preschoolers, every Monday and Wednesday rotating between four households for parents and toddlers, or a daily after-school gathering of teens in the park. Also include who will host each meeting during the initial trial period and a general format for classes (such as working through the poses in this book), following a video, or having different people lead the group in whatever way they choose. Use the template on the next page to organize your thoughts.

5. **Make a list of charter members.** Include their addresses, phone numbers, and e-mail addresses, and make copies for each member.

6. **Have your first meeting!** As you begin your yoga club, you may find that certain things aren't working. You may decide to forego refreshments but later find that a post-workout snack extends the fun. You might begin meeting at different people's houses but find that a central location works better. The person leading the group may decide to step aside to let someone else take over. Let your club change and evolve to stay fun and active. If something isn't working, change it!

The more your club grows and expands, the more modifications you may need to make. Who knows? Eventually one of your members (maybe even you!) may decide to become a certified yoga teacher and you'll have an official yoga class in town at last. Or, your yoga club might be so much fun that it fulfills everyone's yoga needs.

Yoga Club Trial Period Plan

CLUB NAME: _____

MEETING LOCATION: _____

MEETING TIME: _____

MEETING FREQUENCY: _____

WE WILL MEET FOR: _____ (specify trial period length)

HOSTS FOR MEETING DURING TRIAL PERIOD:

_____

_____

_____

_____

_____

_____

HOST DUTIES (providing location, leading class, refreshments, etc.):

_____

_____

_____

_____

_____

_____

WORKOUT FORMAT (book, video, host's choice, etc.):

_____

_____

continues

continued

_____

_____

_____

_____

Yoga + Sports = Fun!

Just because a child is already an athlete doesn't mean he or she can't add yoga to the program. Athletic kids can get a lot from yoga. Yoga is a great way to cross-train, to balance a child's development, and even to ward off sports burnout while maximizing performance. Yoga adds depth, control, polish, vigor, and even a spiritual component to the athletic life of any child, and while a child's sports coach probably isn't a yoga teacher, he or she can become a collaborator in your child's efforts toward overall mind and body fitness. An athlete's yoga teacher can and should also be aware of and supportive of a child's efforts in other physical pursuits, something athletes might consider when choosing a yoga teacher.

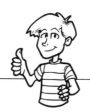

For Kids Only

A yoga club can do more than just practice yoga together. You could take photos and make a collage or a book chronicling the club from its beginning. You could start a yoga book club, reading and discussing books that interest the group. You could take field trips to different areas for inspiration in your practice. You could even organize to get yoga added to your school curriculum.

Yoga as Part of a Balanced Exercise Program

Any sport has certain physical benefits and builds strength and/or flexibility in certain parts of the body. Different sports also have a different effect on the body and the mind. But few sports balance the whole self.

That's where yoga becomes a child's athletic ally. Yoga balances the dominant aspects of a child's favorite sport, whatever those may be.

If a Child's Sport Is ...	Yoga Balances With ...
Intense	Tranquility
Highly competitive	A noncompetitive oasis
Full-contact	Personal space
Teamwork-oriented	Self-direction
Strength-building	Flexibility

118

If a Child's Sport Is ...	Yoga Balances With ...
Rough	Gentleness
Tiring	Invigoration
High-energy	Relaxation

The more a child practices yoga, the more he or she might also notice how much yoga poses are inherent in the movements of other sports and physical activities. Gymnastics, ballet, and running stretches are all borrowed from yoga. Many martial arts include yoga-like movements. Even if the correlation isn't immediately recognizable, all activities designed to move and challenge the human body have aspects in common. That athletic coach and that yoga teacher have more in common in their teaching methods than you might think!

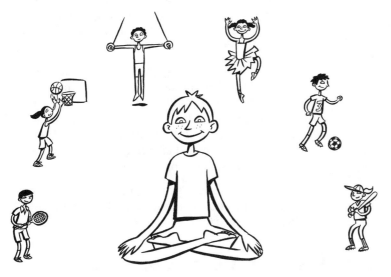

Yoga balances young athletes, complementing any sport—from tennis to basketball to gymnastics to ballet to soccer to softball and more!

No matter what a child's sport, adding yoga can add fun. A child and his or her fellow teammates might even consider warming up or cooling down before or after practice with a group yoga workout. Why not ask the coach about instituting such a routine?

Coaxing Kids to Exercise

Parents, what do you do if your kid doesn't like to exercise? Some kids are uninterested in sports. Some prefer sedentary activities. Or maybe your child just isn't in the mood.

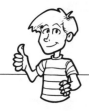

For Kids Only

You might notice that many of the yoga poses in this book look familiar. Jodi's students often tell her they have done certain poses in ballet, gym class, tae kwon do, track, or elsewhere. The poses may have different names when associated with different sports, but technically they are all the same poses.

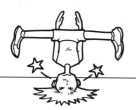

Ooops!

We believe athletes should perform at their best. However, we don't believe athletes should push themselves too far. In the nonviolent, body-cherishing spirit of yoga, we urge kids to refrain from superceding their ever-changing abilities. Even the most well-intentioned yogini sometimes pushes too hard in the heat of competition, but kids who make a conscious effort to be body-aware may be less prone to injury.

The best advice we can give to parents whose children resist exercise is twofold. First, don't push the issue. If you pressure your kids to exercise, they might resist and physical activity will have a negative connotation to them.

You might investigate the source of your child's resistance, however. If your child just doesn't like sports, you can encourage him or her to get involved in a physical activity (like yoga) that doesn't seem to be a sport. Maybe it is the competition or the teams that make your child uncomfortable. Many activities (like yoga!) are noncompetitive and don't involve teams.

Maybe it is the physical effort. Kids who aren't used to physical activity should start slowly and be kind to their bodies. Exercise should be fun and it shouldn't hurt. When kids understand this, they might be more willing to give certain activities a try.

The second part of our advice you've heard before. Be a good role model! If you don't exercise, your kids might feel like they shouldn't have to, either. If your attitude about exercise is one of dread or reluctance, your kids will pick up on that attitude. (A child involved in a yoga class will also have a positive adult role model in his or her yoga teacher.)

Even if your child doesn't do anything else, yoga is a great form of physical exercise. Yoginis are athletes, whether they participate in other sports or not.

Yogini Athletes Reach for Peak Performance

No matter what sport a child is involved with—swimming, football, soccer, tennis, gymnastics, the list goes on—getting involved with yoga will help kids maximize their athletic potential. Yoga keeps the body strong and flexible, which minimizes the chance of injury. Yoga also heightens body awareness, tuning kids in to how their bodies feel as well as teaching them about anatomy, so kids have a better sense of their own bodies. As yoga helps an athlete to grow, mature, and expand his or her awareness, it also helps increase flexibility and balance, and helps the child learn about his or her body.

Yoginis with Special Needs

Everyone can do yoga, even kids who might not think they can. If a child has a learning disability, a physical disability, or is coping with emotional issues, he or she can benefit immensely from a regular yoga practice guided by a professional trained in these areas.

To find a certified yoga therapist who is trained in yoga for children with special needs, see the Web site www.specialyoga.com. There is a page dedicated to certified practitioners that is broken down by state. It's very important that a child with special needs work with a trained professional in the special needs field. This is especially true for those with physical delays.

Yoga and Children with Learning Challenges

Perhaps a child has been diagnosed with attention deficit disorder (ADD) with or without hyperactivity (ADHD), dyslexia, speech impairment, or pervasive developmental delay (PDD). No matter what course of action the parent or child has chosen to deal with learning challenges, yoga can be an excellent adjunctive therapy.

Yoga has several specific benefits for kids with learning challenges. It increases attention and focus, it helps to coordinate the central nervous system through midline movements (more on this in Chapter 25) that use both sides of the brain at once, and it provides an outlet for energy and the physicality some kids need to express. The self-esteem building kids get from yoga is also important for those with learning challenges.

Even if a child hasn't been diagnosed with a learning disability, he or she may learn in a way that is different from his or her peers, making certain academic tasks more challenging than others. In the last chapter, we discussed the seven different types of intelligences. A child's unique combination of dominant intelligence types is well served through an individualized yoga practice that helps your child embrace his or her learning style as well as increasing ability in other learning styles.

For more on yoga for children with learning differences, see Chapter 25.

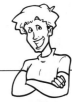

For Grownups, Too!

If your child has a physical, emotional, or learning challenge, he or she may feel self-conscious about group yoga. Private lessons or smaller groups of children with similar challenges can build confidence. The teacher should be knowledgeable and sensitive to learning differences. Once your child is comfortable, he or she can certainly move into a larger, mainstream group, but continue to work with a sensitive teacher.

Yoga and Children with Physical Challenges

Children with physical challenges can also benefit dramatically from a regular yoga practice. Any yoga posture can be modified to meet a child's special needs. Children in wheelchairs, children with varying levels of mobility, sight-impaired or hearing-impaired children, or children with certain health problems that limit their physical movement or range of motion can all do yoga. Some poses involve very small movements, even eye movements. Others involve hands-on yoga in partnership with a parent, caregiver, or yoga teacher.

Parents, if your child has physical challenges, look for a yoga teacher who specializes in working with disabilities. Children with physical challenges have an amazing ability to accomplish the unexpected. Let yoga help to nurture that indomitable spirit.

For more on yoga for children with physical challenges, see Chapter 25.

Samyama: Lifelong Learning

Yoga philosophy includes a concept called *samyama*. Although samyama is a complicated concept, it is also, in some ways, pretty simple. Samyama is a state of mind that results from focusing all your attention and energy on something until you know and understand it completely. Through the guidance of a qualified teacher and their own dedicated efforts, kids can benefit from instituting the concept of samyama in their own lives.

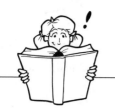

Learn About Yoga

Samyama is a state of being resulting from the complete and thorough investigation of a subject. It is the point when that subject (which could be anything, from yoga to playing the piano) is completely understood. According to yoga philosophy, samyama results from extended contemplation of, focus on, concentration about, meditation on, and study of a subject.

The concept of samyama can be useful to kids, whether they apply it to a yoga practice or to anything else, like math or poetry or long-distance running. Working toward samyama teaches kids concentration, commitment, and how to stick with something until it becomes second nature.

Some kids are interested in everything, and that's great! But the discipline of samyama helps kids concentrate on their interests one at a time, giving them more than just a cursory knowledge of lots of things. What better way for your child to uncover his or her greatest gifts and abilities?

Applying samyama to a yoga practice is an excellent way to get the most out of yoga. How would a child practice samyama? First, a qualified yoga teacher can help a child develop concentration skills and the personal discipline that comes from regular yoga practice. Parents might help their children find lots of age-appropriate reading material on yoga. Parents can read with their children and discuss what they read. Talking about and even drawing the subject will help children explore even further.

Parents, encourage a regular practice each day with varying routines and poses. Help your child find opportunities to talk with other people who know about yoga and might have something to teach. Without pressuring your child, be enthusiastic about his or her long-term commitment to the subject. Your child can spend time thinking and meditating about yoga in addition to searching for knowledge on the subject.

Other ways a child can expand his or her yoga knowledge is to look up relevant Web sites, keep a yoga or spirituality journal, make up and tell or write down yoga stories, and produce yoga-related art. Parents should notice and support their child's efforts. When a child has truly become a yogini expert, she or he will be closer to the experience of samyama.

If a child learns how to pursue goals until subjects are mastered, he or she will have a skill that can be invaluable throughout life. Parents can practice samyama, too. No one is ever too old to stop learning, exploring, investigating, and mastering knowledge. What better way to stay young?

The Least You Need to Know

➤ Resources for finding a yoga class in your area include adult yoga studios, health food stores, holistic health practitioners, pediatricians and nurse practitioners, preschools and daycare centers, the Internet, and the local library.

➤ A good yoga teacher for kids is well qualified, enthusiastic, child-centered, noncritical, and makes each child feel comfortable.

➤ Yoga is a great adjunct to sports, making bodies less prone to injury, balancing the use of the body, and even transforming nonathletic kids into athletes.

➤ Yoga is an excellent therapy for kids with special needs such as learning or physical challenges, because it builds confidence, coordination, and concentration.

➤ Samyama is a state of mind achieved by becoming fully immersed in a subject until it is mastered. Kids who strive toward samyama gain skills that will help them throughout life.

Part 4

Yoga Songs, Play, and Postures

Now the fun really gets going! In this section, we'll show you what to do in your yoga sessions: breathing exercises for energy and tranquility, mantras and chanting for relaxation, meditation, and group fun, and even "handy" ways to hold your hands, to best channel energy back into your body.

Then we'll show you poses, exercises, dances, and games that make yoga with kids such a blast. We'll start with nature poses such as Mountain Pose, Tree Pose, and Rainbow Pose. We'll move on to a menagerie of animal poses, from the barnyard to the aviary, the desert to the jungle, the savanna to the sea. Grownups, don't be shy! These poses are just as good for you as they are for your kids.

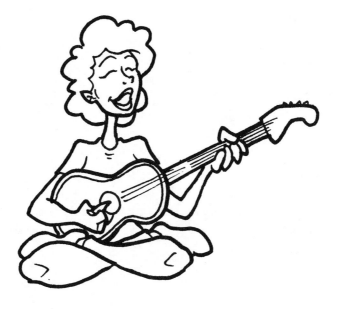

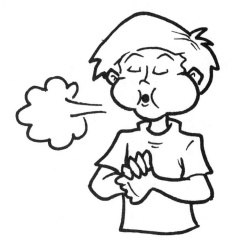

Chapter 10

Chanting and Breathing

In This Chapter

➤ What is prana and what does it have to do with breathing?

➤ How the lungs and heart work

➤ How to sit and stand for better breathing

➤ Fun with mantras and mudras

➤ Breathing into the chakras

➤ Breathing techniques for energizing and calming the body and mind

When people think of yoga, they usually think of the exercises or postures of yoga, but breathing is an equally important part of the yoga experience. It is not only an excellent way to begin any yoga routine, but it can help to stimulate kids when they feel tired or lethargic, focus them when they are feeling scatter-brained or overwhelmed, and relax them when they are tense.

Chanting is also a great way to help kids feel centered. It uses and improves eye-hand coordination and helps the mind to focus—a great exercise for concentration.

Yogini Prana Power

Yoga has a name for the life force energy in our bodies. This energy flows in and out of us, moving through certain channels (according to yogic thought), and also fills our environments. Yoga calls this energy *prana*.

The theory goes that we take in prana when we inhale, suffusing our bodies with this energy. We release prana when we exhale, letting it carry with it negative energies and impurities. The movement of prana in and out of the body is akin to a kind of purification system, and when prana gets blocked in the body or we don't take in enough, our bodies become unbalanced and don't work as well.

What's so special about prana, and why don't we just call it breath? According to yoga, the more prana in the body, the healthier and more alive that body is. Learning to control breathing to take in as much prana as possible is part of the goal of yoga breathing because it is thought that a body suffused with high levels of prana will be not only healthier but more capable of spiritual realization.

This may sound complicated. After all, we just want kids to have fun and learn how to be healthy, right? Actually, whether or not you subscribe to the theory of prana, knowing how to breathe completely and fully is great for your body and your health.

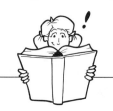

Learn About Yoga

Prana is the Hindu word for the life-force energy in the body (and the environment) that can be taken in and manipulated within the body through special breathing techniques (called pranayama) and energy retention and manipulation techniques (called bandhas).

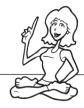

Yoga Stories

How do you picture your lungs? Unlike many believe, lungs aren't hollow, inflatable structures like balloons. They are filled with tissues in the form of bronchial tubes, bronchioles, and alveoli that deliver oxygen to the bloodstream and carry carbon dioxide back out. Nonetheless, the lungs have a great capacity for air. They can hold about eight times the air that people normally inhale. Inhaling more fully to suffuse the lungs with life-giving oxygen and exhaling more completely to clear out all the old, stale air that lies dormant is a great way to keep the lungs in peak condition and the body optimally nourished with oxygen.

People often aren't aware of how to use their breath to its best potential. Learning how to get the most possible benefit from each breath is an amazing skill for a child to learn, one that will serve him or her throughout life. Full and complete breathing builds health, energy, breath capacity, endurance, inner tranquility, and even self-confidence.

Both yogic thinking and Western medicine agree: Breathing is an important mechanism for nourishing the body and cleansing and eliminating impurities. The benefits of breathing exercises and deep breathing for stress management, relaxation, and energy levels are well known, so take advantage of those benefits by learning some fun yoga breathing techniques.

The Breath of Life: What the Lungs Do

Before we begin the real fun, however, let's take a look at what the lungs actually do when you breathe. Knowing what is going on under those ribs can help children to visualize the breathing process and control it more effectively.

Breath really is life. Human bodies need oxygen to survive, and the lungs are the organs responsible for delivering that oxygen to the body, about 12 times each minute and more than 450 million times in an average lifetime!

The air all around us in the Earth's environment is rich with oxygen, the reason we are able to live on this planet. Every time you breathe, air enters your nose or mouth and passes through your *pharynx,* your *larynx,* and through your *trachea.*

The trachea branches into two *bronchial tubes* that, in turn, branch into many more, smaller *bronchioles.* The bronchioles end in clusters of microscopic *alveoli* covered with a web of *capillaries.* When air reaches the alveoli, something interesting happens. It trades its oxygen for carbon dioxide. Oxygen molecules pass through the capillary walls into the bloodstream, and carbon dioxide molecules pass from the bloodstream into the alveoli.

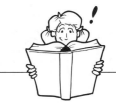

With each exhale, the now-carbon-dioxide-rich air travels back through the bronchioles, bronchial tubes, trachea, larynx, pharynx, and out the mouth and nose. Since carbon dioxide is a by-product of the body, this process is a sort of purification or waste removal system. Pretty efficient!

The trouble is, when people breathe, they usually use only about one-eighth of their lung capacity. When they breathe in polluted air (like cigarette smoke), the mechanisms that trap pollution, bacteria, viruses, and other impurities become temporarily paralyzed and eventually inoperable.

Also, when people don't breathe completely and fully, stale air gets trapped in the lungs. Shallow breathing doesn't deliver nearly as much oxygen to the bloodstream as deep breathing. The reason exercise is great for the lungs is that it forces them to

Learn About Yoga

The **pharynx** connects the nasal passages to the vocal chords. The **larynx** is next, containing the vocal chords or voice box. The **trachea** follows, reaching to the **bronchial tubes** that travel into the lungs. These branch into **bronchioles** which terminate in grape-like clusters called **alveoli** covered with **capillaries,** the tiny blood vessels in which oxygen and carbon dioxide are exchanged.

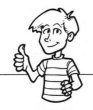

For Kids Only

Babies are born with clean, pink lungs. When people grow older and choose to smoke, their lungs turn into an ugly gray, mottled with black. Air pollution has a similar effect. There are many reasons to avoid smoking, secondhand smoke, and breathing highly polluted air. Keeping your lungs clean, healthy, and the color they were meant to be is just one of them.

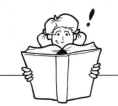

Learn About Yoga

The **diaphragm** is a muscular membrane that separates the chest and abdominal cavities. It is roughly disk-shaped and expands downward when the lungs expand with each inhalation, then moves upward to help push air out of the lungs with each exhalation.

breathe more deeply, taking in and releasing more air than they would if you were sitting watching television or working on the computer.

But exercise isn't the only way to maximize the breathing process. Deep breathing, abdominal breathing, and lots of other fun breathing techniques can have the same effect, and when practiced regularly, will train the lungs to work more efficiently. And that's great for the whole body.

In a Heartbeat: What the Heart Does

Knowing how the lungs work is only half the story when it comes to breathing. As your lungs deliver oxygen-rich air into the body and shuttle carbon-dioxide-rich air out of the body, something else is going on inside the body to bring that carbon dioxide to the alveoli and to distribute oxygen where it is needed. The heart powers this process.

What does the heart have to do with breathing? The lungs deliver the "goods" to the heart, which distributes them to the body. The heart them pumps waste products back to the lungs to be eliminated. The heart and lungs are partners in essential body maintenance.

Breathing exercises and deep breathing can actually slow the heart rate as they promote a relaxation response in the body. They also deliver more oxygen to the bloodstream for the heart to distribute.

Learning to Sit and Stand to Your Best Potential

Breathing exercises aren't just about your mouth and nose and the passageway into your lungs. Your lungs expand and contract as you breathe, and your *diaphragm*, a plate-shaped muscle at the base of your lungs, also expands with the expansion of your lungs.

But what do you think happens if you sit slouched over? Your chest gets all crunched up and your lungs don't have room to expand as well as they could. The same goes for walking with a slouch.

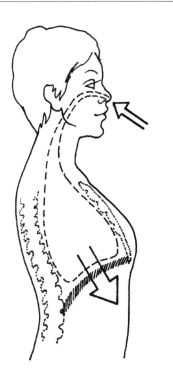 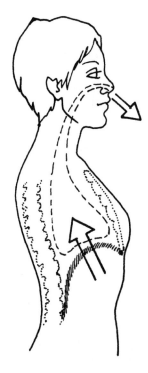

The large diaphragm muscle in your chest moves down when you inhale and releases up when you exhale. Take a deep yogic breath and feel the diaphragm muscle as it moves.

(Drawing by Wendy Frost)

The best way to practice breathing exercises, and also the best way to sit or stand in general, is by lifting your chest and spine and expanding upward, as if you were being gently lifted by an imaginary cord upward from the crown of your head. Remember that straw in your spine that we talked about in Chapter 2? Is the straw crimped, or can air move freely through it? If your lungs, diaphragm, and spinal cord don't have room to work, you can't possibly breathe fully and your body can't work as efficiently.

Ohmmmm, My!

Chanting is an ancient practice probably practiced long before recorded history ever made note of it. According to the ancient Indian scriptures called the Upanishads, mantras originally existed in the primeval ether and were instrumental in forming the universe itself. We know that virtually every culture around the globe and throughout history has made use of some kind of chanting in its religious practices.

Chanting involves more than sound. It also uses rhythm. In her excellent book, *Yoga for the Special Child* (see Appendix B), Sonia Sumar suggests that yoga may have been developed to imitate the effect of natural rhythms on the body and soul. Think of the sound of ocean waves on a beach, the rhythm of bird's singing, water flowing in a stream, or wind blowing the trees.

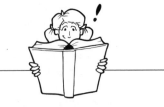

Learn About Yoga

A **mantra** is a sound or group of sounds, like a word or a phrase, that is repeated either out loud like a chant or silently, for the purpose of focusing the mind.

The repetition of certain sounds is thought to provide calming and healing effects on the nervous system and the psyche. Whether performed by cloistered monks thousands of years before or by kids tomorrow, chanting a *mantra*—a sound, word, or phrase—can be an incredibly focusing, calming, or energizing experience. Rhythm and melody are fun additions to mantra chanting, and combined with hand movements and different sound combinations, help to develop concentration, breath coordination, communication, and motor skills.

We think mantra chanting is the perfect preparation for a yoga workout. It facilitates regular, deep breathing as it centers the mind on the workout to come. One mantra we think works well is "hamsa." This is a natural mantra, meaning it is like the sound people make when they breathe naturally. The "ham" is the inhalation (hahm), and the "sa" is the exhalation (sah). Try it a few times: hahmmm sahhhh.

Some people like to use mantras with no meaning, or with unknown meanings, just because they like the sound of the words. Others prefer mantras that are personally meaningful, such as small pieces of religious scripture or words that invoke positive feelings, such as "love," "peace," or "joy."

The symbol for Om represents the sound ohm, *thought to be an approximation of the original sound of the universe, representing the unity of all things.*

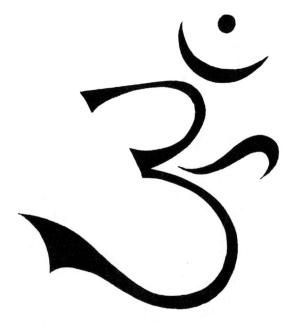

Other popular mantras taken from Hindu Sanskrit include ...

➤ **Om.** Pronounced *ohm,* this sound is intended to imitate the sound of the universe, and symbolizes the unity of all humankind.

➤ **Om Shanti.** Pronounced *ohm shahn-tee,* this mantra is translated as peace and has a joyful sound.

➤ **Om Jothi.** Pronounced *ohm joh-thee,* this mantra means "light."

➤ **Hari Om.** This mantra, pronounced *ha-ree ohm,* is fun to say. "Hari" is one of many Hindu names for the divine being and can be translated as "one who removes all obstacles to spiritual progress."

Kids love to learn the meanings of different mantras, and a little investigation may uncover many more your kids might like to use.

Once you've got a mantra (or more) in mind, you can chant in lots of different, fun ways. Think of it as a game, and a mind and breath warm-up to begin your yoga session. Following are some chanting games parents can play with their children:

➤ **Follow That Mantra.** In this game, you say different mantra combinations in rhythm, and the other person tries to repeat in rhythm. For example, the child says: "Om Jothi Om Jothi Om Jothi Om," and the parent repeats it in rhythm. Then the parent says: "Shanti Peace Om Om," and the child repeats in rhythm. Go back and forth.

➤ **Chant 'n' Clap.** This a game of repetition, too. One person says the mantra as he or she claps, then taps the thighs. In rhythm, the other person repeats the combination. Go back and forth, such as "Hari Om" (with three claps, then three thigh taps) repeated, or "Joy" (clap, then thigh tap) repeated. You can go as fast or as slow as is comfortable, and you can change the pace, such as starting slow and getting faster and faster (prepare to end in giggles!).

➤ **Mantra/Clap Combo.** Take turns making up mantra/clapping combinations. You do one, then the other person copies. Take turns copying each other's combinations. For example, you might say "Peace" (clap over your head), "Love" (clap behind your back), "Joy" (clap in front of you). The other person imitates you, then makes up his or her own. Great for concentration and focus!

➤ **Mantra Union.** Try clapping together, making up your own versions of children's clapping games. For example, you and your partner can say "Om" (clap both your hands with your partner's two hands), "Shanti" (clap your right hand to your partner's right hand), "Shanti" (clap your left hand to your partner's left hand), "Shanti" (clap your right hand to your partner's right hand) and repeat at various speeds. This is a good preface to partner or group yoga because it helps you and your partner to establish a mutual rhythm.

➤ **Mantra Stomp.** Who says chanting has to be peaceful? Get up and stomp your feet to the rhythm of your chosen mantras. Very energizing!

133

Making Up Mantra Songs

Another fun way to chant is to make up your own chants or mantra songs. Some people don't like to be given a mantra by somebody else. Others just like to be creative!

Shorter songs are easiest to chant and to remember. Any phrase, whether made of real or nonsense words, will do. Put the chant to any melody, or just say the words in a rhythm. Some ideas to get you started …

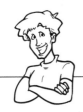

➤ "I love myself, I love myself, I love myself" in a steady rhythm.

➤ "Orange, yellow, green, and blue" (to the tune of the first seven syllables of "Twinkle twinkle little star").

➤ Any word or phrase in any foreign language.

➤ Favorite animal sounds (fun for younger kids), such as "baa baa baa," "meow meow meow," "gobble gobble gobble," "peep peep peep," "moo moo moo."

➤ Any known short prayer or meditation put to a favorite tune.

➤ Any known phrase or line of a song chanted in rhythm without the melody.

For Grownups, Too!

Lots of songs can be borrowed for mantras. Familiar tunes put to different words, or even song snippets, can be perfect for chanting. Some song excerpts we think are fun to use as repeated mantras are: "I love you, you love me" (of Barney notoriety), "Twinkle twinkle little star," and "Abiyoyo, Abiyoyo, Abiyoyo" (from Pete Seeger's story-song).

Handy Mudras

Mudras are hand positions. Technically, mudra means "seal" in Hindu and refers to any purposeful movement or position designed to seal energy inside the body so it doesn't escape. The word is most often used in popular yoga literature to refer to hand positions that connect the fingers, making a sort of circuit for the energy, which would otherwise escape from the fingertips, to travel back into the body.

The hand position kids often imagine when they think of yoga or meditation—index (pointer) finger touching thumb with other fingers gently extended—is a mudra.

Mudras are productive during meditation (sometimes it's nice to just sit and think of your mantra rather than speaking it out loud) and also during deep breathing exercises. One position we suggest is to sit

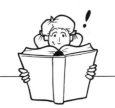

Learn About Yoga

Mudra is the Sanskrit word for "seal" and commonly refers to yoga or meditation hand positions in which fingers and thumb touch to form a "circuit" for re-cycling life energy back into the body.

in Lotus or Pretzel Pose (see Chapter 17) with a straight back, the back of the hands resting on the knees. Allow the thumb and pointer finger to touch lightly and relax the other fingers so they hang slightly open. Breathe!

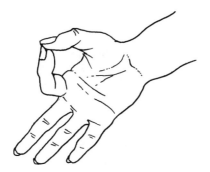

Kids can use the Om mudra when they meditate. The Om mudra represents the energetic union of the self and the divine in a circle.

(Drawing by Wendy Frost)

Breathing Through the Chakras

One final consideration for breathing exercises is the *chakras*. Chakras are energy centers in the body. There are many, according to traditional yogic thought, but seven primary chakras exist along the spinal column, from the base of the spine to the crown of the head.

Each chakra is thought to represent certain energies, although different people will tell you different things about which chakra governs what. We can provide a general guide:

➤ The first chakra, at the base of the spine, is associated with the color red and represents the most primal of our instincts: hunger, anger, and passion.

➤ The second chakra, behind the abdomen, is associated with the color orange and is the source of creation.

➤ The third chakra, behind the navel, is associated with the color yellow and is the source of inner heat that consumes and digests.

➤ The fourth chakra, behind the heart, is associated with the color green and is the source of love, compassion, and empathy.

➤ The fifth chakra, in the throat, is associated with the color blue and is the source of communication.

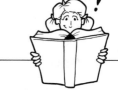

Learn About Yoga

Chakras are energy centers in the body, thought to be concentrated centers of prana, or life-force energy, connected by energy channels. The seven primary chakras are located at the base of the spine, behind the abdomen, behind the navel, behind the heart, in the throat, on the forehead, and at the crown of the head.

Get to know where your chakras are!

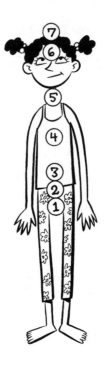

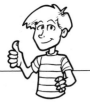
➤ The sixth chakra, on the forehead, is associated with the color indigo and is the source of intuition and perception.

➤ The seventh chakra, at the crown of the head, is associated with the color violet and is the center for spiritual enlightenment.

Of course, not everybody buys into the concept of chakras, but many people, and many cultures, do. These energy centers and their associated channels are the basis for ancient healing techniques such as acupuncture. But, once again, whether or not you believe in chakras, they are something to consider. Visualizing breathing into any of the chakras may help to stimulate the function of that chakra.

For example, perhaps a seventh grader has trouble telling people how she feels. She could visualize breathing into the fifth chakra in the throat, thought to be the center for communication. Or, maybe an eleventh grader is interested in self-realization and spiritual pursuits. He could focus on breathing into the seventh chakra at the crown of the head while visualizing the chakra's color, violet.

Okay, Breathe

Now it's time to try some breathing techniques. Children sometimes have a hard time breathing deeply. Parents, try the following initial breathing exercises with your kids to show them how to breathe deeply, "from the belly."

Belly Breathing

Kids can understand best how to breathe if they have an obvious way to see what they are doing. This exercise uses a prop: Any small, sturdy, light object such as a Beanie Baby, rubber duck, or tissue box will do.

1. Lie on your back, then place your (prop of choice) on your lower tummy.

2. Breathe normally through your nose and watch your prop rise and fall for a minute or two.

3. Sit up and discuss what you saw. Was your prop moving a lot, or just a little, or not at all? Proper belly breathing expands the lower tummy, not just the chest, and will make the prop movement obvious. Shallow chest breathing will result in very little movement of the prop.

4. Try it again. See if you can make the prop move more. Remember to use your breath to move the prop!

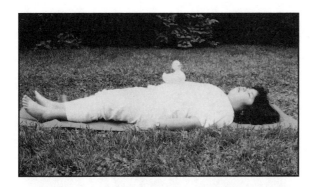

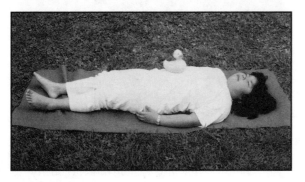

Belly Breathing: Proper slow deep breathing will make this duck bob up and down.

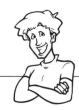

Balloon Breathing

This exercise is a good follow-up to Belly Breathing. It helps kids get an even better sense of how deep breathing feels.

1. Sit on the floor in Pretzel Pose (see Chapter 17) and imagine you have a balloon inside your tummy. Decide what color it is.

2. Interlace your fingers, making a basket shape, and place it over your tummy, imagining you are putting your hands on the balloon.

3. Breathe in through your nose and imagine you are blowing up the balloon.

4. Breathe out through your nose, imagining the balloon deflating.

5. Try to feel the "balloon" with your hands. With each inhale, be conscious of blowing up the balloon as large as possible. With each exhale, imagine deflating the balloon as fully as possible.

6. Continue for a minute or two, then talk about how it felt.

For Grownups, Too!

Unless otherwise specified, all breathing exercises should be done through the nose, a good habit for kids to acquire. The nose has many filtering mechanisms to keep pollutants, bacteria, viruses, and other undesirable things out of the body. However, if your child has a stuffy nose, mouth breathing will work for these exercises. When breathing exercises do specify mouth breathing, it is always on the exhalation only.

Balloon Breathing.

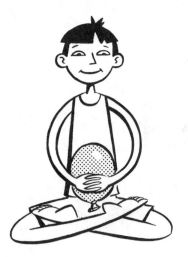

Energizing Breath Exercises

Some breathing exercises are incredibly energizing. Yoga philosophy would say they infuse the body with prana. We would add that these exercises infuse the body with oxygen, helping everything to work better. They also expel stale air, purifying the system. They're great as a way to begin a yoga practice or as a refresher in the middle of a stressful or tiring day—energizing breathing exercises are awesome!

➤ **Bunny Breathing** (designed by Marsha Wenig of YogaKids). Wriggle your nose like a bunny and use your hands, on top of your head, as floppy ears (or put on a pair of store-bought bunny ears). Inhale three times in short, consecutive breaths through your nose, then exhale through your mouth as you make a sighing sound. Repeat several times.

➤ **Wood Chopper.** Stand tall with your legs spread about hip distance apart. Raise your arms over your head and clasp your hands together as if you were holding an axe. Breathe in through your nose and stretch upward, lifting the "axe " over your head. Exhale through your mouth, making the sound "ha" as you drop your arms toward the ground as if letting the axe chop at a piece of wood. Bend at the waist as you lower your arms. Repeat several times, generating momentum in your chopping motion. This is a great exercise for releasing pent-up anxiety and anger.

➤ **Reach for the Sun** (designed by Marsha Wenig of YogaKids). This exercise works well with music, although music isn't necessary. The song "Reach for the Sun" on the YogaKids audio tape is appropriate, or use another sunny song such as "You Are My Sunshine," "Sunshine on My Shoulders," or make up your own! Begin by standing. Inhale through your nose as you raise both arms up overhead as if you were reaching for the sun. Exhale and make the sound "ha" as you pull your arms and hands in toward your upper stomach (this is the area of the chakra associated with the sun, sometimes called the solar plexus). For extra fun, cut out a picture of a sun to hold in your hands as you do this exercise, or hold an object you think is "sunny," such as something sun-shaped or colored a bright yellow.

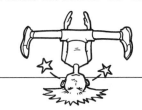

➤ **Lion's Breath.** Sit on your heels with your knees close together (this is a popular meditation position in Japan, sometimes called Japanese Sitting Pose, see Chapter 13). Open your eyes wide like a glaring lion, flare your nostrils, and spread out your hands like they are giant lion paws. Inhale through your nose. Then, exhale through your mouth with a big, fierce, wild roar, opening your mouth wide and extending your tongue as far as possible. See if you can stretch it to touch the

Ooops!

In Japanese Sitting Pose, the yogi sits on his or her heels with knees together. Some people tend to separate their knees, placing the lower legs alongside the thighs. This is particularly hard on the knees and should be avoided. For some, Japanese Sitting Pose is uncomfortable. Sitting with a blanket, pillow, or bolster between the heels can help alleviate the pressure on the knees.

139

bottom of your chin (not everyone's tongue is long enough to do this). Repeat three to five times.

You say Lion's Breath relaxes you instead of energizing you? We believe you! Every person is an individual, and even though we have categorized the breathing exercises in this book as energizing or calming, you may respond differently. Try each exercise for yourself and notice how it makes you feel. This is your best guideline.

Lion's Breath.

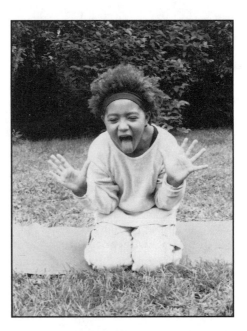

➤ **Breath of Fire.** Sitting in a comfortable position, rest your hands lightly on your stomach. Inhale slowly through your nose. Then, begin to exhale and inhale quickly. Feel your belly pumping to the rhythm of your breathing. Repeat for about 10 inhalations and exhalations, then slowly inhale and hold your breath for a count of 20 (some kids may have to work up to a count of 20). Repeat three times.

Calming Breath Exercises

Calming breath exercises are perfect to wind down a vigorous yoga workout. They are also a great way for your child to de-stress after a hard day or focus when he or she is nervous about something like a test or a performance. These exercises are also beneficial for children who are feeling overstimulated and would benefit from a centering activity.

➤ **Fly Like a Bird.** Stand straight and tall with feet firmly planted and arms hanging at your sides in Mountain Pose (see Chapter 11), or sit in Japanese Sitting Pose (see Chapter 13). Inhale through your nose and extend your arms out to the side, then up over your head. Keep your arms nice and straight but make the movement graceful, as if your arms were wings. Then, slowly exhale through your nose as you lower your wings. Repeat several times until you feel centered.

➤ **Alternate Nostril Breathing.** Extend the fingers of your right hand. Bend your pointer finger (first finger) and tall-man finger (middle finger) into your palm. Keep your thumb, ring finger, and pinkie finger extended. Exhale completely. Press your right nostril closed with your right thumb, and slowly inhale through your left nostril. Close both nostrils and hold for one second. Then, remove your thumb from the right nostril and slowly exhale through the right nostril. Upon full exhalation, inhale deeply through the same nostril. Then close both nostrils, hold for one second, and then exhale slowly through the left nostril. This completes one full round. Repeat several times.

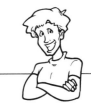

For Grownups, Too!

Make breathing exercises even more fun for your kids with props! Blowing a pinwheel, a tissue, a feather, a small flag, even a kazoo (best for energizing breaths, since the sound of a kazoo isn't particularly calming!) can add variety and spice to a breathing workout.

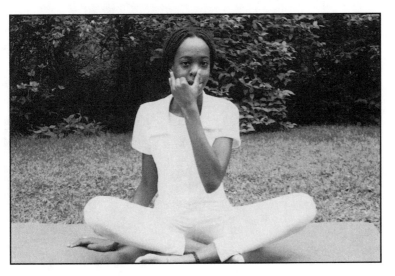

Alternate Nostril Breathing.

The hand position for Alternate Nostril Breathing.

(Drawing by Wendy Frost)

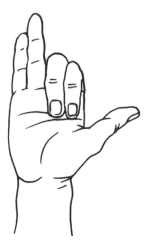

➤ **Breathing Staircase.** This exercise is for two or more children. The first child lies on his or her back with bent knees, feet near his or her bottom. The next child lies down and gently places his or her head on the first child's belly, putting his or her knees and feet in the same position. Children continue in this sequence, each child's head on the previous child's belly, until all are resting with heads on bellies (except the first child, which could also be an adult). Now, everyone closes eyes and listens to the breathing of the person on whose belly they are resting. See if the whole staircase can synchronize its breathing! This exercise is very relaxing and great for unifying a group.

Breathing Staircase.

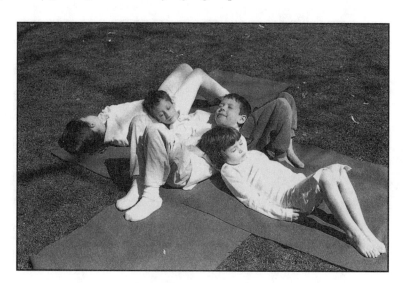

Breathing correctly can contribute to better health, greater energy, and a more profound relaxation. Chanting and other breath-related yoga techniques keep yoga breathing fun, interesting, and rhythmic. Kids who make breathing exercises an integral part of their daily yoga practice will find all of yoga's benefits intensified.

The Least You Need to Know

➤ Prana is the yoga term for life-force energy that the yogi can bring into the body in greater concentration through breathing exercises.

➤ Most people don't use their full lung capacity, but regular breathing exercises can greatly increase the efficiency and effectiveness of one's breathing.

➤ Sitting and standing correctly further enhance the ability to breathe fully and deeply.

➤ Chanting mantras is a great way to focus the mind and warm up the breath before a breathing or yoga workout. Chanting while holding the hands in a mudra position helps to retain the energy generated by chanting.

➤ Chakras are energy centers in the body. The first chakra is the center for primal, instinctual energy; the second for creation energy; the third for digestive energy; the fourth for compassionate energy; the fifth for communication energy; the sixth for intuitive and perceptive energy; and the seventh for enlightenment energy.

➤ Breathing exercises can be energizing or calming, depending on the technique.

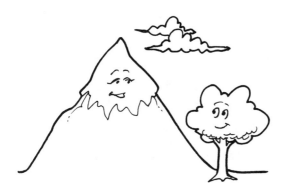

Chapter 11

Nature: You Be a Mountain, I'll Be a Tree

In This Chapter

➤ Kids and nature: naturally!

➤ Learning respect for the natural world

➤ Kids and conservation

➤ Nature poses, from mountains to rainbows

➤ The fun and advantages of a yogini nature walk

Kids and nature are a natural combination. Kids are fascinated by the natural world and their place in it. Whether it's a toddler entranced with a ladybug on the lawn, a grade-schooler wanting to help plant a vegetable garden, or a teenager interested in becoming an ecologist, kids probably have at least a few positive associations with the world on the other side of the window.

Getting in touch with nature is what yoga is all about. Remember, yoga was originally designed to imitate animals and other natural structures and phenomena. Young children do this whether they call it yoga or not.

While not every yoga pose is a reflection of the natural world, so many are that we devote a good portion of the poses in this book to nature poses. In this chapter, we consider the poses that reflect the structures in nature—mountains, trees, flowers, stars, and rainbows. We've also added Butterfly Pose and Frog Pose because, although critters, we consider both to add profoundly to the beauty, sound, and ambience of the natural world.

Discovering Your Yogini Nature

For some kids, pretending is easy; for others, who are very logical and based in reality, it's not so easy. We know one little girl who stares incredulously at her cousin whenever he suggests some elaborate pretend scenario. "We can't play that. That would never really happen!" she insists.

However logical or imaginative (or both) a child may be, he or she can benefit from discovering the natural world within. Parents, use the following questions and activities as a springboard for discussion and imaginative exploration for you and your child. You might be surprised at how your child responds! These questions and activities work for children of any age:

➤ Sit on the grass outside on a sunny day and watch the clouds. What shapes does your child see? What shapes do you see? You might also read the excellent children's book by Charles G. Shaw, *It Looked Like Spilt Milk* (HarperCollins, 1988), for inspiration.

➤ Ask "If you could be any animal, what would it be? Why?" Talk about yourself as an animal, invent a costume to wear so you feel like an animal, and/or draw a picture of yourself as an animal.

➤ Plant a garden. Let your child help plan what vegetables, fruits, and flowers to plant. Don't be bound by tradition. Why not make the garden in an interesting shape, or plant nothing but red fruits and vegetables (strawberries, tomatoes, and radishes), or grow pole beans trained around cornstalks.

➤ Ask "Would you rather be a mountain, a tree, or a star? Why?" Draw a picture of yourself as a mountain, a tree, or a star—or all three!

➤ See how many different kinds of plants you can find in your backyard, nearby park, garden center, or local solarium.

➤ Ask "What are your favorite colors in nature? Where might you see them?" Go on a color walk and point at everything you see in that color.

➤ Make a nature collage. Find objects in nature and glue them in an artistic way to a sturdy poster board or piece of cardboard (found objects unattached to the Earth, only, please—no need to uproot wildflowers or rip leaves off trees! We think of that as a little like pulling the Earth's hair, a metaphor kids can usually relate to). Hang your collage in your yoga space. Or, collect natural objects—pine cones, stones, shells, acorns, and display them on your personal altar.

➤ Pretend you are the earth. What would you say to the people living on you? What would you say to the moon? The other planets and stars?

You can probably think of many other great ideas. The point is to encourage children to see the natural world as part of the self, and the self as part of the natural world. The result? Greater harmony with nature and a greater sense of belonging in the natural world for the child now and throughout life.

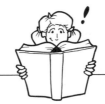

Yoga Stories

Spending time outside is good for a child, but not just because the child is more likely to get exercise, breathe fresh air, and be in contact with nature. Although the dangers of excessive sun exposure are real (your child should wear thoroughly applied sunscreen whenever he or she will be out for more than a few minutes), small amounts of sun exposure are important to help us synthesize vitamin D. People living in climates with very little sun or who stay indoors most of the time are more likely to suffer from vitamin D deficiencies. A few minutes a day with sun on skin is all it takes. (Most types of milk also contain vitamin D because it assists in calcium absorption.)

Respecting the Essence of All Things

Another benefit for getting in touch with the natural world is learning respect for the essence of all things. Yoga philosophy believes that everything in the world, even in the universe, is filled with the same life-force energy. Therefore, everything—other people, animals, plants, ants, even rocks, dirt, and water—deserves reverence.

We believe the earth as a whole deserves respect as well, and one way children can actively participate in caring for their planet is by learning about ecology and conservation. Recycling, reducing consumption, picking up litter, and other conservation-related projects are great opportunities for kids and parents to work together toward a shared concern. Kids who learn about ecology often embrace the concept with fervor. Parents should encourage their children's enthusiasm by getting involved themselves. A few ideas for projects parents and children can do together …

> ➤ If your community doesn't have curbside recycling, visit the neighbors and offer to pick up their newspapers, plastics, cans, or other recyclables. Haul what you collect to your neighborhood recycling center.

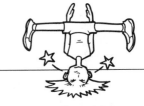

Ooops!

If you live in a large city, pay attention to pollution warnings. Playing outside when the air is polluted is hazardous for children, especially those with asthma, allergies, or other respiratory ailments. Pollution lowers the body's resistance to illness and can exacerbate a number of health problems. Pollution levels are most likely to be high on hot, hazy, humid, windless days.

➤ Make a list of ways your family can produce less trash, such as buying refills for cleaning products and juice in concentrated form, and by making more food at home instead of buying the packaged versions (healthier, too!). Implement one item on the list each week.

➤ Organize a group of kids to patrol the park for litter. (Have kids wear gloves for safety and germ control.)

➤ Collect used magazines and deliver them to a local doctor's office or library.

➤ Pick out and plant a tree in your yard.

➤ Ask your kids to be on "nice day" alert. When the weather permits, your kids can remind you to turn off the heat or the air conditioner and open the windows.

➤ Drive less. Organize family hikes, bicycle trips, and walks around the block instead of drives across town to the mall.

➤ Ask your kids to come up with ways for your family to consume less and live more simply. Kids tend to be inventive and may come up with ideas you would never have considered, such as giving only homemade presents for Christmas, using newspaper as gift wrap, buying clothes in only two colors so everything matches, purging toys and sending the excess to Goodwill, a local shelter, or a daycare center in need. Remember, although the "official" Earth Day is only once a year, your family can make every day Earth Day!

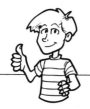

For Kids Only

Whether or not you've ever been tempted to squish a bug, you might really enjoy the book *Hey, Little Ant,* by Philip M. Hoose (Tricycle Press, 1998). This fun, rhyming book tells the story of an ant who begs a boy not to squish him. It might make you think about the importance of all life, no matter what size. The ending of the book will really get you to think for yourself.

Children who learn respect and reverence for the natural world tend to be kinder, more accepting, and more loving with their fellow human beings. They may also learn to be less materialistic, more resourceful, more concerned with social and environmental justice, less selfish, and able to think on a larger scale: How will the earth look when I have kids? How can I improve that picture?

We're not saying conservation efforts will effect such a change in every kid, but such efforts do provide a value system for kids that they can relate to. There is the outside world, right in front of them. They can change it for the better, or for the worse.

Nurturing the naturally loving and care-taking spirit in children is one of the most powerful things parents can do to help their children be happy in the world. And don't worry if a toddler is obsessed with squishing bugs. With the right encouragement, direction, and learning, this too shall pass.

Nature Play

Let's get down to some serious (but fun!) business. We think few things are more fun than nature play. Whether that means climbing a tree, counting stars, or pretending to fly like a butterfly, nature is full of inspiration. Where better to start than with an imitation of one of the most basic and inspiring structures of Earth: the mountain.

Mountain Pose (Tadasana)

Mountain Pose is designed to help the yogini feel the strength, solidity, and power of a great mountain. It is the perfect beginning pose for a yoga practice because it helps stabilize the body and focus the mind.

Mountain Pose teaches proper posture and helps to strengthen the back, making it straight and strong. It also puts the mind into an alert state.

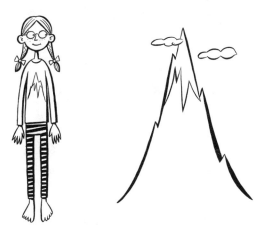

Mountain Pose.

1. Stand with both feet parallel and close together, hands hanging by your sides.

2. Focus your eyes on an object in front of you and try to remain still.

3. Imagine you are strong and tall like a mountain. Not even the strongest wind could blow you over!

➤ **For More Fun:** Parents, test your child's concentration by pretending to be a bird flying around the mountain, or take a blanket and shake it to make wind against the mountain, so kids are challenged to keep focused and not be distracted.

➤ **For Even More Fun:** If you live near a mountain or even a hill, or if you can drive to one easily, hike with your child to the top and sit for awhile. Together, try to feel the energy of the mountain. Notice everything you can about it—ground cover, wildlife, its shape, its slopes and dips. Even try Mountain Pose up there! Incorporate that feeling into your next yoga practice.

Tree Pose (Vrikshasana)

Tree Pose is a balance pose that takes some practice. This kind of practice is fun, however. Kids think it is great to try standing on one foot, especially since falling over is half the fun! Also, there are so many kinds of trees, kids enjoy choosing which tree to be.

Tree Pose strengthens the back and legs. It improves the sense of balance and can help synchronize both hemispheres of the brain. It also improves concentration.

Tree Pose.

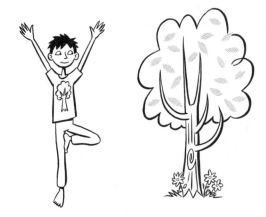

1. Begin by standing in Mountain Pose (the previous pose). Focus on something in front of you, to help maintain your balance.

2. Spread your toes and imagine you have roots growing out of your feet, anchoring you to the ground.

3. Slowly bend one leg and place the sole of that foot on the inside of the standing leg, anywhere between the ankle and knee, as if your bent leg is a crooked branch.

4. Raise your hands in front of you and place your palms together in front of your heart, a position called Namaste Pose.

5. Slowly lift your arms over your head and separate your arms and hands.

6. Spread your arms wide like branches and hands like leaves. Feel the branches and leaves pulling you up to the sky while, at the same time, your roots ground you to the Earth.

7. Hold for as long as you feel comfortable and then slowly lower your foot to the floor and perform the pose with the other leg raised.

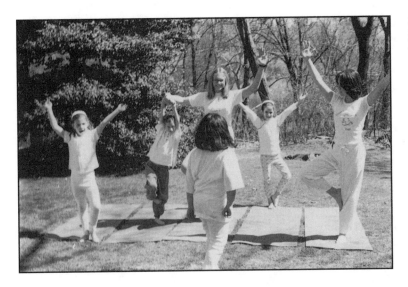

Spread your arms like branches. Play "Small Tree, Tall Tree, 1, 2, 3."

➤ **For More Fun:** What kind of tree are you? An elm? A palm? What about an apple tree? Maybe someone would like to pick some apples off you. Allow a hungry giraffe (see Chapter 14) to come and eat some leaves off your branches. Can you keep your balance?

➤ **For Even More Fun:** If you feel balanced enough, you can gently wave your branches, as if it were a breezy day. Then, maybe the breeze gets stronger. How would a forest look in a windstorm? Gather with a group of friends, each holding Tree Pose, then imagine a slight wind comes up. The wind gets stronger, and stronger, and stronger, until it is a cyclone. How much can the trees thrash before they topple? (Make it a controlled topple, please!)

➤ **For Even *More* Fun:** Play "Small Tree, Tall Tree, 1, 2, 3" (a game adapted from the book *Yoga for Children*, by Mary Stewart and Kathy Phillips, Fireside, 1993). This game is similar to "Red Light, Green Light, Go." All kids except for one go to the far side of the room. The chosen child, at the opposite end of the room, closes his or her eyes, turns around to face away from the group, and says the rhyme "Small tree, tall tree, 1, 2, 3!" During this time, the children in the group take small steps. Upon hearing "1, 2, 3" each child lifts

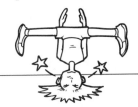

Ooops!

Balance poses are great fun, but they require concentration. They also require good sense! If you start to fall out of Tree Pose, especially if you are pretending to be a tree in a windstorm, please put both your feet back on the ground. There is no benefit in falling over while standing on one foot, and you could injure yourself.

up a leg and assumes Tree Pose. This game is not a race to be the first one to get to the caller—*no winners, no losers.* Everyone gets a turn to be the caller.

Frog Pose (Malasana)

Kids think of frogs as bouncy creatures that hop around the garden or the edges of ponds, but sometimes, frogs sit perfectly still. Kids can play leapfrog, but they can also do Frog Pose for a different kind of frog experience! Frog Pose strengthens the leg muscles, aids constipation and digestion, and works concentration and focus.

1. Squat down with your heels close together and reach toward the ground. Some may be able to touch the ground, some may not. Go at your own pace.

2. When you feel balanced, slowly raise one hand at a time to Namaste Pose, with palms together in front of the heart.

3. Stay still here for as long as it feels comfortable.

➤ **For More Fun:** Ready? Jump! Croak! Catch a fly!

➤ **For Even More Fun:** Play the song "Jeremiah Was a Bullfrog" (actually called "Joy to the World") while squatting or jumping in Frog Pose. (Look for *Jeremiah Was a Bullfrog,* by Hoyt Axton, Youngheart, 1998.)

➤ **For Even *More* Fun:** Play leapfrog. Form a line, with everyone crouched down, heads lowered. The person at the back of the line begins by jumping over the line of people (pretend they are the lily pads) until he or she gets to the front of the line and then turns into a lily pad. Next frog!

Butterfly Pose (Baddha Konasana)

Now it's time to get down on the floor and stretch those hips. Imagine you are a beautiful, playful butterfly and your legs are the butterfly wings, gracefully flying in the wind. Kids vary widely in how far they can lower their knees in Butterfly Pose, a measure of the flexibility in their legs and hips. Anyone can do this pose, however. Lowering your knees only slightly still reaps the benefits, which include mobilization, stimulation, and increased flexibility of the knee and hip joints.

1. Come down into a sitting position on the floor or the ground.

2. Bend your knees, draw your feet in toward you, and place the soles of your feet together.

3. Hold your feet with your hands to connect the butterfly wings (your bent legs).

4. Slowly flap your "wings," lifting and lowering your bent legs.

5. Continue for as long as you are having fun!

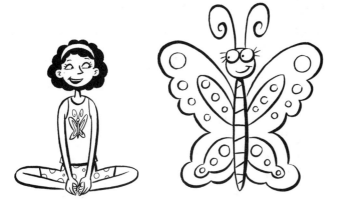

Butterfly Pose.

➤ **For More Fun:** Imagine you are taking off from a tree branch, flying away to a magical place, or anywhere you would love to go—a park, a beach, a carnival, or never-never land! Use your arms as antennas to help you get to your destination.

➤ **For Even More Fun:** Try Extended Butterfly. Begin in Butterfly Pose, then gently lean back onto your tailbone (coccyx). Hold on to your feet and extend your legs, opening your wings until your legs are straight (keep hold of those feet). Now you are really flying high!

➤ **For Even *More* Fun:** Think about a butterfly. It starts as a caterpillar, then spins a cocoon of silk around itself. Later, it emerges transformed. When you have some time alone, try wrapping yourself in a blanket like a cocoon and thinking about what you would like to grow into someday. Then, throw off your blanket. You are already transforming!

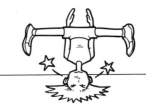

Ooops!

Some kids are very flexible, or hypotonic, in their hips and can easily rest their knees on the floor in Butterfly Pose. That doesn't mean they shouldn't bother with this important pose! These children should still practice the pose because it will strengthen the muscles in this area. Butterfly Pose builds both flexibility and strength, whichever the child needs.

Flower Pose

Flowers add beauty, color, texture, shape, and fragrance to the natural world. Flowers come in so many different forms, just like kids! Flower Pose stretches the shoulders, arms, and hips. It also strengthens the abdominal and back muscles, as well as the mind.

1. Begin by sitting in Butterfly Pose.

2. Place your hands in the space in between your feet and groin. Walk your hands out underneath your shins and take hold of your feet, so that your legs are resting on your arms and your hands are holding your feet.

3. Gently lean back onto your "sitz bones" and raise your feet off the ground. Try to keep your feet together.

➤ **For More Fun:** What kind of flower are you? How do you smell? Allow someone to come near you and inhale and exhale your scent. Mmmm!

➤ **For Even More Fun:** While in the pose, take hold of a pinwheel, either with your hands or with your toes! Try a breathing exercise, like Breath of Fire. Can you make the pinwheel spin while holding Flower Pose?

➤ **For Even *More* Fun:** Try a group Flower Pose, to make a garden of flowers. Gather at least three friends and sit closely in a circle, with everyone in Flower Pose. As you lift your feet up and balance, take hold of your neighbor's hands. Try to have everyone balance together.

Star Pose

This relaxing, meditative pose is a nice counter pose to the invigorating Butterfly Pose. It is excellent after a stressful day in helping you regain a clear-headed, alert, wakeful, energized state. Kids can imagine they are sparkling like shining stars in a clear night sky.

The benefits of Star Pose include flexibility in the arms, back, hips, and ankles. Star Pose is also a modified inversion, which means your head is down and blood flows into your brain. This helps to clear the mind.

Star Pose.

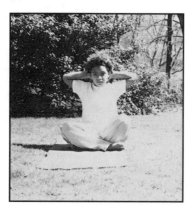
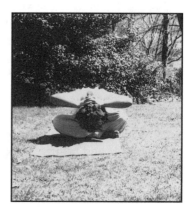

1. Begin in Butterfly Pose.

2. Interlace your fingers to form a basket shape, then place your locked hands behind your head, stretching your elbows out to the sides.

3. Slowly lower your head and arms down toward your feet.

4. Breathe through the pose as you lower your upper body.

5. Relax in this pose for as long as it feels good.

➤ **For More Fun:** Ask a friend, parent, or sibling to count and name or touch the points on your star!

➤ **For Even More Fun:** As you rest in Star Pose, sing or listen to the songs "Twinkle Twinkle Little Star" or "When You Wish Upon a Star."

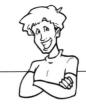

For Grownups, Too!

On a clear mild evening, spend some time outside with your child after dark, star gazing. Talk about what stars are—bright balls of gaseous energy—and how far away they are. Talk about why they twinkle (the interference of the atmosphere) and what they inspire in people. Find constellations, invent your own, and then spend some quiet time in celestial contemplation.

Rainbow Pose (Vasisthasana)

Rainbow Pose is a more difficult balance pose that builds both strength and concentration. It is also beautiful and empowering. When kids master this one, they feel as bright and colorful as a real rainbow!

Rainbow Pose activates the entire body, opening up the ribs on each side as it strengthens the arms, legs, and torso. It also improves balance and concentration.

1. Begin in Downward Facing Dog Pose (see Chapter 12), with feet and palms flat on the floor, hips raised and head lowered so the entire body forms an upside-down V.

2. Slowly roll your body to the right, dropping your hips so your body forms a diagonal line from head down to feet. Your left hip is over your right and your left leg rests on your right leg. Your feet should be stacked one on top of the other with ankle bones touching. This takes strength—if you can't get it right away, just go as far as you can.

3. Slowly bring your left arm off the ground and up to your left hip so you are balancing on your right arm and right leg (the ground is the long side of the triangle).

4. When you feel balanced and comfortable here (maybe not today, but someday), raise your left arm to the sky.

5. Hold this balance for a few seconds (or longer) and imagine you are a glowing, shining, bright rainbow in the sky.

6. Slowly roll back to Downward Facing Dog Pose, bringing your left arm and left foot back to the floor. Rest here for a moment.

7. Roll to the left and repeat on the other side.

8. Rest in Mouse Pose (see Chapter 12).

Start in Downward Dog Pose (upper) and move into Rainbow Pose (lower).

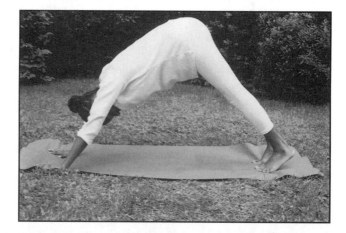

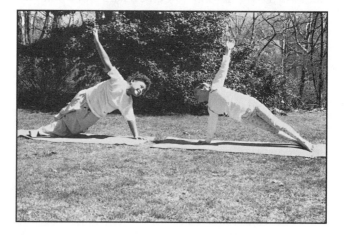

➤ **For More Fun:** To help you focus and hold the pose longer, focus on each of the colors of the rainbow, one by one, while in Rainbow Pose. You can even chant the colors out loud: red, orange, yellow, green, blue, indigo, violet. Imagine your rainbow brightens with each recited color.

➤ **For Even More Fun:** Dress in your most rainbow-ish clothes for Rainbow Pose.

Take a Yogini Nature Walk

Parents, one way to structure yoga nature poses is to take an imaginary nature walk, just you and your child, or with a group of yoginis. Venture out into the imaginary woods, the beach, the rainforest, the savanna, or anywhere else your imagination desires. Stroll around. What do you see?

As you observe your environment make sure to include the pose corresponding to what you see. For example, you are hiking in the mountains. Climb all the way to the top of the mountain, and when you reach the peak, take a look around. Be still in Mountain Pose just like the mountain range around you. When you are ready to move on, walk toward a big tree. Do the Tree Pose and be a part of the forest. If the sun is shining on your nature walk, do a Yoga Sun Dance.

Yoga nature poses are the substance and essence of yogini nature walks, prompting a personal connection to the natural world as well as stimulating yogini imaginations. If a child doesn't know a pose for the things he or she imagines, why not make one up together? The point is to help children delve into their imaginations and practice being one with nature.

Weather permitting, you might wind down your yoga workout with a real nature walk. A nature walk doesn't have to be in the deep wilderness. A park, a nearby trail, or even a stroll around the neighborhood can all provide opportunities for observing and appreciating the natural world. Some things for you to look out for …

➤ What different kinds of trees do you see? Notice the different shapes of the tree outlines, their colors, the textures of their bark, their leaves. Are they covered in buds or are the leaves ready to drop? Are they bare or blossoming? Do they move in the wind or stand still?

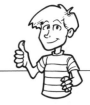

For Kids Only

Did you notice the colors of the rainbow are the same as the seven chakra colors from the last chapter? As you hold Rainbow Pose, you might consider, one by one, each color and the energy it represents: red for basic instincts, orange for creativity, yellow for energy consumption, green for compassion, blue for communication, indigo for intuition, and violet for spiritual enlightenment.

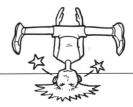

Ooops!

Always dress appropriately for a nature walk, with shoes that support and protect feet, and with sunscreen and a hat for skin protection. If you'll be walking through high grass or in a wooded area, wear long pants and a hat to guard against ticks and other biting insects. And, depending on where you go and how long your walk will be, don't forget to carry water and a snack!

➤ Notice the lay of the land. Is the landscape around you flat, rolling, dramatically rising or dropping? Are the slopes gentle or jagged? What is the ground cover? Grass? Weeds? Rocks? Gravel? Cement and lawns? A carpet of pine needles?

➤ What wildlife do you see? Birds and squirrels? Deer and hawks? Farm animals? Ducks? Minnows in a lake? Crickets and ants?

➤ What nature sounds do you hear? Wind in the trees? Rustling weeds and grass? Birds singing? Bugs chirping? What other sounds? Cars? People?

➤ Describe the sky. Blue and cloudless? White and fluffy? Darkening? Is the sun rising, setting, or bright overhead? Can you see the moon today?

➤ In the middle of your nature walk, enjoy a few moments of silence. Have everyone sit, preferably not on cement or any human-made structure but right on the earth, the grass, or a tree (dress appropriately). No talking! Just listen and observe. After 5 or 10 minutes, talk about what you felt, thought about, or noticed.

We believe nature is a truly abundant source of life-force energy and creativity. A yoga practice as well as a life steeped in nature and in frequent touch with the natural world is sure to be richer, simpler, and more harmonious.

The Least You Need to Know

➤ Everyone is part of the natural world, and the natural world is part of us. Getting in touch with the nature within us helps to harmonize the soul and cultivate respect for nature, animals, and other humans.

➤ Learning about ecology and conservation can help kids become less wasteful, more resourceful, more caring, less selfish, and more concerned with preserving the Earth for future generations.

➤ Nature poses are great fun. Mountain Pose, Tree Pose, Flower Pose, Frog Pose, Butterfly Pose, Star Pose, and Rainbow Pose all reflect things in nature and strive to capture some of their energy.

➤ Combine all the nature poses you know in a yogini nature walk. Stroll through the natural setting of your choice. Whenever you see a mountain, a tree, a star, a rainbow, or a butterfly, pause and do the pose.

➤ A nature walk can be a nice way to wind down a yoga practice.

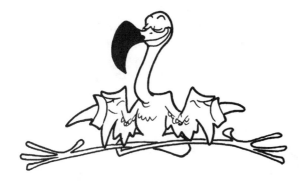

Chapter 12

What Animal Are You?

In This Chapter

➤ Getting in touch with your animal nature

➤ Learning from animals through animal play

➤ Go country with farm and domestic animal poses

➤ Take flight with bird poses

Kids love to be animals. Remember that scene from the classic movie, *Miracle on 34th Street,* when little Susie learned, for the first time, how much fun it was to pretend to be a monkey? Something about animals fascinates kids. Soft, silky cats are sure-footed. Big growling grizzly bears are powerful. Antelopes are lightning-fast. And birds can fly!

In the next few chapters, we'll help children explore their animal natures with lots of fun poses and animal play. And don't think grownups are immune. If you're a grownup, just because it's been a long time since you've kicked up your heels like a bucking bronco doesn't mean it isn't still really, really fun!

Discovering Your Yogini Animal Nature

If you're a parent and your child has ever visited the zoo or a farm or even a pet shop, you've probably witnessed firsthand his or her fascination with the animal kingdom. But how often does your child think of his or her own animal nature?

Animals are more than just fellow sentient beings on the planet Earth. They are a lot like us, and we are a lot like them. We can do lots of things most animals can't do, but then again, animals can do lots of things we can't do—humans aren't very good at breathing underwater, soaring through the clouds, burrowing through the earth, or running as fast as a speeding car.

What do we have in common with animals? Not sharing a language, we may never know the complete answer to this question, but why not explore our own animal natures to try to answer the question for ourselves?

The following activities can help children get in closer touch with the animal within (because every child has an animal within!):

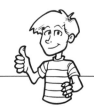

For Kids Only

It's fun to spend some time quietly observing a cat or dog. How does it stretch when it wakes up from a nap? How does a dog swim? How does a cat rub itself against your legs? How does its expressions change, its ears move, its tail wag or twitch? See how much you can notice about your favorite dog or cat, and how much you can imitate.

➤ Invent an animal! What two animals could be combined for an all-new animal? A giraffe-lizard? A fish-cat? A possum-moose? Draw a picture of the animal, give it a name, or try to act out how it would move and what sound it would make.

➤ If a child could be any animal, what would he or she choose to be? Why? Talk about it. What animal does a child picture his or her parent to be?

➤ Play the animal sound game (a kind of chanting): The child says an animal sound: "Moo." The parent repeats it, and adds another: "Moo, baa." The child repeats and adds another: "Moo, baa, meow." Continue on until somebody can't remember the order. This is lots of fun in a group, going around the circle.

➤ Parents, challenge your child to walk around on all fours (hands and feet or hands and knees, whichever is more comfortable) for as long as possible during an at-home day. You might throw in an occasional "Nice doggy" or "Good kitty" as your child scampers around at your feet. The game is over when your child resumes a bipedal stance. (Now is it your turn?)

➤ Play "Animal Hour." Each day of the week (or one day a week), a child can choose a different animal, then can spend one hour thinking about, pretending to be, and learning about that animal. For example, young kids might spend time experimenting with positions a cat might make, making cat sounds, stretching, purring, and practicing cat movements. Older kids might spend the day researching giant tortoises and inventing yoga movements and positions that capture the spirit of their animal.

➤ Choose a totem, which is a personal animal a child (or any individual) can identify with. The child should choose an animal he or she feels a special bond with—the friendly dog, the trickster coyote, the majestic eagle, the quiet mouse, the playful otter. Parents, talk to your child about the qualities of that totem animal, and which of these qualities your child sees reflected in himself or herself. You might even involve the whole family. Everyone chooses a totem animal, then makes a special picture of the animal to mount on a totem pole made from a paper towel or wrapping paper tube. A family totem pole! Display it with pride.

And of course, doing yoga animal poses is a great way to get in touch with the animal inside everyone. When kids do animal poses, they should focus on imagining what it is like to really be that animal. How does the animal move? What sound does it make? What is it thinking? Be one with your animal. How is that animal similar to something in you?

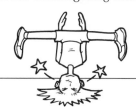

Learning from Animal Behaviors and Movements

Doesn't it feel great to really stretch like a cat or a dog when you wake up in the morning? To climb a tree or a jungle gym like a monkey? To burst out into song like a bird? To lie in the sun like a lizard or leap through the water like a dolphin?

We can all benefit from watching, learning about, and imitating animals. They aren't so different from us, and they have a lot to teach us about living in the moment, practicing simplicity, and the simple joy of being.

Ooops!

Even though a child may be getting in touch with the animal within, be aware that he or she may not be ready for the responsibility of having a pet. Having a pet is a big responsibility only an older child or a grownup should assume. While kids can handle certain duties, adults must make sure the duties are accomplished.

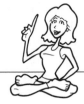

Yoga Stories

Animal trivia is fun and fascinating. Here are a few animal fun facts we like (taken from the Useless Facts Library, www.southhouse.com/useless/factlib1.htm):

➤ A hippo can run faster than a man.

➤ A kangaroo can hop 30 feet in one leap.

➤ A lion's roar can be heard from five miles away.

➤ A snake has no ears but picks up sound waves with its tongue.

➤ A giraffe can clean its ears with its 21-inch-long tongue.

➤ A hummingbird weighs less than a penny.

➤ A group of larks is called an exaltation (that's also what we would call a group of yoginis!).

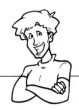

For Grownups, Too!

Many adults and children are allergic to pets and can't have them in their homes. That doesn't mean your child can't have plenty of exposure to animals, however. An outdoor zoo, an aquarium, a park or forest, even the Nature Channel are all good sources for animal observation. And remember, never touch a wild animal or put your hand in the cage of a zoo animal!

Animal Play at Home and on the Farm

Let's get ready for some animal fun. Of course, you can't be a farm animal without first getting to the farm! Sit upright with legs extended in front and hands on a pretend steering wheel in Driving My Car Pose (see Chapter 15) to travel to the farm. (Parents, you can hop in the backseat.) Or, assume Boat Pose (see Chapter 15) and row there! Or, ride your bicycle (see Chapter 17).

Or, rest on your back and imagine taking flight. There's the farm, stretched out on that acreage below. Coming in for a landing ....

Cat Pose (Bidalasana)

Just about every farm has a cat. Slipping in and out of the shadows, balancing on fences, leaping over garden gates and purring for attention, cats are amazing, flexible, graceful, resilient creatures that know how to stretch, play, and relax with the best.

Cat Pose improves circulation in the spine, elongates the spinal column, relieves gas, and improves digestion.

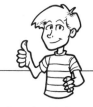

1. Get down on all fours and spread out your paws (that is, your fingers). Make sure your hands are directly under your shoulders and your knees are directly beneath your hips.

2. Round your back and let your head curl downward and in toward your lower body so you are looking toward your belly.

3. Tuck your tailbone (coccyx) down and under.

4. Really stretch that spine, like a Halloween cat!

5. Follow with Cow Pose (see the following section).

For Kids Only

Do you think animals can do yoga? If you watch a cat for awhile, you might begin to believe they can! The flexibility, suppleness, graceful movements, and superb balance cats regularly display makes them seem like little feline yogis. However, it might be more accurate to say that humans do yoga so they can move more like a cat!

➤ **For More Fun:** On the stretch, meow like a cat. Experiment with different tones. Are you a Siamese cat? A scaredy cat? A kitten? A growly tomcat?

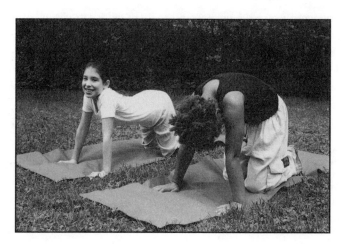

Yoginis practice Cow Pose (left) and Cat Pose (right).

Cow Pose

Have you ever watched a cow standing, relaxed, chewing its cud? Cows have a casual hanging dip to their backs, as if the weight of their bellies bows their spines just a bit. This pose is the counter pose to Cat Pose and works well in conjunction, going back and forth between the two poses.

Cow Pose has the same benefits as Cat Pose, since it is really the other side of the same pose.

1. Start in Cat Pose (on all fours, fingers spread out, hands under your shoulders, back rounded, head down).
2. Inhale and arch your back so your tummy reaches down toward the ground.
3. Lift your chest up, pressing firmly into the ground with all of your hand.
4. Gaze upward. Try to assume the expression of a cow.
5. Move back into Cat Pose. Repeat about four times, back and forth from Cat Pose to Cow Pose.

➤ **For More Fun:** Moo like a cow as you perform the pose.
➤ **For Even More Fun:** Allow a friend or younger sibling to pretend to milk you!

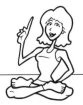

Yoga Stories

The cow is traditionally considered a sacred animal in India, cherished for its giving nature. Cows give both milk for drinking and cooking, and dung, which is used for fuel. Symbolically, the cow represents the giving nature for which humans should strive. Because cows are considered sacred and so highly valued in India, we like to give Cow Pose a special reverence. As you perform Cow Pose, think about the giving nature of the cow and take a moment to honor this animal that has served humans so well for thousands of years.

Downward Facing Dog Pose (Adho Mukha Shavasana)

What's a farm without a dog? We admit not everyone likes dogs, but we think dogs are great—friendly, forgiving, playful, companionable sources of unconditional love. Dogs also know how to stretch, and this well-known yoga pose strives to imitate a nice, deep doggy stretch.

Downward Facing Dog Pose strengthens and stretches the back, arm, and leg muscles. It also tones the kidneys and refreshes the mind as it allows blood to flow to the head. This pose wakes you up! Try it in the morning. (Your dog does!)

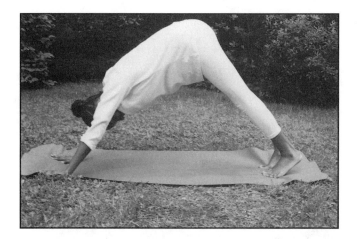

Downward Facing Dog Pose.

1. Get down on all four paws (hands and knees), front paws (fingers) spread wide.

2. Drop your head down so your ears are between your arms.

3. Curl your toes under your feet and slowly begin to raise your knees off the floor and reach your "tail" upward and back, straightening your back legs until you feel a nice stretch in your muscles and hamstrings (the tendons along the backs of your legs).

➤ **For More Fun:** Bark like your favorite dog! Are you a Dalmatian atop a fire engine? A fancy poodle prancing down the avenue? A watchdog alerting the family to visitors?

➤ **For Even More Fun:** Go for a walk! Have someone pretend to be the dog walker, and walk you around the room. Decide how long the leash is (pretend leashes only, please), and approximately where you will go. "Dogs," try to pay attention to where your "owner" is leading you! You might even lift your leg to go ... you know what! Or, have a friend or sibling "train" you to do some doggy tricks like sit, shake, lie down, and roll over. Jump through a Hula-Hoop! You might even beg for a treat (pretend treats, or even a small cube of cheese or bread). The Dog Pose fun could go on for hours.

➤ **For Even *More* Fun:** Have a younger sibling crawl under you as you hold Dog Pose.

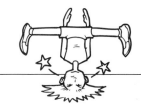

Ooops!

Kids love dogs, but dogs that aren't used to children may get nervous and could even bite. Many children get bitten by dogs each year. Parents, to help prevent your child from getting bitten and perhaps developing a fear of dogs, teach your child to never approach a strange dog and never pet a dog on a leash without first getting permission from the owner.

Mouse Pose (Pindasana)

Mice are nice! They scamper but they also know how to relax, hunkered down and cozy in their mouse houses. Mouse Pose is a good pose to wind down a series of more vigorous poses, or even just a quiet way to rest if you are feeling tired from Sun Dance, lightheaded from an inversion, or just generally out of sorts. It is also the perfect complement to any backbending pose.

Mouse Pose relieves tension, calms the body and the mind, synchronizes both hemispheres of the brain, and gives all the internal organs a gentle massage with each slow, relaxing breath.

Mouse Pose.

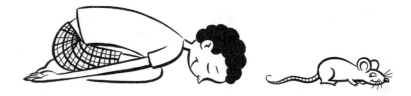

1. Bringing your knees and feet together, sit back on your heels with your arms at your sides. Make sure your feet are flat without toes curled under.

2. Slowly bend forward and allow your forehead to rest on the floor. If this is uncomfortable, place a firm pillow under your forehead.

3. Allow your arms to stretch back behind you, toward your feet, palms facing up and resting near your feet.

4. Hold this relaxing pose for 30 seconds to 1 minute. This is a resting pose, so enjoy the rest!

➤ **For More Fun:** Try to make your body as small as possible in Mouse Pose, then hold the pose as quietly as possible. Yes, quiet as a mouse! Imagine you are a tiny mouse hiding in a small crack.

➤ **For Even More Fun:** Play "Cat, Mouse, Dog," a variation of the classic "Rock, Paper, Scissors" game. Three participants close their eyes then assume Cat Pose, Downward Facing Dog Pose, or Mouse Pose. Open your eyes, make your animal sound, and see what happens, depending on who is what. Dogs chase cats, cats chase mice, mice escape from dogs. Act out the results!

Birds of a Feather

Birds capture our human imaginations like few other creatures. How fantastic and amazing that a bird can fly! Although none of the following yoga bird poses will *actually* allow you to fly, they can certainly help you to feel something of a bird's energy and form. Will you choose to be a goose flying south for the winter today? Perhaps a bright green parrot soaring over the jungle canopy, a finch in a great aviary at a zoo, or a robin nesting in a tree? And we certainly advocate *imaginary* flying whenever possible!

Flamingo Pose

How many legs does a flamingo use to stand? Only one! Flamingo legs are as skinny as sticks but their three long, forward-pointing toes and a stabilizing hind toe help them to balance. You can balance like a flamingo, too! You may not have a hind toe, but you've got a nice stable foot.

Flamingo Pose strengthens balance, stretches the hip flexor and quadriceps, opens up the entire body, and improves posture.

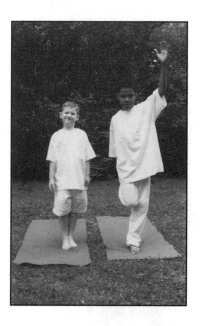 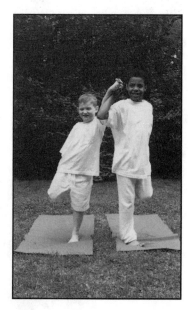

Move from Mountain Pose into Flamingo Pose.

1. Stand in Mountain Pose (see Chapter 11) and look at an object in front of you to help your balance.
2. When you feel balanced, slowly bend one knee and raise your foot behind you until it is pointing toward your backside.
3. Grasp your raised foot with the hand on the same side of your body.
4. Reach your opposite arm and hand high in the air, as if it is the flamingo's long, curvy neck.
5. Return to Mountain Pose and repeat on the other side.

167

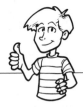

For Kids Only

Flamingos come in a rainbow of reds, from pale pink to vermilion, depending on their type. If you think flamingos are beautiful or you particularly enjoy Flamingo Pose, why not collect a few flamingos for your bedroom or your personal altar? Collecting is fun, and flamingo collectibles are easy to find. Try garage sales, flea markets, thrift shops, and just about anywhere in Florida, where flamingo paraphernalia abounds.

This yogini wears an eagle beak to help get into the spirit of Eagle Pose.

➤ **For More Fun:** When holding Flamingo Pose, imagine you are standing on your flamingo leg in a Florida lagoon among tropical flowers and fellow flamingos. Relax and feel the humid air. Smell the heavy, wet, swampy smell. Listen to the sound of the water.

➤ **For Even More Fun:** Make or buy a flamingo nose to wear while doing this pose.

Eagle Pose (Garudaasana)

The majestic eagle is one of the largest and most imposing birds. While Eagle Pose imitates the eagle as it sits solemnly and silently on a cliff overseeing its domain, we also encourage kids to practice soaring like an eagle around the room, wings outspread, moving in a grand, slow, and regal manner.

Eagle Pose strengthens the ankles and calves, exercises all the arm and leg joints, and removes stiffness from the shoulders. Being a balance pose, it also develops the concentration.

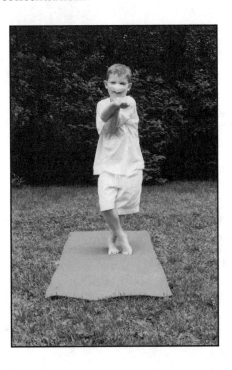

1. Begin in Mountain Pose (see Chapter 11). Look at something in front of you to help you balance.

2. Spread your eagle wings (arms) out to the sides, then place one arm over the other and spiral them around each other until your palms touch, a position called Namaste.

3. Bend your knees and raise one foot off the ground. Spiral it around your standing leg as best you can, hooking your foot around your opposite lower leg.

4. Try to remain balanced on one leg in this position. (It gets easier the more you do it.)

5. Return to Mountain Pose and perform the pose on the other side.

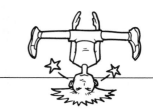

➤ **For More Fun:** Play the song "Fly Like an Eagle" by the Steve Miller Band while you practice this pose.

➤ **For Even More Fun:** As you hold Eagle Pose, imitate the whistling shriek of the eagle. If you don't know what eagles sound like, you can listen to the eagle's call on the Web site of the American Eagle Foundation at www. eagles.org/moreabout.html.

Ooops!

Protect your joints, especially your knees, in Eagle Pose. Don't force your leg to wrap around the other leg farther than is comfortable. Listen to your body and don't exceed your limits.

Pigeon Pose (Ekapada Rajakapotasana)

No matter where you live, you've probably seen the ubiquitous pigeon. Although they may seem ordinary, pigeons are extremely intelligent creatures with many interesting characteristics and have been used over the years for many purposes including the delivery of messages across vast distances. Pigeons have a unique shape and stance that Pigeon Pose strives to imitate.

Pigeon Pose stretches the arms, back, hips, and legs.

1. Get down on all fours, with hands below your shoulders and knees below your hips.

2. Slide one knee forward so it rests on the floor between your two hands, pointing slightly away from the corresponding hip.

3. Rest the shin of your bent leg on the ground and angle your foot over and in front of the opposite hip, keeping your foot flat.

4. Gently slide your other leg back behind you, keeping that foot flat, too.

5. Place your fingertips by your sides on the floor and gently look upward, arching your lower back.

6. Hold for a few seconds, then walk your hands out in front of you and rest your forehead on the floor.

7. Hold for about 20 seconds, then walk your hands back up, returning to all fours.

8. Repeat on the other side.

Pigeon Pose.

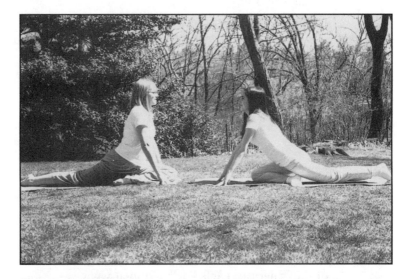

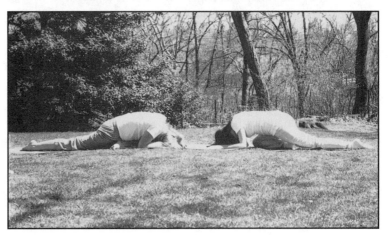

➤ **For More Fun:** Have a friend or sibling pretend to throw breadcrumbs in front of you. Peck at them like a pigeon pecks.

Swan Pose

The lovely, graceful, snow-white swan is well-known to kids through the story of the ugly duckling, who turned into a magnificent swan at the end, to the surprise of his duck family. Swan Pose imitates the grandeur and beauty of the swan.

Swan Pose releases tension in the lower back, strengthens the upper back and neck muscles, expands the rib cage, and helps relieve gas and constipation.

1. Lie down on your tummy with your arms perpendicular to your body, as if you were spreading your wings.

2. Place your forehead against the ground, then gently inhale.

3. Exhale as you lift the forehead, the chin, the chest, and the arms off the ground.

4. Hold for five to eight seconds, imagining your raised upper body is the elegant long neck of a floating swan.

5. Lower slowly back into the starting position, then repeat a few more times.

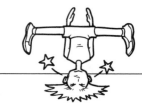

Ooops!

If you have a history of knee problems (unusual for young kids but older kids involved in athletics sometimes sustain knee injuries), perform Pigeon Pose only under the guidance of a certified yoga teacher. Or just skip this pose.

Swan Pose.

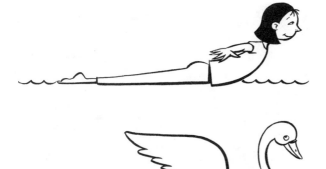

➤ **For More Fun:** Sway your raised upper body as if you were gliding to-and-fro on a calm, sparkling lake.

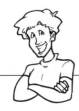

For Grownups, Too!

It's probably best to avoid the "Ugly Duckling" story when your child is feeling insecure about appearance. As beautiful as you find your child, he or she may not want to hear any story with the word "ugly" in it. Keep in mind your child's delicate ego. A better suggestion when your child is feeling down? "Let's do some yoga. How about Swan Pose?"

Seagull Pose

Seagull Pose takes two: a grownup and a child. It mimics the seagull's lazy flight over the water.

Seagull Pose massages the internal organs of the torso, promotes digestion, eases gas and constipation, and builds confidence. It's fun to fly!

1. Lie on your back (the adult) with knees bent, feet raised off the floor toward your child.

2. Have your child stand with his or her tummy against the bottoms of your feet.

3. Take both child's hands and using them for support, slowly straighten your legs to lift your child off the ground. Keep hold of your child's hands so his or her arms are outstretched like seagull wings.

4. Sway your legs gently back and forth so your child can "fly."

5. Come in for a landing: Slowly bend your knees and lower your child to the ground. Rest in Mouse Pose (described earlier in this chapter).

Seagull Pose.

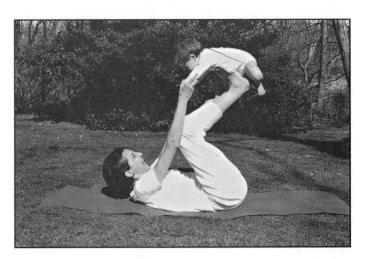

➤ **For More Fun:** Your child can screech like a seagull while you make ocean or wind noises.

Crow Pose (Bakasana)

Moving from the sublime to the cacophonous, we find a pose celebrating the confident, noisy, and rascally crow. This is a very difficult balance pose but if you can learn to achieve it, you will feel just like a proud, saucy crow sitting on a telephone wire.

Crow Pose bestows strength and confidence on the yogini who masters it. Crow Pose specifically strengthens the hands, wrists, and arms, and improves concentration.

Crow Pose.

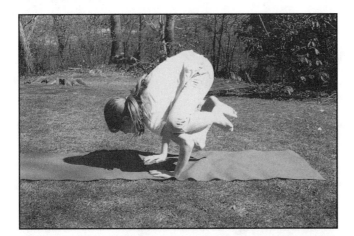

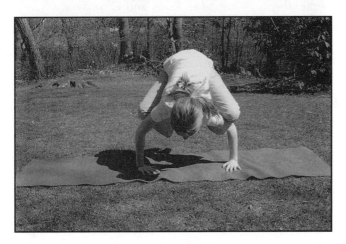

1. Squat down and place your hands on the floor in front of you. Look at something in front of you to help you balance.

2. Bend your elbows and ease your shins onto your upper arms, using your arms like a shelf.

3. Once you feel stable, shift your weight forward so your shins rest completely on your arms with feet off the floor. Pretty impressive!

173

4. Don't be frustrated if you can't do this pose right away. It truly is challenging, even for experienced yoginis. Give yourself plenty of time to develop your strength and balance, and be patient.

➤ **For More Fun:** Once in Crow Pose, let loose some robust "caw-caws."

Young yoginis may feel they have experienced the animal kingdom galore, but we're not finished yet. Read on to the next chapter for even more fun animal poses!

The Least You Need to Know

➤ We all have a little animal in us. A child can discover his or her animal nature through yoga.

➤ Animal games and activities like building a family totem pole or observing and imitating a family pet increase a child's respect and reverence for creatures other than humans.

➤ Fun yoga farm poses include Cat Pose, Cow Pose, Downward Facing Dog Pose, and Mouse Pose.

➤ Birds are an inspiration, and many yoga poses are based on birds, including Flamingo Pose, Eagle Pose, Pigeon Pose, Swan Pose, and Crow Pose.

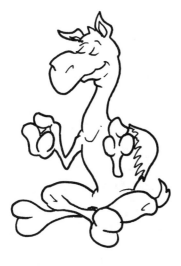

Chapter 13

Exploring the Desert

In This Chapter

➤ Creatures of the desert

➤ Stretch like a snake

➤ Hoot like an owl

➤ Calm as a camel

➤ Roadrunner, poised for action

➤ Comical cacti

Wild animals! What child isn't fascinated by them? The desert is home to some of the most fascinating, unusual, and inspiring wild animals in nature. Desert creatures have adapted to the desert's harsh, dry, severe conditions in many amazing ways, including sleeping during the day and hunting at night. Desert plants are unique, as well, with their thick flesh and sharp spines.

Learning from and imitating the creatures and plants of the desert is fun, educational, and potentially enlightening for kids, teaching them what life could be like in an entirely new environment.

Every child has something of the untamed spirit of the wild within, and this chapter gives kids an opportunity to revel in the wildness of the desert, while gaining strength, flexibility, and concentration.

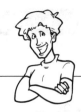

For Grownups, Too!

We're guessing you probably don't have a pet cobra or camel at home, and although you might have a small one in a pot, your house probably isn't populated with cacti. However, many cities have excellent, humane zoos and wildlife parks you and your family can visit to watch wild animals in their natural habitats. Take a field trip and encourage your kids to observe the way wild animals move.

Destination: Desert

Before we get wild, we must first get to our destination. Remember how you got to the farm in the last chapter, by car, or boat, or on foot through the fields? How will you arrive in the wild desert? Perhaps you would like to take a Jeep. Try Driving My Car Pose again (see Chapter 15), or ride your bike (see Chapter 17).

Make Like a Snake

Here we are, deep in the heart of the desert. You can see for miles out here (when the sand isn't blowing), and you might not see any desert creatures at first, but they are all around. Let's pretend to be some of them!

Baby Snake Pose

This pose is also known as Baby Cobra Pose and it is a great introduction to the world of desert creatures. Baby Snake Pose stretches and elongates the top of the spine, allowing for better posture and helping to keep it flexible and healthy. It stretches the throat, chest, abdomen, and shoulders, and strengthens the muscles of the back. Baby Snake Pose also tones the kidneys.

Baby Snake Pose.

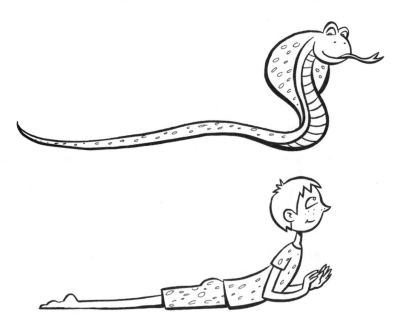

1. Lie on your stomach with your legs close together, as if you are a long, slithery snake.
Remember, snakes have only one tail, so try
to keep those feet near each other.

2. Place your forehead on the mat, and rest
palms face down next to both sides of your
chest.

3. Inhale through your nose, then exhale.

4. As you exhale, slowly lift your head and
chest, gently arching your upper spine.

5. Lift your hands off the mat, keeping them in
position near the chest, and hold for a few
seconds.

6. Lower gently back to the starting position,
then repeat a few times.

➤ **For More Fun:** As you raise your head, chest,
and arms up, "hisssssss" like a baby snake.

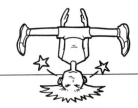

Ooops!

The snake poses involve resting
the forehead on the ground.
Not being a snake, you might
not feel comfortable resting your
forehead on the grass or a hard
floor. You can adapt this pose by
resting with your arms down by
your sides and your head turned
one way or the other, alternating
between poses. Or, make a pillow with your hands to cushion
your forehead.

Mother Snake Pose (Bhujangaasana)

Mother snakes are bigger than babies are so they can get into positions that are just a
little more challenging. That doesn't mean only moms can do this pose, of course!
This pose is also called Mother Cobra. Mother Snake Pose has the same benefits as
Baby Snake Pose. It also gives the internal organs a gentle massage when you breathe
slowly while holding the pose. This action helps rid the body of waste.

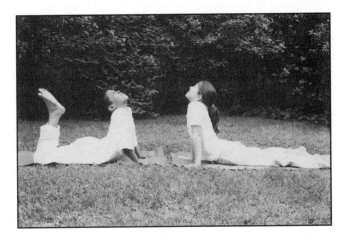

*Father Snake meets Mother
Snake.*

177

1. Begin as in Baby Snake Pose, lying on your stomach with your legs and feet close together.

2. Place your forehead on the mat with your palms on the floor next to both sides of your chest.

3. Inhale through your nose, then exhale.

4. As you exhale, slowly lift your head and chest, gently arching your upper spine, as in Baby Snake Pose.

5. Using your hands pressed firmly into the mat, lift up your body even farther until your entire spine arches.

6. Hold for a few seconds, then gently lower into the starting position.

7. Repeat a few times.

➤ **For More Fun:** As you lift your head, chest, and body, "hissssss" like a mother snake. This would, of course, be a slightly louder hiss than you made for Baby Snake Pose.

➤ **For Even More Fun:** Using your arms, pull yourself around the room, slithering like a snake, looking for some food.

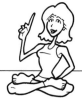

Yoga Stories

Cobras are large, venomous snakes found in many parts of the world including India, Thailand, the Philippines, Malaysia, southern China, and Africa. Cobras have loose skin around their heads that they fan out into a hood when threatened. The hood is most prominent in the common cobra, the snake most often used by snake charmers. Although it causes many deaths in India each year, the cobra is regarded as a holy animal and rarely killed. The king cobra is the longest venomous snake in the world, averaging 12 feet in length but known to grow as long as 18 feet.

Father Snake Pose

This pose is the most challenging snake pose, using the entire body from head to toe. Once again, it isn't just for dads, it's for everyone! Also called Father Cobra Pose, Father Snake Pose stretches the entire front of the body, strengthens the arms and back, and tones the kidneys.

1. Begin by doing Mother Snake Pose.

2. When you are in the raised position, move your hands gently, one at a time, about five to six inches in front of your body. Try to keep your hands in line with where they were at the beginning. You are simply moving them forward.

3. Bend your knees and lift your feet toward the sky.

4. Gently bring your head back toward your feet and look up at the sky.

5. Try to reach your feet and head toward each other. Go slowly and breathe!

6. Hold for a few seconds, then gently lower back into the starting position. Repeat a few times.

➤ **For More Fun:** Hiss like a big Cobra and slither your tongue in and out.

➤ **For Even More Fun:** Have someone pretend to be a snake charmer. Put on some sultry Egyptian music. Lie on the floor in the beginning position, forehead on the floor, hands next to your chest. Have the snake charmer wrap a scarf around his or her head, then sit in Pretzel Pose (see Chapter 17) in front of the cobra. As the snake charmer pretends to play a flute or recorder (or plays a real one), slowly rise up into Baby Snake Pose, Mother Snake Pose, then all the way into Father Snake Pose, swaying with the music.

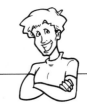

For Grownups, Too!

What's in a name? Other yoga books, videos, classes, martial arts, or even gymnastics or ballet classes may use many of the poses in this book, but with different names. Yoga pose names often change and in this book, we give names to the poses we think kids will enjoy, but these names certainly aren't fixed. If your child likes a different name for a pose, by all means, rename it!

Wise and Wonderful

The wise old owl and the wonderfully humped camel are two fascinating desert creatures that are great fun to imitate. Pretend to perch, hoot, and fly, or stretch into the shape of a camel's hump with these fun poses.

Wise Owl Pose

Watch out, snakes—there's an owl on the loose! Owl Pose imitates an owl keeping watch over the desert at night from a tall perch. Are you observing the desert in darkness, or are you looking for a nice dinner? Owl Pose tones the ankles, knees, and hip joints, opens the chest, increases flexibility in the shoulders, and is good for concentration. It also makes you feel wise!

This pose was invented by four-year-old Angus Adamson, son of your co-author, Eve, who like a typical mommy is quite proud of her inventive yogini. One afternoon, Angus climbed on the flat back of a small chair, crouched, tucked his arms neatly behind his back, placed his palms together, hooted twice, and proclaimed himself to be in Owl Pose.

Owl Pose.

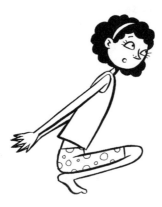 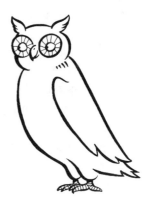

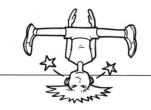

Ooops!

Camels can go for several days without drinking water, but people can't. Kids should drink lots of water (about 64 ounces per day for teens). Water keeps the body hydrated, cleansed, and lubricated so it works more efficiently. However, children under two shouldn't drink so much water that it compromises their milk intake.

1. Stand with feet about shoulder-width apart, then slowly squat all the way down, keeping feet pointing straight ahead and flat on the floor. (Some kids might find it easier to squat while standing on just the balls of their feet.)

2. Bring your arms behind you as if they were folded wings.

3. Touch your fingertips or, if you are able, clasp your fingers and palms together, fingers pointed down toward the floor.

4. Open your eyes wide and gaze around you, rotating your head from left to right.

5. When you see your prey, or are simply ready to stretch your wings, jump up as you open your wings (lift your arms out to the sides) and pretend to fly around the room.

➤ **For More Fun:** Hoot like an owl as you survey your surroundings, and as you fly around the room.

➤ **For Even More Fun:** If your balance is steady enough, try this pose on the seat of a chair or other raised surface where you can survey the lay of the land below.

Camel Pose (Ushtraasana)

Maybe you arrived in the desert on your camel. Now you can *be* a camel! One-humped camels, also called dromedaries, have been used for thousands of years for transport of goods from one place to another.

Camel Pose keeps the spine healthy and flexible. It stretches the throat, shoulders, chest, stomach, and thighs. It also strengthens the back, tones the kidneys, and opens the chest, which is great for people with asthma or bronchitis.

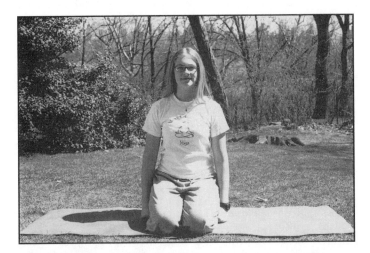

Move from Japanese Sitting Pose (top) into Camel Pose (bottom).

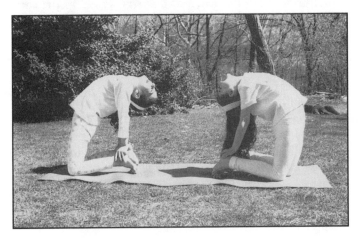

1. Begin in Japanese Sitting Pose, a position in which you sit on your heels with your knees bent and legs together.

2. Lift your body up off your heels and curl your toes under. This allows for a close reach. (Once you are comfortable in this pose, you can try it with your feet flat on the floor.)

181

3. Look back toward your heels and, one at a time, take hold of each ankle. Don't let your feet come off the ground.

4. Press your hips forward and if you are comfortable, look up, letting your head relax back.

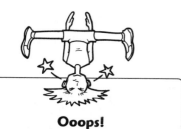

Ooops!

If you have neck problems or serious back problems, avoid Camel Pose, or perform it only under the supervision of a certified yoga instructor.

5. Hold for a few seconds.

6. Press your hands, one at a time, into your lower back and come back up to an upright position.

7. Lower your body forward into Mouse Pose (see Chapter 12) for a nice counter stretch.

8. Repeat one more time.

➤ **For More Fun:** Imagine you actually have a hump, like a camel has. How would it feel to carry a person across the desert? What else might you carry on your back? See if you can really carry something on your hump. We suggest something lightweight like a Beanie Baby.

Desert Still Life

Imagine a desert scene: a stretch of sand, a towering cactus with long spines and crooked arms, and a sleek roadrunner with its crown of feathers, as still as the cactus, poised to dash away at any moment. You can create the scene with the following poses.

Roadrunner Pose

Roadrunners are the fast-as-lightning birds that run along roads or across the sand. Remember the roadrunner cartoon? Wile E. Coyote never stood a chance catching this speedy desert denizen. This pose, however, mimics the roadrunner as it stands still, waiting for a good reason to dash away (or waiting for the coyote to get *almost* close enough!). Roadrunner Pose stretches the front of the legs, the hips, and the back.

1. Begin in Downward Facing Dog Pose, hands and feet on the floor, head down, hips raised up (see Chapter 12).

2. Lunge forward, moving one of your feet up between your hands. Keep the other leg extended, reaching back with the heel. (If this is too difficult, rest your knee on the ground.)

3. Hold for a few seconds, then return to Downward Facing Dog Pose.

4. Switch legs, doing the pose on the other side.

5. After you have lunged with both legs, rest for a few seconds in Mouse Pose (see Chapter 12). Then try it again!

➤ **For More Fun:** Instead of returning to Downward Facing Dog Pose in between lunges, jump back and forth between the lunges, switching leg positions with each jump. Imagine you are running as fast as a roadrunner.

➤ **For Even More Fun:** As you hold Roadrunner Pose or jump back and forth in the above variation of Roadrunner Pose, make the sound of the roadrunner in the cartoon: "beep-beep!"

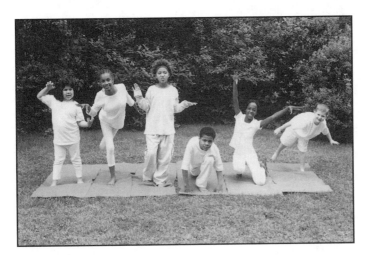

This yogini roadrunner is surrounded by cacti. Can you spot him ready to run?

Cactus Pose

Cacti are sharp and prickly. Look at some pictures of cacti in the desert and notice how many prickles and funny shapes different types of cacti have. Cactus Pose puts kids in touch with each body part and enhances balance.

1. Be a cactus! Bend your elbows and knees into points. Use your fingers and toes as cactus spines. What about your ears, nose, tongue, elbows, and toes? Anything can be a prickle!

2. Balance in different cactus positions.

➤ **For More Fun:** Have a friend or parent come near you and touch one of your cactus thorns to see how sharp it is. Younger kids especially enjoy a convincing "Ouch!" from an adult.

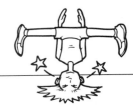

Ooops!

If you choose to try the jumping version of Roadrunner Pose, stay light on your feet and keep your knees from extending beyond your toes to avoid stressing your knee joints. Ideally, your thigh should be parallel with the floor and your knee should form a right angle.

The desert is an endless source of inspiration, with its many creatures, unusual geography, and strange plants. Don't feel limited by the poses in this book. Feel free to make up your own desert poses to add to the ones we've described here. What about Tarantula Pose? Sidewinder Pose? Lizard Pose? Hawk Pose? Butte Pose? Sand Dune Pose? Tumbleweed Pose? Let your imagination travel the desert sands. And don't forget to have a glass of water when you're finished! Pretend it came from a desert oasis.

The Least You Need to Know

➤ The desert is a great source of ideas for yoga poses.

➤ Snakes are desert creatures imitated in yoga for centuries. You can be a Baby Snake, a Mother Snake, or a Father Snake.

➤ Perch on a pretend tree branch in Wise Owl Pose.

➤ Stretch into Camel Pose.

➤ Stay poised for action in Roadrunner Pose.

➤ Get creative as a prickly cactus in Cactus Pose.

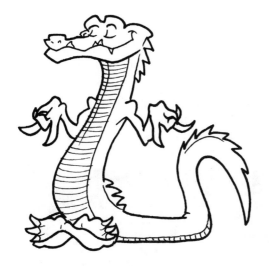

Chapter 14

Exploring the Wild

In This Chapter

➤ Walk on the wild side with wild animal poses

➤ Be a bucking bronco, a deer, a unicorn, a giraffe, or an antelope

➤ Walk like a bear, swim like a shark, or snap like a crocodile

➤ Watch out: *T. rex* ahead!

➤ You Tarzan!

Kids love to imagine nature in all its untamed glory, whether its creatures are from the desert, the jungle, the savanna, or the sea. Some wild animals may seem vicious by human standards—the fierce crocodile, the giant grizzly bear, the ravenous shark, and the notorious (if extinct) *Tyrannosaurus rex* (*T. rex*).

Other wild creatures seem calm, almost tranquil, completely at ease in nature—the swift deer and swifter antelope, the towering giraffe, and the mythical unicorn. This chapter is full of fun, exciting, and untamed wild animal poses, so get ready to get wild!

Hooves and Horns

This section is full of ungulates—that is, animals with hooves. Some move fast, some move slowly. Some lope smoothly across the savanna (giraffes) and others kick up their heels with gusto (donkeys). They are all great inspiration for yoga poses.

Bucking Bronco Pose

The bucking bronco is a powerful animal brimming with energy and strength. Kids of all ages enjoy this fun pose, which provides them with an opportunity to burn up excess energy or let off steam.

Bucking Bronco Pose strengthens the arms, wrists, and back, and even gives the heart a good workout because it is a cardiovascular exercise. It is also a modified inversion, bringing fresh blood to the head and helping to clear the mind.

Bucking Bronco Pose.

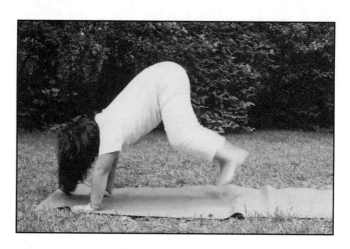

1. Begin in Downward Facing Dog Pose (see Chapter 12).

2. Bracing your upper body to support your weight, kick your feet up in the air, one at a time, as if you were a bucking bronco kicking its back legs into the air. Try to switch your legs in midair.

3. Repeat about 10 times, then rest in Mouse Pose (see Chapter 12).

➤ **For More Fun:** The easier this pose becomes, the faster and higher you can kick. Faster kicks make for an even more intense cardiovascular workout.

➤ **For Even More Fun:** Make the sounds of a bronco snorting and toss your head while you try to toss your rider!

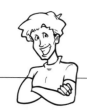

For Grownups, Too!

Some kids love to try handstands, often long before they are able to do them well. You can "spot" your young child, however. As your child kicks up in Bucking Bronco Pose, catch your child's feet and support him or her in an inverted position for a few seconds. This helps build the arm strength necessary for your child to do a handstand independently someday, and prevents injury.

Deer Pose (Marichyasana)

The elusive deer knows how to listen, move quietly, and dash away when danger approaches. Deer Pose trims the waist, relieves backaches and stiff necks, and improves appetite.

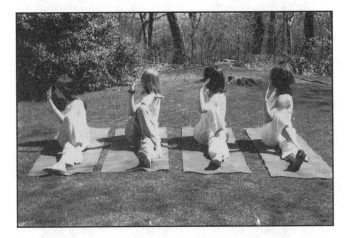

Deer Pose.

1. Sit with your legs straight in front of you, then bend your right leg, knee raised, and place the sole of your foot on the opposite side of your outstretched leg.

2. Twisting at the waist, bring your left arm over your bent knee and look over your left shoulder.

3. Look cautiously around as if you were a deer in the night, keeping your eyes wide open.

4. Come back to center, switch legs, and twist in the opposite direction.

➤ **For More Fun:** Have a friend or sibling growl or make a noise like a crackling twig. Untwist, lower your leg, and dash away as silently as possible.

Unicorn Pose

Who says unicorns don't exist? There you are, in Unicorn Pose! If you imagine it, you can be anything you want to be. Unicorns have horns in the middle of their foreheads, right in the place the ancient yogis believed was the center of our imagination and intuition (the sixth chakra). Imagine growing a unicorn horn, and enjoy a fantasy world of your own creation. Unicorn Pose strengthens the abdominal, leg, and arm muscles and elongates the spine.

Unicorn Pose.

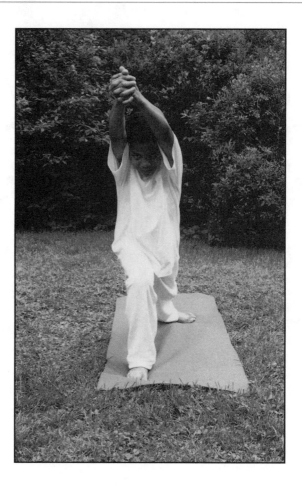

1. Begin in Downward Facing Dog Pose (see Chapter 12).

2. Lunge one foot forward so it rests between your hands, just like in Roadrunner Pose, but this time, drop your back foot so only the sole of your foot is on the floor.

3. Slowly raise your hands up to your bent knee and when you feel balanced, reach your arms out in front of you, placing your palms together.

4. Keep your head and ears in between your outstretched arms and hold for a few seconds.

5. Return to Downward Facing Dog Pose, then repeat on the other side.

6. Lower yourself into Mouse Pose (see Chapter 12) to rest.

➤ **For More Fun:** Make a unicorn horn to wear during this pose. Be creative! Use glitter, ribbons, or anything else that looks magical.

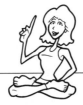

Yoga Stories

The unicorn is a mythical animal that has, since the Middle Ages, been symbolic of purity and innocence. The unicorn is represented in the artwork of many ancient civilizations from Asia and Europe in tapestries, woodcuts, and illuminated manuscripts. The unicorn has also been mentioned in the writings of Aristotle, Pliny, Aelian, and the ancient Greek physician, Ctesias, who described the unicorn as an "Indian wild ass." Some believe the idea of the unicorn may have evolved due to misrepresentations of the rhinoceros. Described as a savage fighter when cornered, the unicorn is also gentle and tame with the innocent. Its fleet-footed movements and pure spirit are a fitting model for the practicing yogini.

Giraffe Walk

Giraffes are tall all around—tall legs, tall big bodies, and of course, those towering necks. This pose is inspired by the height of the mighty giraffe. Giraffe Walk Pose stretches and strengthens the feet, toes, ankles, and calves. It extends and opens the entire body. It also improves balance.

The Giraffe Walk.

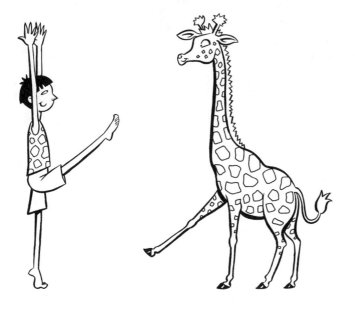

1. Stand tall, on your tippy toes.

2. Reach your arms up straight over your head, palms open and facing each other, fingers pointing up.

3. Walk around the room, lifting one leg at a time, as high as possible straight out in front of you, without bending your knee.

➤ **For More Fun:** Have one person be a tree (see Tree Pose in Chapter 11 for a description). The other person walks like a giraffe over to the tree and eats some leaves off the tree. Yummy!

Antelope Dash

When it comes to speed, the antelope is second only to the cheetah (and possibly a few species of gazelle). A mere human would quickly be outdistanced by an antelope, but that doesn't mean we can't pretend! Antelope Dash benefits gross motor control (motor control that governs large movements, like running and jumping) and strengthens the arms, wrists, legs, and ankles. To avoid obstacles, try to do this pose outside or in a large, open space indoors.

Antelope Dash.

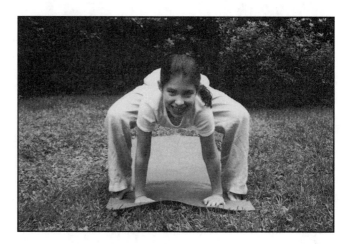

1. Begin Downward Facing Dog Pose (see Chapter 12), but with your hands close together on the ground.

2. Starting slowly, jump both feet forward on either side of your hands, in a leapfrog-like motion.

3. Next walk hands out in front of you keeping them close to each other. Now again, jump both feet forward on either side of your hands, in a leapfrog-like motion.

4. Move faster and faster, increasing your speed until you are moving at a gallop, with your feet coming forward on either side of your hands. Find a rhythm and balance.

5. Slow down and stop gradually.

➤ **For More Fun:** Have a stampede! With a group of friends, pretend you are grazing in a field. One person looks up suddenly, as if he or she heard a noise. Then, everyone takes off in one direction, stampeding across the grass.

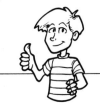

For Kids Only

Antelope Dash is pretty strenuous, but kids find it much easier than adults do, maybe because kids are smaller or lower to the ground, or maybe because adults have been walking upright for a few more years. If your parents join your antelope herd, you may have to slow down your pace so they can keep up!

Beware: Wild Animals Ahead!

A foray into the land of fierce creatures, anyone? Wild animal poses are a great way to release pent-up energy, even built-up anger. They also give kids a sense of power and confidence.

Bear Walk

Bear Walk imitates the movements of a lumbering bear foraging for food. Bears may look cute and furry, but they are very large and powerful animals with great strength. This pose builds strength in yoginis, too! It also works gross motor control, strengthens the arms, wrists, legs, and ankles, and because it uses both sides of the body in opposition, it helps to coordinate the central nervous system.

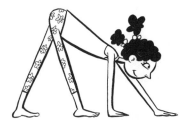 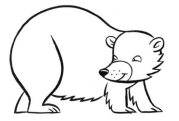

Bear Walk.

1. Begin in Downward Facing Dog Pose (see Chapter 12).

2. Slowly begin to walk around the room, moving opposite hands and feet (step forward with your right arm and left leg, then with your left arm and right leg).

3. Keep walking with arms and legs mostly straight. Try to feel like a bear moving through the forest.

➤ **For More Fun:** "Grrrrooooowwwwl!" like a hungry bear!

➤ **For Even More Fun:** Pretend you are searching a forest for honey. Your friends could be the trees. Any honey in that belly button? What about under that knee or elbow? Snuffle around.

Shark Pose

Watch out: Hungry sharks are patrolling the water! Some scientists consider sharks to be the ultimate animal. Sharks are strong, powerful, efficient, and focused on their primary goal in life: eating! This pose can give kids a sense of power, strength, and purpose. Few things are more invincible than a shark! It also adds flexibility to the spine and neck, opens the chest, and stretches the shoulders.

Shark Pose.

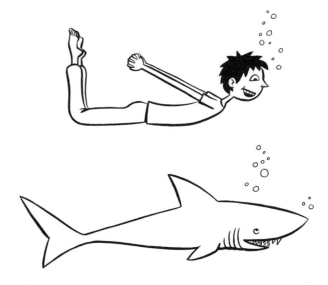

1. Keeping your knees and feet together, lie on your stomach and bend your knees so your feet point up toward the ceiling. Imagine your feet are your tail fin.

2. Bring both arms behind your back, clasp your hands, and straighten your arms behind you, lifting your hands as high as possible to form that notorious shark fin that sticks out of the water.

3. Lift your head up and gnash your teeth. Chomp!

➤ **For More Fun:** Wiggle from side to side as if you are a shark swimming through the water.

➤ **For Even More Fun:** Put on some ocean wave music while you do this pose.

Crocodile Pose (Makaraasana)

Never smile at a crocodile (as the "Peter Pan" song goes) … unless that crocodile is really a yogini! Crocodiles are fearsome creatures indeed, and one species of crocodile is the largest reptile on earth! Crocodile Pose can make yoginis feel powerful and strong, too. Crocodile Pose strengthens the muscles of the back and neck, tones the hamstrings, and helps to keep the spine healthy and flexible.

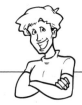

For Grownups, Too!

If you are trying to encourage a more gentle spirit in your household, you can turn Shark Pose into Porpoise Pose. Same form, but you and your child can be porpoises jumping, diving, and swimming through the ocean. No chomping required!

1. Begin on your stomach on the floor as in the snake poses, forehead on the ground, legs close together (this time your legs are the crocodile's tail).

2. Place your hands behind your head, extending your elbows out.

3. Inhale through your nose, then exhale.

4. On the exhale, slowly lift your elbows, head, and chest. You may not be able to lift very high at first, but even an inch or two is great!

Crocodile Pose.

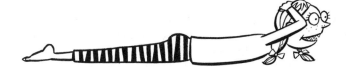

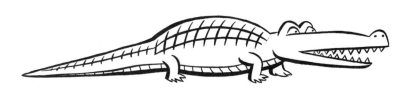

➤ **For More Fun:** Have a friend, parent, or sibling walk in circles around you as you prepare for Crocodile Pose. When you are ready, have them come near you. Lift your head, chest, and arms and growl "Grrrrrr!" like a ferocious crocodile.

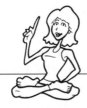

Yoga Stories

Alligators may be more common in the southern United States, but crocodiles can be found all over the world. Many (often contradictory) stories exist about how to tell alligators and crocodiles apart—which is bigger, meaner, louder, or shows more teeth. When it comes to size, however, the crocodile is the winner. The largest reptile in the world is the Estuarine or saltwater crocodile found in Australia and Asia. For more on crocodile size, see the Crocodilian Biology Database at www.flmnh.ufl.edu/natsci/herpetology/brittoncrocs/cbd-faq-q2.htm. For more information on crocodiles and alligators, including a chance to hear real crocodile sounds, check out the Crocodilians Web page at crocodilian.com/.

Alligator Pose

Don't feed the alligators, or they might feed on you! The alligator is a ferocious reptile with a large mouth, plenty of sharp teeth, and a powerful tail. You can be an alligator, but in this pose, to get a really good bite radius, use your legs for the mouth and your arms for the tail. Alligator Pose mobilizes the hip joints, strengthens the leg muscles, and gives the arms and shoulders a nice stretch. Depending on how fast you chomp, it can also get pretty aerobic.

Alligator Pose.

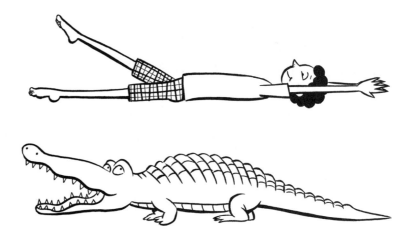

1. Lie down on the floor on your back, arms up to cover your ears, palms together, fingers pointed. Your arms are the alligator's powerful tail.

2. Bring your legs together, feet pointed. Then, slowly lift one leg, pretending it is the alligator's large, ferocious mouth.

3. "Chomp" your leg back down. Then raise the other leg and lower it. Chomp chomp! Go as fast as you can.

➤ **For More Fun:** Tape some white paper "teeth" to your inside legs.

➤ **For Even More Fun:** Let a friend or sibling try to crawl through the alligator's jaws without getting chomped.

T. Rex *Pose*

Preschoolers and grade-schoolers seem particularly fascinated with dinosaurs, but dinosaurs can capture the imagination of yoginis of any age. The *Tyrannosaurus rex* is perhaps the most famous of the giant reptiles, and lots of fun to imitate. This pose captures the powerful and intimidating approach of a *T. rex*. It stretches the backs of the legs, encourages flexibility of the spine, strengthens the neck, and makes kids feel they are truly creating a powerful impression!

1. Stand up straight with your feet about shoulder-width apart.

2. Bend over at the waist and grab your ankles with your hands, keeping your legs straight. If you can't reach your ankles, hold your legs as close to your ankles as is comfortable.

3. Begin to stomp around the room like a huge dinosaur. (Watch where you're going!)

➤ **For More Fun:** After each five steps, let go of your ankles/legs, rise up with claws (hands) raised, and roar! Then it's back down, hands on ankles, for more stomping fun.

➤ **For Even More Fun:** Have a friend, sibling, or parent provide a background rhythm or bang a drum for your stomping: "Boom boom. Boom boom. Boom boom." Stomp to the beat. Hold your *T. rex* roars for two or three beats.

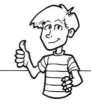

For Kids Only

If you love dinosaurs, why not invent more dinosaur poses? Visit a museum or the library for ideas. Examine each picture or display and invent a pose that looks like that dinosaur.

Tarzan Holler

By now you yoginis must surely feel like masters of the jungle, so it's time to express your inner confidence and wild spirit with a nice, long, loud Tarzan Holler. This exercise is part yoga pose, part breathing exercise. It stimulates the esophageal glands, promotes inner confidence and self-esteem, helps to blow off steam and release anger or excess energy, and is a whole lotta fun! (But make sure you do this exercise in a place where the noise won't bother anybody!)

1. Stand strongly, knees slightly bent as if ready to spring onto the next passing jungle vine.

2. Inhale deeply, then let out a loud Tarzan "aaaaaaaaaah, ee-aaaaaaaaaaah, ee-aaaaaaaaaaaaah!"

3. As you vocalize, beat (gently please) on your upper chest to make the sound vibrate, in the manner of the great apes, and of course, like Tarzan himself.

4. Keep yelling until all your air has been exhaled, then inhale deeply and do it again. And again! Do it as long as it is fun (or as long as the other members of your household can stand it!).

➤ **For More Fun:** If you have access to a playground or gymnasium with a climbing rope (and the people in charge don't mind the occasional loud sustained noise—ask permission first, please), try this exercise while swinging on a rope. You can't beat on your chest while swinging, but you can still do the Tarzan yell.

➤ **For Even More Fun:** Do a Tarzan Circle Holler! Form a circle with a group of friends. One person starts the Tarzan Holler, then sustains it while the next person starts, then the next. Keep going until the whole circle is yelling and beating their chests. Then the first person stops, then the second, and so on, until only the last person is left. This exercise is fun and helps to synchronize a group. It can be a nice way to get energized prior to a group yoga practice.

After all these animal poses, you grownups might need a rest, but we say, let's keep on going! Turn to the next chapter for poses on the move, where your children can learn techniques for yoga movements, marches, dances, and salutations.

The Least You Need to Know

➤ Wild animal poses help kids get in touch with their wild sides!

➤ Wild animal poses help kids release excess energy or help to generate energy in kids who need it. They also give kids a feeling of strength and power.

➤ Many wild animals have hooves and horns. Try Bucking Bronco Pose, Deer Pose, Unicorn Pose, Giraffe Walk, and Antelope Dash.

➤ Fierce creatures make for fun poses, too. Try Bear Walk, Crocodile Pose, Alligator Pose, Shark Pose, *T. rex* Walk, and the Tarzan Holler.

Part 5

Super Yoginis on the Move and Staying Still

Time for even more yoga poses kids love. In this section, we'll show you lots of great movement and rhythm poses, including our kid-friendly version of the traditional yoga Sun Salutation, which we call the Yoga Sun Dance. Some of the other fun-for-kids poses in this section include Roller Coaster Spin, Volcano Blast, and the "Ants Go Marching" March.

We'll also help your child target special areas, such as strength-building, enhanced flexibility, and motor coordination. Challenging poses for advanced yoginis also build self-confidence.

Partner and group yoga poses come next. These are fun activities for yoga clubs, classes, or parties. Last but not least, we teach you all about Shavasana, yoga's most essential peaceful pose, featuring deep relaxation and guided imagery designed just for kids.

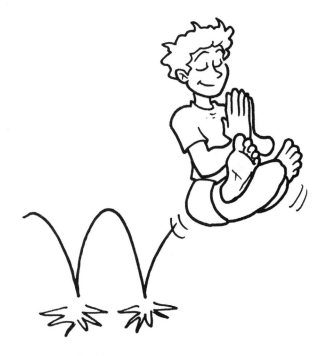

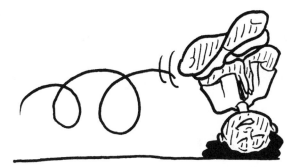

Chapter 15

Kids on the Move

> **In This Chapter**
>
> ➤ The world is full of movement!
>
> ➤ Getting in touch with your unique rhythm
>
> ➤ Yoga vinyasa, also called flow series
>
> ➤ Yoga dances, games, and other rhythmic movements

Many of the exercises in this book have been named "poses," but that term can be misleading. "Pose" sounds like something that stands still. When Madonna sings, "Strike a pose," we strike a pose and hold it … right?

But as you may have noticed, many of our poses include lots of movement. Cat Pose, Cow Pose, Seagull Pose, the snake poses, Bucking Bronco Pose, Alligator Pose, and Owl Pose, to name a few, are hardly stationary.

But in this chapter, we're *really* going to get going. Yoga is more than poses—it is motion, rhythm, movement, and dance. Turn up the music, start tapping your foot, and let's get moving!

Finding the Yoga Groove

Our environment is full of movement. If you want stillness, you may have to look at a photograph because the world is constantly in motion. Leaves blow across the street, clock hands tick out the seconds, tree branches sway in the wind, cars drive by, birds sail across the sky under the ever-changing clouds.

And people! Well, we all know people can't stay absolutely and completely still, even if they try. Hearts beat, blood circulates, breath flows, eyes blink, muscles contract, and eventually, we can't help talking, stretching, gesturing, and smiling.

Of course, we move because our bodies are meant to move, even though sometimes we forget to move as often as our bodies would like. The yoga movements in this chapter include *vinyasa,* which is a flowing series of postures, and lots of other fun movement games and dances. They give you specific movements and activities to try again and again. Are you bored? Have nothing to do? Read this chapter so you can

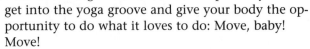

get into the yoga groove and give your body the opportunity to do what it loves to do: Move, baby! Move!

Who's Got Rhythm?

Who's got rhythm? Everybody! Every kid has his or her own rhythm. Some kids naturally move at a fast-paced tempo, always go-go-going. Others seem to move at a leisurely pace. Some meander, taking time to relish the joys of the life. Still others move with a slow and measured intent. We aren't referring to anything as simple as a child's normal walking pace. We mean his or her very rhythm of life, the pace at which a child moves, thinks, feels, responds, comprehends, and experiences the world.

A child's natural rhythm can't be measured by any instrument, but why would you want to measure it? No rhythm, no approach to life, no internal drummer, clock, or beat are better or worse than any others. Knowing one's own individual pace is the important thing. Embracing one's internal rhythm and inner sense of movement can help anyone feel comfortable, self-assured, and confident.

The yoga movements in this chapter are perfect for helping children get in touch with their own rhythm because the movements aren't performed at any prescribed pace. The child should choose the song and the tempo—the right tempo for a child is the one that feels most comfortable for a particular exercise.

The Equilibrium of Motion

Every child has a different internal rhythm, but some children have a harder time being in touch with that rhythm. Some kids get going too fast and have trouble

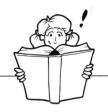

Learn About Yoga

Vinyasa is a Hindu word referring to multiple yoga poses that are synchronized with breathing and strung together into a flowing motion. The Yoga Sun Dance (coming up in a moment) is an example of vinyasa. In contemporary Western yoga classes, vinyasa is often referred to as "flow" or "flow series."

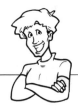

For Grownups, Too!

Spend some time outside with your child playing Motion Detector. Sit quietly in a secluded spot and see how many things you can see moving. Call out what you see, or make separate lists, then compare your lists.

slowing down to a more comfortable pace. Other kids have trouble "revving up their engines" and, although they might do better moving and living at a higher energy level, habit or other factors have stalled them. For example, children with special needs often have very high or very low energy levels.

Yoga movements are a good way to address these imbalances, helping kids to get in touch with the rhythm that works best for them. Because yoga works for all children, it can energize kids who need a little help boosting their energy, and it can help slow down kids who need a little assistance putting on the brakes. Remember, yoga is all about balance. Kids whose rhythm of life has become un-balanced can regain their equilibrium through yoga movements.

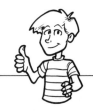

For Kids Only

This book contains only one true vinyasa or flow series of yoga poses, but that doesn't mean you can't make up your own! What about a Dance for the Birds using your favorite bird poses, or a Desert Dance, stringing together your favorite desert creature poses from Chapter 13? Your imagination is the only limit.

The Yoga Sun Dance (Surya Namaskar)

The Yoga Sun Dance, or Sun Salutation, as it is often called, is a popular and widely known yoga vinyasa that you can find in almost any book on yoga poses. Many yoga teachers have their own variations on this exercise or teach different versions. This version is kid friendly, although adults can benefit from it as well.

The Yoga Sun Dance is a way of thanking the sun for coming out every day, for pro-viding us with warmth and light as well as its many other beautiful gifts. The Yoga Sun Dance stretches the entire body, preparing you for other yoga exercises. It devel-ops strength, flexibility, alertness, and coordination. It is a great cardiovascular exer-cise and it builds internal heat for further practice. We'll stop there, but the benefits of the Yoga Sun Dance are endless. After doing it a few times, you'll understand be-cause you will feel so great!

The Yoga Sun Dance.

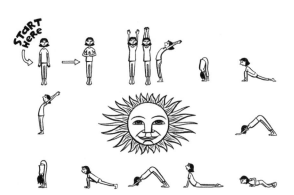

1. Begin in Mountain Pose (see Chapter 11).

2. Inhale as you bring your arms up and out to the sides.

3. Exhale and bring your palms together in front of your heart, the position called Namaste Pose.

4. Inhale and bring your arms up over your head, crossing your thumbs above your head, gently arching your back and looking up toward your hands.

5. Exhale and slowly lower your linked hands, arms and upper body, in one motion, forward and down so that you hang over in a forward bend. Let your knees bend just enough so you can place your hands, palms face down, on the floor on either side of your feet.

6. Inhale and step your right leg back behind you so you are in a lunge, as you were for Roadrunner Pose (see Chapter 13). Keep your chest lifted and look forward or slightly up. Exhale deeply. If this position is too strenuous, you can drop your knee to the floor.

7. Inhale and step your left leg back, raising your hips so you are in Downward Facing Dog Pose (see Chapter 12).

8. Exhale and lower your knees, chest, and chin to the ground, then inhale and slide forward through your arms until you are in the Mother Snake Pose (see Chapter 13).

9. Exhale, curl your toes under, and lift your hips back into Downward Facing Dog Pose.

10. Inhale, step your right foot forward, and return to Roadrunner Pose.

11. Exhale, step your left foot forward, and return to a forward bend.

12. Cross your thumbs, then reach them out and up overhead and slightly behind you, creating a gentle arch in the back.

13. Return to Mountain Pose with your hands together in front of your chest in Namaste Pose.

14. Repeat the entire series on the other side, this time stepping back with your left foot first.

15. When the full series (both sides) is complete, stand in Mountain Pose for a few seconds and listen to your breath. Then do it again! We recommend one to five full rounds.

➤ **For More Fun:** As you move through each pose, make the sound of the appropriate animal. For Roadrunner Pose, make the "beep-beep" sound from the roadrunner/coyote cartoons. Bark like a dog in Downward Facing Dog Pose. Hiss like a snake in Mother Snake Pose. When you end in Mountain Pose, you might even imitate the gentle sound of wind through the trees on a mountaintop.

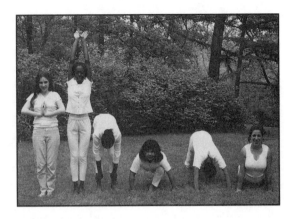

Jodi and sun dancers demonstrate the poses of the Yoga Sun Dance.

➤ **For Even More Fun:** Place a picture of the sun or of something sunny in front of you as you do this dance, to help you remember that you are thanking the sun.

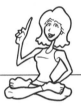

Yoga Stories

People have been thanking the sun for thousands of years as the bringer of light, warmth, and life. Without the sun, plants couldn't grow, nobody could see anything, and there wouldn't be any people because the Earth would be too cold to live on. In fact, our whole solar system wouldn't even exist because "solar" means "sun" and the sun is the center of the entire system. Even before people realized that the planets revolved around the sun instead of the Earth, they recognized the sun's great and essential importance in the life of the Earth. We think that's worth a daily Yoga Sun Dance (or two)!

Go, Go, Go!

The exercises in this section are less formal than an organized sequence of yoga poses, but they are just as much fun. Yoginis, keep moving through this workout and you'll be assured a great time!

Yoga Dancing

Yoga Dancing is a great energizer and lots of fun, allowing for individual movement and expression. Yoga Dancing generates energy, lets kids expend excess energy, and adds a sense of joy to the day.

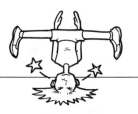

Ooops!

While vigorous exercise during the day can help kids sleep better, vigorous exercise right before bed can actually make some kids too energized to sleep. Every child is different, so experiment with what works best. If the Yoga Sun Dance works in the evening, great! If kids have a hard time settling down right after exercise, schedule yoga practice for earlier in the day.

Try Yoga Dancing with or without music. Some songs we enjoy are "Sabre Dance" by Khachaturian (we like the version on the CD entitled "More Classical Music for People Who Hate Classical Music"), "Shake Your Sillies Out" by Raffi, and "Dancing Mood" from "Disney's Sebastian—from *The Little Mermaid*."

1. Hold out your right hand, and shake it. Don't move anything else but your right hand.

2. After a few seconds, include your right arm in the shaking movement, so both your arm and hand are shaking and shimmying.

3. Now get your right shoulder into the groove.

4. Next, extend your left hand and start shaking it.

5. Get your left arm into the act, then your left shoulder.

6. Shake and shimmy with your whole upper body, trying to keep your lower body relatively still.

7. Add your neck and head, shaking and bobbing to the rhythm.

8. Now begin to rotate and twist your waist to the beat. Then, let your hips feel the rhythm.

9. Time for your right leg! Move and shake your right foot, then right lower leg, then your entire right leg.

10. Your left leg is last but not least. First the foot, then the lower leg, then the whole leg.

11. Now you are really gettin' down! Twist, shake, and boogie with your entire body. Let every inch of you feel the music and the freedom of moving in whatever way you want to move.

➤ **For More Fun:** Put on some disco-dancing clothes (raid your parents' wardrobe!) and ask a friend or parent to flicker the lights like a strobe light. Boogie-woogie the night (or the afternoon, or the morning) away!

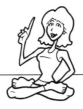

Yoga Stories

Yoga Dancing is based on an ancient meditation ritual, sometimes called ecstatic or trance dancing, where people dance wildly to release their excess energy so they'll be better prepared for meditation. The dancing itself is also a sort of meditation, allowing the self to move with complete freedom, shaking loose old ideas and preconceptions to break into a more enlightened consciousness. We don't suggest children need to consider anything so serious, however. Have fun, be free, but try to let go of stress, worry, and all the "shoulds" and "musts" and "have tos" in life, if just for a few minutes.

Roller Coaster Spin

Kids love roller coasters, Ferris wheels, merry-go-rounds, and other carnival rides because they twirl, spin, dip, zoom, and make the whole world seem to tip and twirl. Roller Coaster Spin mimics this excitement, building internal energy and increasing gross motor coordination. Even though this exercise gives kids the sensation the ground is moving, it actually helps kids to feel more grounded, centered, and organized.

For this exercise, choose a space free from obstacles you might bump into, and stop if you start to feel dizzy or as if you might lose your balance.

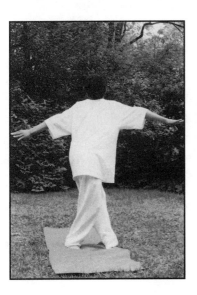
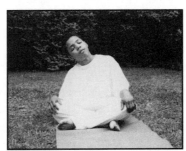

Take a spin in Roller Coaster Pose!

1. Stand in Mountain Pose (see Chapter 11), then slowly turn in circles, picking up your pace at a comfortable speed. Feel free to extend your arms out to the sides as you spin.

2. Continue spinning until you have had enough, then carefully sit with your legs crossed in Pretzel Pose (see Chapter 17).

3. Close your eyes and imagine you are on a roller coaster. Feel the ground moving beneath you!

➤ **For More Fun:** As you sit with your eyes closed, raise your arms up in the air like some people do on real roller coasters.

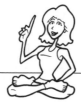

Yoga Stories

Spinning is more than just fun for kids. It is an ancient spiritual ritual practiced by several cultures. The most famous of these is probably the Whirling Dervishes, a branch of the Sufi religion (which is itself an offshoot of Islam). The Whirling Dervishes, also known as the Mevlevi Order, were founded in the thirteenth century Ottoman Empire by the mystical poet Rumi. Whirling Dervishes wear long white skirts that fan out when they spin. They extend their arms with the right palm facing up to receive energy from above, and the left hand facing down to pass energy into the earth. In the words of Rumi, "A secret turning in us makes the universe turn."

Flopping Rag Doll

Rag dolls are floppy and look about as relaxed as a doll can get! In this pose, surrender to complete relaxation by taking on the characteristics of a rag doll like Raggedy Ann or Raggedy Andy.

Flopping Rag Doll is an inversion, so it sends fresh blood to your brain, helping to clear the mind. It stretches and elongates the spine and neck. Flopping Rag Doll also releases tension and stress, helping the body to relax.

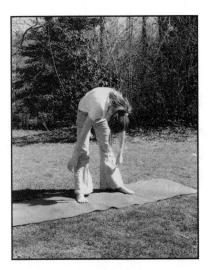

Flopping Rag Doll.

1. Stand with your feet slightly apart, arms reaching way up over your head.

2. Stretch your torso as you inhale, then exhale and flop over, bending at the waist. Allow yourself to make a sound of release: "aaaaahhh" or "haaaahhh" or "phoooohhh!"

3. Allow your arms, hands, and upper body to relax completely. Try not to control your movement. Instead, let your body surrender all by itself.

4. When you come to complete stillness, roll up slowly with your chin into your chest.

5. Repeat several times.

➤ **For More Fun:** What else is floppy that you could imitate in this pose? A scarecrow? A floppy teddy bear? A marionette?

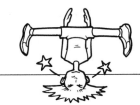

Ooops!

When rolling back up in Flopping Rag Doll, move slowly, as if stacking spinal vertebrae on top of each other one at a time. This movement should be practiced carefully and slowly without straining the spine. Children's backs should be treated with care.

Volcano Blast

An exploding volcano is one of the most spectacular displays nature has to offer: glowing hot lava blasting out of the top of a mountain! Volcano Blast lets kids symbolically blow off steam by pretending to be an exploding volcano. This movement is great for relieving stress and can be useful for kids with built-up frustration, anger, and energy. It also loosens and mobilizes the shoulder joints. (This pose was created

207

by Blake Vissing, who stars in the *YogaKids* video, referenced in Appendix B, and who performs this pose on the tape. The pose was inspired by movements Blake found himself making naturally to relieve stress while rehearsing for and filming the tape.)

Erupt from Namaste Pose to Volcano Blast!

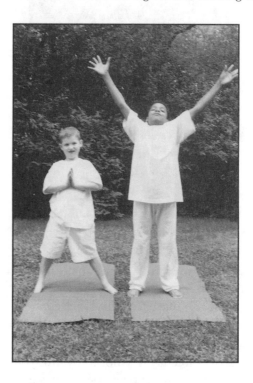

1. Begin in Mountain Pose (see Chapter 11) with hands placed in front of the chest, palms together, in the position called Namaste Pose.

2. Breathe in; then breathe out as you jump your feet apart.

3. Imagine you are a volcano ready to explode. Feel the building heat.

4. Get ready, get set, and go! Inhale deeply, as if preparing the hot lava to explode. Then, exhale fully and loudly, like a burst of lava and steam: "paaaaaaahhhhh!" As you exhale, throw your hands and arms up to the sky. Explode your volcano by spreading your arms out to the sides until they come all the way back down.

5. Return your hands to Namaste Pose and repeat until you feel your volcano is fully erupted.

➤ **For More Fun:** Add more sound effects to your exploding volcano!

➤ **For Even More Fun:** Imagine your volcano exploding with things besides lava. What about an explosion of butterflies? Peanut butter? Beach balls? Maple syrup?

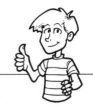

"The Ants Go Marching" March

You probably remember the old song: "The ants go marching one by one hurrah, hurrah …," sung to the tune of the old Civil War song, "When Johnny Comes Marching Home Again" (to hear it, go to members.tripod.com/~Randy_T/johnny.html). In this version, the lyrics are a little different:

"The ants go marching one by one, hurrah, hurrah, the ants go marching one by one hurrah, hurrah, the ants go marching one by one, the little one stopped to suck his thumb, and they all go marching down to the ground to get out of the rain, boom boom boom …." Then repeat with "the ants go marching two by two, the little one stopped to tie his shoe …" and continue for as long as desired, with new rhymes for each number. Make up your own!

This game is lots of fun. We all know ants are tiny, but they are also very persistent! This game promotes concentration and body awareness, as well as aiding good posture.

For Kids Only

Do you have a room in your house where you're allowed to climb on the furniture, or access to a yard or park with lots of big rocks, stumps, and roots? If so, play Hot Lava! In this game, everyone must keep moving, but nobody can touch the floor or ground because it's covered with hot lava. You can place pillows, short sturdy chairs, and other things to step on around the room. No standing still!

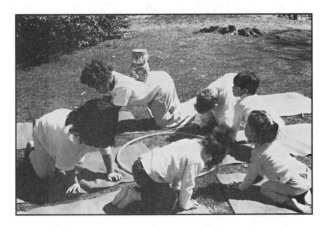

Which ant is carrying the food home?

1. All the kids kneel down onto all fours and form a circle. Kids can kneel around a Hula-Hoop to help keep the circle's shape.

2. Inside the middle of the circle (or inside the Hula-Hoop), place a plate containing some food for the ants, such as granola, breadcrumbs, or a sliced banana.

3. All the kids look at the food and crawl around the circle to the beat of the music. This is a slow crawl. Keep your eyes on that food, as if you were salivating in anticipation of your feast!

➤ **For More Fun:** An adult or friend can call out different directions, such as "backwards!" or "sideways!" and the ants must then change directions.

➤ **For Even More Fun:** Remove the Hula-Hoop and place the food on one ant's back. The ant should try to crawl very carefully across the room, carrying its food on its back to its fellow ants. (Be careful not to spill or you might end up with real ants!)

➤ **For Even *More* Fun:** Play or ask someone to sing the song "The Ants Go Marching."

Driving My Car

Okay, we know, a car is hardly something from nature, but yoga is adaptable, and cars are part of our culture, so why wouldn't they inspire a yoga pose? Driving My Car is a fun and different way to move around a room, a yard, or a park. It increases motor coordination and strengthens the lower body.

Driving My Car Pose.
Vroooooom!

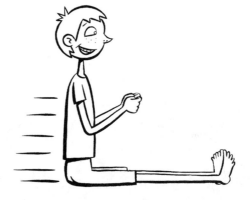

1. Sit on the ground with your legs out in front of you. Imagine your right foot is on the gas pedal and your left foot is on the brake pedal.

2. Fasten your seatbelt, start the engine by turning an imaginary key, then take hold of an imaginary steering wheel in front of you.

3. Move your "sitz bones" (those two bones you can feel under you when you are sitting) alternately forward to move yourself (and your "car") forward. Don't let go of the steering wheel or you might get a ticket!

➤ **For More Fun:** Use a paper plate for a steering wheel, or design your own steering wheel to hold while driving. Test out the horn. "Beep beep!" Rev the engine. "Rrrrrr, Rrrrr!"

➤ **For Even More Fun:** Try to drive in reverse, turn corners, do a K-turn, even parallel park!

➤ **For Even *More* Fun:** Have a friend sit in the passenger seat. See if you can "drive" in synch, moving together forward and backward, keeping your car seats in line. This takes concentration and helps to build focus and trust.

Rock and Roll

This movement is fun, aerobic, and a great way to loosen up a tight spine or massage pulled back muscles. It's a nice way to balance out a pose that arches your back (like Bow Pose in the next chapter) and also a great way to get your body warmed up for the day when you first wake up in the morning. Rock and Roll massages the spine and improves gross motor coordination.

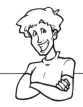

For Grownups, Too!

You can teach your kids more about conservation by explaining all the ways in which driving a car releases pollutants into the environment (emissions, leaking fluids, disposed oil), uses up natural resources (gas and oil), and makes noise. Think of creative ways to spend your days without driving. Can you walk? Ride bikes? Just stay home and do a yoga car ride?

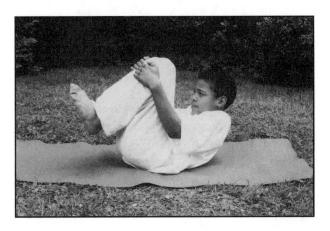

Rock and Roll Pose.

1. Sit down and bring your knees to your chest. Wrap your arms around your legs, holding onto your shins, so your body forms a ball.

2. Rock backward on your spine as you breathe, then roll back up to your original sitting position. See how well you can control the rocking and rolling. Can you rock in rhythm?

➤ **For More Fun:** Sing one of your favorite rock and roll songs as you perform this exercise, or play it on your stereo. Can you roll to the beat of your favorite song?

211

➤ **For Even More Fun:** Spell out the letters in your name for each full rock and roll you do. Too easy? Try saying the alphabet. Recite the alphabet backward! Count to 100!

Boat Poses

Boat Poses are a fun way to pretend you are out on the water, relaxing in the sun and enjoying the salty sea air or the sun on your favorite lake. The first boat pose is Sailboat Pose, for a single yogini. Imagine you are out on the ocean, drifting in the breeze, with nothing but bright blue water and sky, warm wind, and the sound of the waves. Sailboat Pose increases balance and concentration, strengthens the abdominal and leg muscles, and calms both the mind and body.

Sailboat Pose.

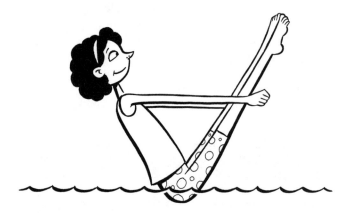

1. Sit with your legs bent and the soles of your feet on the floor.
2. Gently tilt backward and lift your feet up off the floor, straightening your legs as much as you can so you are balancing on your bottom. Your legs should be at a 45-degree angle from the floor.
3. Stretch your arms out in front of you, parallel to the floor, to help you balance. Your body should form a V-shape, with your legs as one side, your body as the other side of the V.

➤ **For More Fun:** When you feel balanced, raise your arms overhead as if they were the mast for your sail.

➤ **For Even More Fun:** Sing "Sailing, Sailing, Over the Ocean Blue" as you hold this pose.

➤ **For Even *More* Fun:** Let a younger sibling sit on your tummy and ride the boat. See how long you can balance!

The second Boat Pose is for partners, and since two can row a boat more easily than one, we call it Row Boat Pose. Row Boat Pose strengthens the stomach muscles and stretches the inner thighs, hips, shoulders, and back. It also helps two people learn to work together, increasing trust and camaraderie.

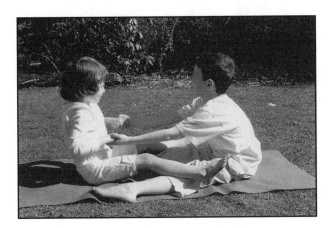

Row Boat Pose (for partners).

1. Sit facing a partner and open your legs into V shapes.

2. One person gently places his or her legs over the other person's shins.

3. Hold hands and begin to row your boat by leaning forward and backward.

4. After a few rows switch leg positions so the other person's legs are on top, and row some more. Have fun and don't be afraid to paddle with all your might!

➤ **For More Fun:** Sing "Row, Row, Row Your Boat" in a round, one person coming in after the first person says the first "boat." If you have more than one boat of partners, your whole group can do a round, each pair coming in after the previous "boat" has sung a full line.

➤ **For Even More Fun:** Pretend the boat is sinking and you are on the rescue team! Both partners lie on their backs and use all their strength to help each other up and out of the sinking ship.

After all this movement, yoginis may be ready to slow down and work on some yoga poses with less movement (but still plenty of power!), the subject of the next chapter.

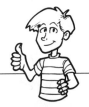

For Kids Only

The next time you're in the bathtub or the swimming pool, float on your back and imagine you are a real boat. Feel the water around you. Let yourself bob up and down. Where are you going? What *is* riding on your boat? Are you on the sea, the lake, or a river?

213

But for now, let's do one more Yoga Sun Dance!

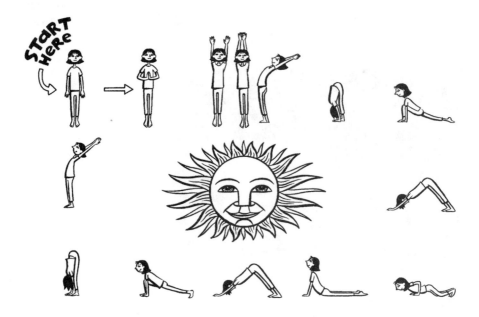

The Least You Need to Know

➤ Yoga isn't just about static poses, it's about movement and energy.

➤ Everyone moves to his or her personal rhythm of life.

➤ A vinyasa, or flow series, is a series of yoga poses strung together with specific breathing patterns. The Yoga Sun Dance is among the most well-known of the classic yoga vinyasa.

➤ Yoga movements needn't be a structured series of poses. They can be just plain fun, with games and movements like Yoga Dancing, Roller Coaster Spin, Flopping Rag Doll, Volcano Blast, "The Ants Go Marching" March, Driving My Car, Rock and Roll, and Boat Poses.

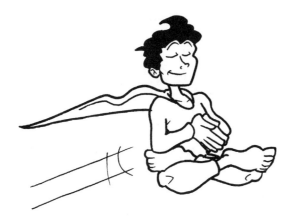

Chapter 16

Super Yogini!

In This Chapter

➤ The value of holding yoga poses

➤ Strong yoginis!

➤ Heroic yoginis!

➤ Flexible yoginis!

This chapter is full of power poses to make yoginis feel strong, flexible, body-confident, and assertive. Although most yoga poses build strength and flexibility in one way or another, the poses in this chapter are specifically divided into those that are particularly strength building, and those that particularly increase flexibility.

Strength and flexibility go hand in hand, like two sides of a mountain, like the sun and moon, like yin and yang (the complementary energies that flow through the body and the universe). Together they create a feeling of confidence and well-being that will help kids achieve maximum power!

While not every pose in this chapter is held perfectly still, they are designed to work the body in stillness rather than through movement.

Yoginis Holding Their Own

Holding yoga poses has several powerful effects. It builds strength because the muscles must work to maintain the body's position in the pose. It builds flexibility because the body holds itself in ways that stretch and elongate muscles and tendons. Holding

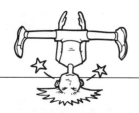

Ooops!

Just because a specific pose requires you to hold still, instead of moving aerobically, doesn't mean it's easier. Many yoga poses that are held are challenging. If you can't hold a pose at first, frustration or even injury may result if you try to push beyond your physical ability. Remember, treat your body gently and proceed comfortably!

yoga poses builds confidence because if the child is focused and still, it is clear when progress happens. Yesterday, the child couldn't quite hold the pose, but today, *she can!*

Once a yogini moves into these poses, he or she may choose to pause and really pay attention to how the pose feels.

Yogini Strength

These poses build strength in both mind and body. They increase muscle tone by lifting and manipulating the body's own weight rather than the weights found in a gym on a weight machine.

But these poses do more than work muscle. They build mental strength by imparting a sense of power and force. By power and force, we don't mean violence and aggression. We mean strength, assertiveness, vibrant health, and the confidence to go out into the world and shine your light!

Hero Pose (Parvatasana)

Who is a hero? You are, of course! This pose lets you sit straight and tall, displaying the confidence befitting of a hero. Even kids who don't feel particularly confident can gain a feeling of strength and power by sitting in Hero Pose. Before trying this pose, have an open discussion about what it means to be a hero.

Hero Pose helps to straighten a rounded back, open the chest, strengthen the arms, and add flexibility to the wrists.

Jodi and yoginis practice Hero Pose.

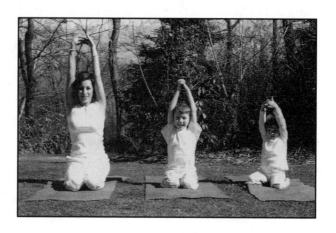

1. Sit in Japanese Sitting Pose (Chapter 13) or Pretzel Pose (Chapter 17). Think about having a strong mind and a strong body.

2. Imagine your spine is elongating, getting taller and taller. Raise your arms out to the side, then up over your head.

3. Interlace your fingers to make a basket with your hands, then turn the basket inside out so your palms face the ceiling with your fingers still entwined. (If this sounds difficult, practice the hand position before starting the pose.)

4. Focus on something in front of you for about 15 seconds. Think about strength and being a hero.

➤ **For More Fun:** Post a picture of your hero somewhere in view so you can look at your hero as you do this pose. Better yet, if your hero is available, ask him or her to sit across from you so you can look at the real thing!

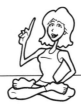

Yoga Stories

What is a hero? In mythology, a hero was a figure famous for acts of strength and bravery, such as Hercules, Achilles, or Perseus. In literature, a hero is the main character of a story. A hero is also a sandwich you buy at the deli! Children may have different answers or may be unsure about how to answer the question. Is a hero the same as a superhero—someone who can fly, shoot fireballs, or catch "bad guys"? Is a hero someone who performs good deeds or saves someone's life? Maybe a hero is anyone you admire, such as a parent or teacher, author or artist, athlete or actor. Parents, listen to your child's response without criticism, then express your own idea of heroism, too.

Superperson Pose

It's a bird. No, it's a plane. No! It's *Super Yogini!* This pose lets you pretend you are flying through the air, just like Superman and Wonderwoman. It also tones the kidneys, strengthens the entire back and spine, and works those gluteal muscles (you know, the ones you sit on!).

Superperson Pose.

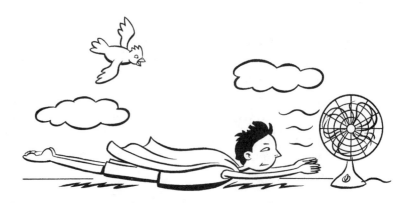

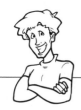

For Grownups, Too!

Sometimes parenting is tough and adults can lose perspective. Are you trying too hard to be a "super parent"? After talking with your kids about their definition of a hero, consider what qualities really make someone a "super parent." What is really important to you and your family? What are your priorities? How might you focus on those and let some of the less important details fall away?

1. Lie on your stomach with your legs together and forehead on the floor, as if you were about to do one of the snake poses (see Chapter 13).

2. Stretch your arms out in front of you and rest them on the floor.

3. Slowly inhale and exhale through your nose.

4. On the exhale, slowly lift up your arms, head, chest, and legs. Try to keep your arms and legs straight, without bending at the joints.

➤ **For More Fun:** Pretend you're flying through the sky, and as you hold this pose, imagine what disaster you are flying off to avert. Who or what are you saving?

➤ **For Even More Fun:** Put on a cape (a scarf or a towel tied loosely around your neck works great). For an even more realistic effect, do this pose in front of an electric fan. Feel the wind rushing by you as you shoot through the sky. Yogini to the rescue!

Warrior I Pose (Virabhadrasana I)

Don't let the name fool you. A warrior pose is a classic yoga pose that, though originally based on fighting stances, is used to impart strength and confidence, not violence. Warrior poses are a great remedy for kids who are feeling sapped of confidence, power, or strength.

Warrior I Pose was originally designed to mimic the warrior holding a sword overhead. Without resorting to weaponry, try to feel the strength and confidence of a warrior with a powerful, awe-inspiring sword. The sword could represent the strength of love, joy, strong values, good character, or talents. Warrior I develops strength, stamina, and stability in the entire body. It increases flexibility in the front of the groin area, the hips, back, and shoulders. It also opens the chest.

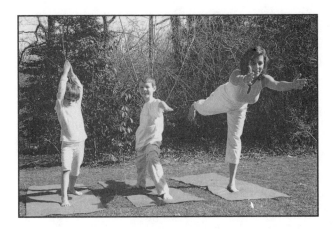

From left to right, yoginis and Jodi practice Warrior I Pose (left), Warrior II Pose (center), and Warrior III Pose (right).

1. Begin in Downward Facing Dog Pose (see Chapter 12).

2. Step one foot forward in between your two hands so you are in a lunge position or Roadrunner Pose (see Chapter 13).

3. Drop your back foot so the sole of your foot is flat on the floor and angled slightly out. You should be able to draw an imaginary line from the heel of your front foot to the arch of your back foot.

4. Keep your extended leg straight and your bent leg close to a right angle without extending your knee beyond your toes.

5. Raise your chest up and extend your arms over your head and look forward. Clasp your hands together and reach your pointer fingers up toward the sky. Do a gentle backbend, and gaze up.

6. After a few seconds, lower your arms and place your hands on either side of your forward foot. Step back into Downward Facing Dog.

7. Repeat with the other leg.

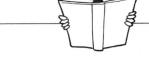

Learn About Yoga

The Sanskrit name for a warrior pose is **virabhadrasana,** pronounced *vee-rab-hah-DRAH-sah-nah.* *Vira* means "hero," *bhadra* means "auspicious," and *asana* means "pose," so the word could be translated as "heroic auspicious pose."

➤ **For More Fun:** Imagine your energy and power streaming all the way up to the sky from your fingertips! While holding Warrior I Pose, as you clasp your hands and point your pointer fingers toward the sky, be immovable and undistractable, with the focus and concentration of a great warrior! Imagine that coming out from your two fingers are the colors of the rainbow. Feel how strong the colors can feel as they pour out of you!

➤ **For Even More Fun:** Hold a flashlight in your hands and point it straight up. Imagine this is your light energy force.

Warrior II Pose (Virabhadrasana II)

Warrior II Pose imitates the stance of a warrior getting ready to throw a spear. The front hand lines up the target as the back hand extends, ready to throw. However, we like to think of the spear as symbolic of each person's special light, talents, and energy. Throw your own light out there, into the world!

Warrior II is very powerful and a great self-confidence booster. It opens the groin and chest, improving breathing and increasing circulation. It stretches the inner thigh muscles and strengthens the buttocks, as well as leg, upper thigh, abdominal, shoulder, and arm muscles, and the arches of the feet.

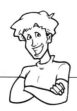

For Grownups, Too!

Talk with your child about the meaning of the word "warrior." What does the name imply beyond "fighter"? In what ways does your child consider himself or herself a warrior? Together, try to think of ways your child can be a warrior that doesn't involve aggression, but instead involves assertiveness, standing up for beliefs, working for justice, and building personal integrity.

1. Begin in Warrior I Pose.

2. Open your arms out to the sides so they are parallel to the ground. Extend forward the arm that is on the same side as your forward leg (which should be bent at approximately a right angle). Extend the other arm straight back behind you. Both palms should face the ground.

3. Look out over your front arm and gaze at the spot just over your middle finger. Feel the strength, concentration, and power of the warrior.

4. Move into Downward Dog Pose, then repeat on the other side.

➤ **For More Fun:** Make Warrior II into an energizing movement exercise. Move into Warrior I and inhale deeply. Move into Warrior II and shout: "Yah!" on the exhale. Go back and forth from Warrior I to Warrior II, inhaling and "Yahing." Very energizing!

Warrior III Pose (Virabhadrasana III)

A warrior must have strength, coordination, and confidence, as well as the focus to accomplish difficult physical feats. Warrior III Pose is a balance pose that builds such strength, coordination, and confidence. Warrior III also develops the concentration tremendously, as it strengthens the legs, hips, back, and heart, and tones the kidneys.

1. Begin in Mountain Pose (see Chapter 11).
2. Raise your arms up above your head with palms facing each other.
3. Take a small step forward with one foot and slowly lower the front of your body until your torso is approximately parallel to the floor. Find a spot in front of you and fix it in your gaze to help you balance.
4. As you lower your body, raise your opposite leg behind you until it is in line with your body, also approximately parallel to the floor, and extend your arms in front of you. (If you can't lift your leg very high, that's fine. Just go as high as you can. The more you do it, the more strength you will build.)
5. As you balance on your standing leg, try to imagine that your arms and raised leg are connected so they form one long straight line from fingertips to big toe. Hold for a few seconds.
6. Slowly lower your arms and back leg, then bring your torso upright again, back into Mountain Pose.
7. Repeat on the other side.

➤ **For More Fun:** As you balance, imagine you are flying through the air! You might even look at a photograph or a picture of a beautiful outdoor scene and pretend you are flying right through it, or face an open window as you do this pose.

➤ **For Even More Fun:** Instead of flying, pretend you are swimming! See if you can do some swimming strokes with your arms without falling over. It takes even more concentration and strength.

➤ **For Even *More* Fun:** If you loved the Yoga Sun Dance and like to create your own vinyasas, or flow series of yoga poses, try stringing together the warrior poses (you can experiment with the order) for a powerful, confidence-inspiring Warrior Dance. Warrior Dance is a powerful way to start your day. What a send-off!

Table Pose

It is great fun to pretend to be a piece of furniture. Don't ask us why! Kids enjoy taking turns being the table, and if parents decide to give it a try, young children might even enjoy climbing on the table! Table Pose strengthens the arms, legs, and abdominal muscles.

221

Jodi balances a water bottle on this yogini "table."

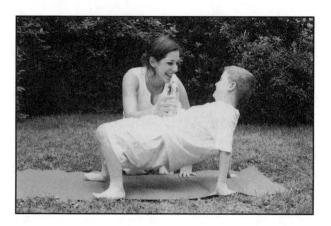

1. Sit with your knees slightly bent and your feet out in front of you. Place your hands right behind you, facing either toward you or away from you, whichever is more comfortable.

2. Slowly lift your hips as you look up at the ceiling or back behind you (if that's comfortable).

3. Try to lift your hips so that your stomach and chest are parallel to the floor, and your arms and legs are perpendicular to the floor (the "table legs").

4. Make sure to spread your weight evenly between your hands and feet. Try not to press only into your arms or just into your heels and feet.

➤ **For More Fun:** Have a picnic! Ask some friends to come over and set your "table" with plastic plates and bowls. What will you serve? Use pretend food or save small cereal boxes, or any other lightweight containers. Allow them to eat while you, if comfortable, look back behind you for ants.

➤ **For Even More Fun:** Allow a friend or younger sibling to be an ant and do "The Ants Go Marching" March (see Chapter 15) under your table. Or, your friend or sibling could be a snake slithering under you.

Slide Pose (Purvottanasana)

The possibilities for fun with Slide Pose are endless, and the strengthening benefits are significant in this pose, too. Slide Pose strengthens the legs, arms, buttocks, and abdominal muscles.

1. Begin by sitting with your legs close together and out straight in front of you, hands just behind you, facing either toward you or away from you, palms down.

2. Slowly lift your hips and thighs off the ground, evenly distributing your body weight onto your hands and feet.

3. Point your toes and try to keep your legs as straight as possible, so your body forms a diagonal line from your shoulders down to the floor.

Slide Pose.

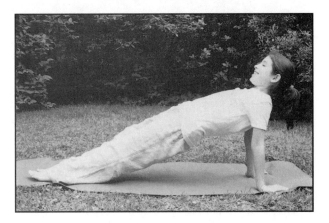

➤ **For More Fun:** Ask a friend, parent, or sibling to roll a medium-sized ball (smaller than a basketball, bigger than a baseball) down your slide. "Weeeeee!" Rolling a ball down your slide will help you to tell whether your slide is sturdy and straight. If the ball bounces off rather than rolling straight down, try to straighten your body and legs even more.

Handstand Pose (Adho Mukha Vrikshasana)

Remember Bucking Bronco Pose in Chapter 14? That exercise was a preparation for Handstand Pose. Handstand is a challenging inversion pose. Many kids don't yet have the arm strength to support themselves in a handstand, even with their feet balanced on a wall. It's best to have an adult spotting for this one.

Handstand floods the brain with fresh blood, clearing the mind and increasing sharp thought. It also strengthens the arms and adds flexibility and strength to the wrists. Achieving Handstand Pose builds great confidence, too!

For Grownups, Too!

Lots of the poses in this chapter, including Bridge Pose, Slide Pose, and Wheel Pose, are great exercise for parents, too, and provide the perfect space for your young child to crawl underneath you. A playground made out of a parent! You might even let your child make you into a tent house with a sheet. Just make sure to warn your child when you're coming down.

Handstand Pose.

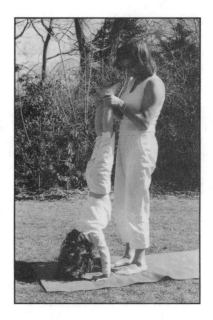

1. Begin in Downward Facing Dog Pose (see Chapter 12) with your hands one or two feet from a wall.

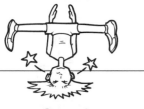

Ooops!

Because inversions send large quantities of blood to the brain (the reason they increase clear thinking), yoginis should ease out of them gradually, allowing body fluids to settle in and redistribute themselves.

2. Kick your legs up until your body is completely inverted, and rest your feet, legs straight, against the wall. Ask an adult to stand nearby or hold your feet to steady them if necessary. (Many kids find it difficult to stay in the right position, especially before they are old enough to be in grade school.)

3. Hold for a few seconds. As you get more comfortable and stronger in this position, you can hold for longer periods of time.

4. Come down slowly and spend a few minutes in Mouse Pose (see Chapter 12). If you stand up too quickly, you might get dizzy or feel faint. Give your body time to readjust to being right side up.

➤ **For More Fun:** Have an upside-down conversation! Ask a friend to sit in front of you as you do Handstand Pose. Talk to him or her while you're upside down. Try to act as if you are right side up. Is it harder to talk? Hard not to laugh?

Yoga Flexibility

Almost every yoga pose increases flexibility one way or another; however, the poses in this section are very focused on flexibility. No, you don't already need super flexibility to try these poses. The point is to build your flexibility by practicing these poses regularly.

These poses also help to increase mental flexibility, challenging your mind to consider new and different ways of moving and being.

Untying Knots

What is a knot? Parents, ask your child and discuss the possibilities. Kids, imagine what it would be like to be all tied up in knots. That's the basis for this pose (developed by Marsha Wenig of YogaKids). If kids imagine they are all tied up in knots, then go through the process of untying the knots, the effect is a loosened, free feeling. Untying Knots increases body awareness and physical and mental flexibility.

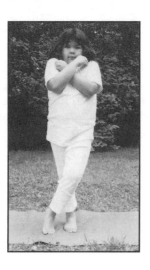 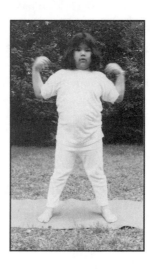

Untying Knots Pose.

1. Stand up and "tie" your body in "knots." Wrap one leg around the other, twist your arms, cross all your fingers, cross your toes (if you can), even your tongue and eyes can look like they are in a knot! Hold the tied-up pose and really feel what it is like to be all knotted up!

2. Beginning with your hands (so you can use them to untie the rest), slowly untie each knot.

3. After your hands, go to the top of your head and pluck out all the imaginary knots in your hair.

4. Slowly move down your body and make sure to "untie" every part.

5. Once you've untied your entire body, you should feel loose as a goose. Notice how different you feel from when you were all tied up! Move your body around the room freely and relaxed.

➤ **For More Fun:** Pretend your back is all tied in knots. Ask a friend, parent, or sibling to help you untie all the knots on your back you can't reach.

➤ **For Even More Fun:** With a group, make a circle and untie all the imaginary knots on the back of the person in front of you. Then switch directions.

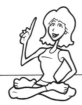

Yoga Stories

When people say their muscles are in knots or that they have knots in their necks, they don't really mean their muscles are literally tied in knots. They mean they have a stiff, contracted muscles. When you touch a contracted muscle on the surface of the skin, however, it sometimes does feel like a rope tied in a knot! Muscles can contract or tighten and stay that way for awhile if they are overused or not properly stretched after exertion. We also get knots in our muscles when we are feeling lots of stress. That is why it's so important to develop muscle flexibility along with muscle strength.

Twister Pose (Supta Parivartanasana)

This relaxing pose gently twists the spine, almost as if you were wringing out all the tension in your spine. This is a nice pose to help kids wind down after a strenuous workout. It feels so good to relax on the floor in a nice stretch that increases flexibility of the spine and back muscles.

Twister Pose also relieves tension in the lower back and hips, tones the abdominal area, frees the chest and shoulders, soothes the spine and neck, improves digestion and elimination, and is overall a wonderful pose for increasing flexibility of the torso.

Twister Pose.

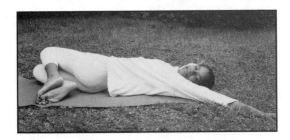

1. Lie on your back with your knees bent into your chest, and your outstretched arms resting on the floor, perpendicular to the body.

2. Allow your knees and legs to fall gently and slowly to one side. Try to keep your knees stacked one on top of the other.

3. Slowly turn your head to look in the direction opposite your knees, for a spinal twist.

4. Hold for about one minute, really relaxing into the twist.

5. Straighten your neck; then slowly bring your knees back to the center.

6. Repeat on the other side.

➤ **For More Fun:** Place an object that has special meaning to you, something you love to look at (a photograph, a memento, a souvenir from a great trip, a letter from a loved one, or a favorite toy), on both sides of you so that when you turn to each side, you can see the cherished item.

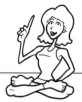

Yoga Stories

Your backbone is really made up of 26 small bones (vertebrae) that form a column supporting your head and body, attach to your ribs, and protect your delicate spinal cord. You have 7 cervical vertebrae in your neck, 12 thoracic vertebrae along the main part of your back, 5 lumbar vertebrae in your lower back, 1 sacrum (a large, roughly triangular bone at the base of your spine), and 1 coccyx (tailbone), a little pointed bone that marks the end of your spinal column. Your vertebrae have discs of spongy material between them for cushioning and for helping them move freely.

Bow Pose (Dhanurasana)

Bow Pose mimics the shape of an archery bow. The arms are the straight part of the bow, and the rest of the body forms the string, pulled back taut, ready to shoot an arrow. This pulling motion, created by holding the feet with the hands, is the mechanism for the flexibility-increasing power of Bow Pose. Bow Pose expands the chest and lungs and keeps the spine limber, healthy, and full of energy. This pose is excellent for digestion, but should not be done on a full stomach.

Bow Pose.

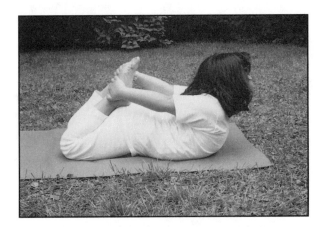

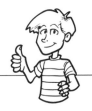

For Kids Only

Bow Pose is great for stretching out stomach muscles after doing sit-ups. Sit-ups contract the abdominal muscles and Bow Pose elongates and loosens them for a more balanced abdominal workout.

1. Lie on your stomach with your legs close together, forehead on the mat, as if you were preparing for one of the snake poses.

2. Bend your knees, lifting your feet. Reach your arms behind you and take hold of your ankles.

3. Exhale and slowly lift your head and chest up while keeping hold of your ankles. Keep breathing as you pull on your feet and lift your chest higher, putting tension into your "bow."

➤ **For More Fun:** As you hold Bow Pose, rock back and forth on your stomach.

➤ **For Even More Fun:** While holding Bow Pose, gently roll over to your side, then come back up into Bow Pose, then roll to the other side.

Sandwich Pose (Paschima Uttanasana)

What is your favorite sandwich? Peanut butter and jelly? Grilled cheese? Avocado and tomato on rye? Whatever it is, in this pose, a child can become a sandwich, which is really just a fun way of envisioning the classic yoga forward bend. Sandwich Pose stretches the legs, the back, the neck, and sends fresh blood to the brain. It encourages flexibility of both mind and body!

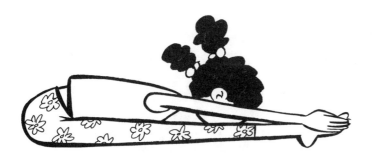

*Sandwich Pose.
Mmmmm—good!*

1. Sit down with your legs straight out in front of you and your upper body per-pendicular to your legs. Imagine that your legs are a slice of bread which you will use to build your sandwich, and your upper body is another slice which you will use later to close the sandwich. Decide what kind of sandwich you will make.

2. Why, look! All the sandwich ingredients are *way* up high on the very top shelf, almost out of reach. But you can do it! Reeeeeeeach up with both hands to get your first item.

3. Spread the first ingredient over your toes, ankles, shins, knees, and thighs. In other words, spread it on your bread slice. Is it cheese? Veggies? Peanut butter?

4. Now reeeeeeeach up to get the next sand-wich item. Turkey? Mayonnaise? Jelly?

5. Put sandwich fixings on your legs by touch-ing each body part (recite them out loud as you go, if you like), to cover the entire slice of "bread." Continue the sequence of reach-ing to get an ingredient and then spreading until your sandwich is full.

6. Now put the two slices of bread together! Try to put the piece of bread on your upper body on top of the piece on your lower body. Reach your hands straight up overhead, then lower yourself down, down, folding your whole body in half at the hips.

7. Reach your hands toward your toes as you put the top part of your sandwich on the bottom part. If you can't reach your toes, place your hands on your shins. Smoosh your sandwich really tight!

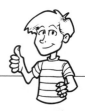

For Kids Only

Are you stuck in a peanut-butter-and-jelly rut? Sandwiches make a great healthy snack, and they can also be a source of endless taste and nutritional vari-ety. Try these combinations: peanut butter and pear slices; light cream cheese and shredded carrots; cheddar cheese and apple slices; almond butter and dried apricots; or mashed white beans with tomatoes and a little fresh basil. See Chapter 23 for more ideas.

229

➤ **For More Fun:** Once your sandwich is put together, ask a parent, friend, or younger sibling to pretend to gobble you up! Yum!

Bridge Pose (Setu Bandha Sarvangaasana)

Bridges are fun to build, especially when the only building material you need is your own body! Bridge Pose forms a bridge with the body as it increases flexibility in the spine and builds strength in the thighs and buttocks as it opens the chest.

Bridge Pose.

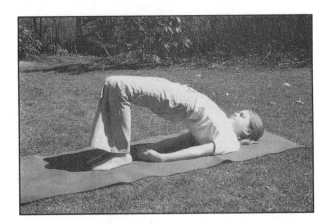

1. Rest on your back with your knees bent and feet close to your bottom.
2. Place your arms next to your body and down by your sides. Imagine that there is a chain tied to your belly button that will help to raise the drawbridge.
3. Slowly, feel the chain lift up your stomach, hips and thighs until the bridge rises off the floor. Press into the floor with your hands and feet.
4. Slowly lower the bridge down, then try it again.

➤ **For More Fun:** Let someone drive a toy car or boat under the bridge.
➤ **For Even More Fun:** Maneuver your shoulders closer together so you can interlace your fingers together under your hips to form a basket. Pretend your hands are a large ship sailing under the bridge.
➤ **For Even *More* Fun:** Let a younger sibling be a water snake, eel, or even a barge and slither under the bridge.

Wheel Pose (Urdhva Dhanurasana)

Wheel Pose forms the shape of a wheel, perhaps slightly sunk into the ground like one of those old wagon wheels. It is a challenging and flexibility-enhancing pose that corrects rounded back and shoulders, increases spinal flexibility, and improves breathing.

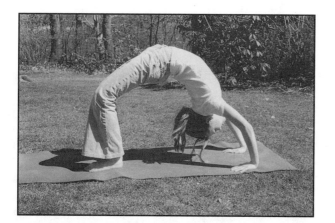

Wheel Pose.

1. Position yourself as if you were going to do the Bridge Pose, only this time, place your hands behind your shoulders with your elbows reaching up to the sky, palms on the floor.

2. Press into your hands and raise yourself up to the top of your head, then push yourself up off your head so that you're standing on your hands and feet.

3. Hold for a few seconds, concentrating on keeping your body in a curved shape.

4. Slowly come down by tucking your chin into your chest and lowering your body back to the ground.

5. Rest for a few minutes on your back, bringing your knees into your chest.

➤ **For More Fun:** While holding Wheel Pose, if you feel balanced, slowly and gently lift one leg up so your toes point to the sky. Lower, then try the other leg.

➤ **For Even More Fun:** Allow someone to roll something on wheels underneath you.

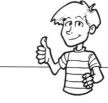

For Kids Only

When is a Wheel Pose not a Wheel Pose? When it's a Bridge Pose! The terms "Wheel Pose" and "Bridge Pose" are often interchanged. Many of Jodi's students call Wheel Pose Bridge Pose because that's what they call it in gymnastics or other movement classes. Whichever name you are most comfortable using is just fine. We are flexible about our asana names!

X Pose

X marks the spot for a super stretch! X Pose lets you form a giant letter X with your body. This pose feels great, especially after hard exercise or a stressful day. X Pose stretches the entire body to its maximum capacity, toning and elongating the muscles and increasing flexibility all over. You might even feel an inch or two taller after doing this pose!

231

1. Lie on your back with your arms and legs split apart to form a giant letter X with your body.

X Pose.

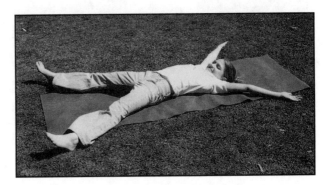

2. Imagine being gently pulled in four directions, as if someone were tugging on each arm and each leg. Stretch! Hold for a few seconds and then relax and try it again.

➤ **For More Fun:** Ask a few friends to gently pull on your arms and legs (gently!).

➤ **For Even More Fun:** Do X Pose standing up. Form a long X line with your fellow yoginis.

➤ **For Even *More* Fun:** Now that you have made the letter X with your body, what other letters could you make with your body? Could you spell out your name? The whole alphabet?

After honing strength and flexibility, parents and children can prepare to work on co-ordination and a few special yoga challenges to increase confidence.

The Least You Need to Know

➤ Yoga poses that are held in stillness (as opposed to movement poses) build strength and flexibility in a way that's different from movement poses.

➤ Hero Pose, the warrior poses, and other power poses also strengthen self-confidence.

➤ Yoga strength-building poses use the body's own weight to build muscle strength.

➤ Yoga flexibility-enhancing poses elongate, stretch, tone, and increase mobility in muscles and joints.

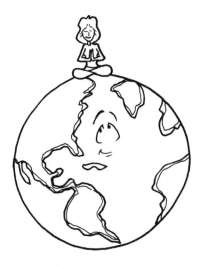

Chapter 17

Yoginis on Top of the World

In This Chapter

➤ Mind–body synchronicity

➤ Yoga poses to build coordination

➤ The classic yoga Lotus Pose with variations

➤ Other yoga poses to build confidence

In this chapter, yoginis get the chance to tackle some coordination-enhancing poses that make both sides of the body—and the brain—work in concert. From eye exercises to a pose based on the old-fashioned windmill calisthenics, coordination poses can help a child's whole self—body, mind, and spirit—get into balance.

Then we have some extra-challenging yoga poses, including the classic Lotus Pose. Challenging poses are fun and boost self-confidence immensely when they are achieved or when a child makes progress toward achieving them. Coordination-enhancing poses are excellent for helping the entire mind and body work together.

Yoga Coordination

Many different yoga poses and exercises help to build coordination by working opposite sides of the body in tandem, or by moving different parts of the body at the same time. Yoga exercises that work both sides of the body at the same time (called bilateral movements) or that involve working both sides of the body across the body's midline (called midline movements) also work both sides of the brain at the same time, encouraging the complete coordination of body and mind. (The concept of midline movements is based on the work of Paul E. Dennison, Ph.D., and his program, *Brain Gym*.)

Remember, the right side of your brain controls the left side of your body, and vice versa. When you use both sides of your body and brain at once, the whole system learns to work effectively in tandem.

The Eyes Have It

Eye exercises might not seem like bilateral movements at first, but even though your eyes are relatively close together, they are on opposite sides of your body, so working them both uses both sides of the brain. This exercise is great for relieving eyestrain. It strengthens the eye muscles and develops mental concentration as well as eye-hand coordination.

If a child has an eye problem, such as a wandering eye, they should certainly see an eye doctor. In addition to proper medical care, however, this exercise is an excellent therapy for many eye and vision problems.

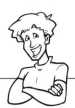

For Grownups, Too!

Puberty and growth spurts can make kids feel less than graceful, but these coordination glitches are only temporary. If your child gets frustrated with a sudden lack of normal coordination, the best course of action may be to explain that the condition is temporary, to be reassuring, and to not make a big deal about it. A regular yoga practice can also help.

Eye exercise.

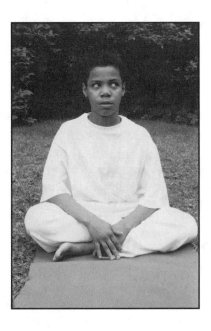

1. Warm up your eyes by making circles. Without moving your head or neck, look as far up
   as you can, then all the way around your pe-
   ripheral vision. Go one and then the other
   way. Rest your eyes.

2. Now be a clock watcher! Pretend you have a
   large clock in front of you. First look at the
   12, then the 1, 2, 3, and so on, working your
   way all the way around the clock. Remember,
   try not to move your head or neck, just your
   eyes!

3. When you are finished, blink a few times,
   then go the other way, from 12 to 11, 10, 9,
   and so on, all the way back to 1.

4. Rub your hands together vigorously, to generate heat (something Jodi calls "Healing
   Hands"). Close your eyes, then gently place
   the palms of your hands on your eyes, sending them energy and allowing them to rest.

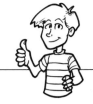

For Kids Only

If your eyes feel tired after a long study session, computer session, or a little too much time in front of the television, try a few of the eye exercises in this book, or simply look up, down, right, left, and then do a few big circles with your eyes. You might also rest them using an eye pillow (see Chapter 19).

➤ **For More Fun:** Try this exercise either alone or with a partner. Find a favorite
object, a flower, a crystal, or any other small item pleasant to look at. Either
hold the item yourself or ask a friend to hold it up in front of you. Move the
object around within your field of vision. Follow the object with your eyes,
but without moving your head.

➤ **For Even More Fun:** Ask a partner to draw letters or numbers with the object.
The person following the object must guess what the letter or number is.
(Remember, the person moving the object should make the figure backward so
it will appear correctly to the observer.)

Toe-Ups

Toe-Ups? Sound a lot easier than push-ups, don't they? Actually, Toe-Ups are pretty
tough. They involve working and moving the toes one at a time, and that's pretty
tricky, a real exercise in fine motor control and coordination. Toe-Ups also help with
concentration and mind-body coordination because it takes a lot of focused mental
power to stick with this one. (This exercise was designed by Jodi's colleague, Deb
Donefrio, C.Y.K.F.)

*Jodi and a yogini
practice Toe-Ups.*

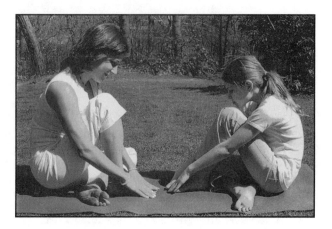

1. Sit with your bare feet flat on the ground.

2. Gently press your toes into the ground.

3. Now, starting with whichever foot you want, keep all your toes pressed into the ground except your big toe, and try to raise your *big toe only*. You can use your hands to hold down your other toes.

4. Place your big toe back down, and try to raise only your second toe. (This is super tough!)

5. Continue with each toe, trying to raise each one individually and using your hands to hold down your other toes whenever you need to.

6. Try the other foot.

➤ **For More Fun:** Challenge yourself! Try to lift all your toes *except* your big toe and pinkie toe. That's right, just the middle ones.

➤ **For Even More Fun:** Make up your own combinations. Raise the second and third toe only? Do both feet simultaneously? Tap your big toe and then your fourth toe, alternating? The choice is up to you.

Windmill

Windmill Pose coordinates both sides of your brain with both sides of your body in a fun and effective movement that mimics those large, wooden, old-fashioned windmills. Windmill is a midline movement that increases body awareness and gross motor coordination.

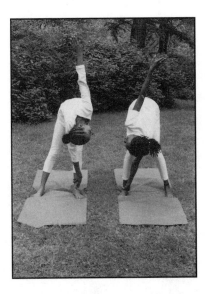

Windmill Pose.

1. Stand in Mountain Pose (see Chapter 11), then jump your legs apart so they are straight and wide enough to give you a firm, stable base.

2. With feet facing forward stretch out with one arm and then reach down to touch your opposite foot as you raise your other arm straight up to the sky.

3. Hold for a few seconds, then switch and do it the opposite way. Pick up the speed when you feel comfortable.

4. Repeat 15 to 20 times, or until you feel tired.

➤ **For More Fun:** Have someone wave a paper fan or stand in front of an electric fan turned on low. Pretend you are moving and turning with the wind.

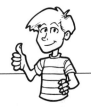

For Kids Only

You probably already know how to do a great exercise that uses both sides of your body at once, coordinating both sides of your brain: skipping! Skip down the street, around the park, or in the yard, swinging your arms, for an energizing and mind-body-coordinating exercise.

Crossovers

Crossovers is another midline movement that coordinates both sides of the brain with both sides of the body. It benefits gross motor coordination and has a centering, synchronizing effect on the mind and body.

Crossovers.

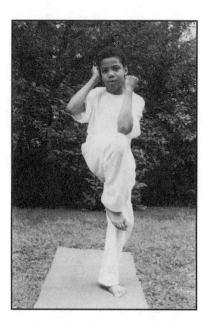

1. Begin in Mountain Pose (see Chapter 11).

2. Lift one knee, then the other, alternating until you have a rhythm going, like a march in place.

3. When the knee lifts feel comfortable, raise both arms out to the sides and bend your elbows. Make fists that point toward the sky.

4. As you raise each knee, lower the opposite elbow toward the raised knee. Your arm will cross over your torso.

5. Once this movement is comfortable, switch to bending your knee, but raise your foot behind you, tapping each foot with the opposite hand behind your back.

➤ **For More Fun:** Ask someone to be the "caller," calling out when to tap in front and when to tap in back. When the caller says "front," tap in front. When the caller says "back," switch to the back. Try not to miss a beat!

➤ **For Even More Fun:** Try this movement to music. First pick a slow or moderately paced song, then a faster song, and a faster song. See how fast you can do it! Challenge yourself.

Bicycle Pose

This pose allows you to experience the fun of bicycling, no matter what the whether! The scenery is limited only by your imagination! Bicycle Pose is a good cardiovascular exercise. It also benefits gross motor coordination and strengthens the legs and abdominal muscles.

1. Lie on your back with your legs and feet in the air, arms down by your sides.

2. Move your legs and feet as if you were pedaling a bicycle. Try to make big circles as you go around and around.

➤ **For More Fun:** Imagine you are riding somewhere in particular. The desert? The farm? The playground? Deepest Africa? Picture the scenery.

➤ **For Even More Fun:** Pedal backward!

➤ **For Even *More* Fun:** Once you get comfortable with the pedaling motion, try different speeds. Imagine pedaling through thick mud … slow! Uh-oh, now it's raining. Pedal fast! Ride uphill … so slow! Time for the downhill … whoosh!

Yoga Confidence

Nothing builds confidence like personal achievements, and these are what the following challenging poses are designed to inspire. While we don't want anybody trying a pose that is too difficult (because that can result in both injury and frustration), we do encourage yoginis to work toward these poses, bit by bit, as goals.

Pretzel Pose

We add this basic sitting pose here—a pose we've already mentioned frequently throughout this book—because it is a precursor to the more challenging Lotus Pose. Pretzel Pose is a good position for sitting on the ground in just about any situation. It builds hip flexibility. Parents can prompt a kid to sit in this pose by calling "Criss Cross Applesauce!"

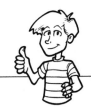

For Kids Only

You might sometimes feel frustrated if you can't get a pose right away, but many yoga students who aren't able to do certain poses at first can do them within time. You'll feel proud of yourself if you stick with it until you see progress, and that doesn't take long!

1. Sit on the floor and cross your legs so they feel comfortable and look like a pretzel.

2. Keep your back straight and tall. Hold the pose for as long as you like.

➤ **For More Fun:** This is the perfect pose in which to eat a healthy snack. Pretzels, anyone?

➤ **For Even More Fun:** While you sit in Pretzel Pose, ask someone to trace your lower body onto a large sheet of drawing paper or butcher paper. Then stand up and fill in the shape to make it look like a pretzel. Color it and pretend to eat it!

Lotus Pose (Padmaasana)

The Lotus Pose is probably the most famous of all the yoga poses. Yogis are often depicted in Lotus Pose, immersed in deep meditation, and when kids achieve this pose, they tend to be filled with pride and elation! In Lotus Pose you look as if someone has tied your legs up in a knot. It requires well-developed hip flexibility that most people have to work toward (although naturally limber people can do it right away).

Lotus Pose teaches correct posture. It is such a stable sitting pose that it almost automatically adjusts your body to sit in the most natural and healthy position. It keeps the mind alert and feels refreshing. It also keeps your knee, hip, and ankle joints flexible, strong, and healthy.

Lotus Pose.

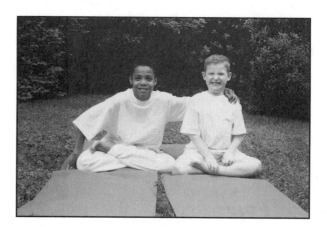

1. Begin by sitting in Pretzel Pose.

2. Take hold of one of your feet and gently raise it onto the opposite inner thigh. The sole of your foot should be angled upward.

3. Sit with a tall back. This is called Half Lotus. Rest here for a minute or two. Stay with this position for as many yoga practices as it takes to feel very comfortable before you move to the next step.

4. When Half Lotus feels comfortable, gently lift your other foot to its opposite thigh so that both feet are resting on opposite thighs.

5. Keeping your back straight, shift on your sit bones until you feel the most balanced and centered position. Rest here for a minute or two.

6. When you become very comfortable in Lotus Pose, you can use it as a meditation pose or as a handy (and attention grabbing) way to sit just about anywhere it is appropriate.

➤ **For More Fun:** Do the Lotus Walk! When in full Lotus Pose, rock forward until you are standing on your knees. Can you "walk" on your knees?

➤ **For Even More Fun:** Cross your arms behind your back and grab each big toe with the hand on the same side. You are twisted so many times here that it seems like you are grabbing the opposite toe, but if you "untie" the whole lotus you'll see that right hand grabs right toe and left hand grabs left toe. Pretty fancy!

➤ **For Even *More* Fun:** In the full Lotus Pose, press your palms down to the floor by your sides, then lift your body up off the floor. Swing your lower body back and forth through your arms. Weeee!

Candle Pose (Sarvangaasana)

In this pose, the body is inverted and lifted into the air. This is a fun pose and it feels just great to be upside-down! Candle Pose is a nice inversion with all the great health benefits of inversions, including increased clarity of thought and a nice rest for the legs and feet. Candle Pose also tones and strengthens the neck and shoulders and stimulates the thyroid gland. It's also a great confidence builder.

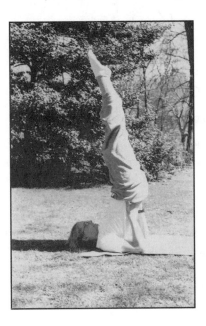

Candle Pose.

1. Begin by rolling in a ball and rocking back and forth on your rounded back, in Rock and Roll Pose (see Chapter 15).

2. Slowly swing your legs up and over your head. You don't need a lot of speed. This movement is easier when slower and more controlled.

3. Reach your legs toward the sky and place the palms of your palms pressing on your lower back, elbows resting on the floor, to support your body in the inverted position.

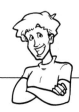

For Grownups, Too!

Parents tend to be on their feet all day long. A nice rest in Candle Pose can be rejuvenating to both mind and overworked feet!

4. Hold this pose as long as you feel comfortable.

5. Come down slowly, easing your hips toward the ground with the support of your hands and roll down, one vertebra at a time.

➤ **For More Fun:** Pretend to light the wick of the candle (your feet!) and sing "Happy Birthday to You," "Happy Anniversary to You" (it could be the anniversary of just about anything!), or just "Happy Day to You!" Don't forget to blow out the candles as you slowly roll down.

➤ **For Even More Fun:** Pretend you are a candelabra with two candle holders by opening your legs into a V shape.

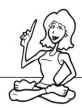

Yoga Stories

Any pose that turns your body upside down (called an inversion) is great for your health. As you walk around during the day, blood and other fluids tend to move downward toward your legs and feet. Inversions flip gravity's effect so that it pulls up (sort of!), allowing blood and fluids to flow in the opposite direction, supplying your brain and the other upper reaches of your body. It lets muscles and bones hang in the opposite direction. It gives feet and legs a break from holding body weight. Inversions also promote growth; improve the functioning of vital organs, glands, and nerves; and help relieve constipation, headaches, coughs, and colds. For better health, why not do an inversion every day?

Plow Pose (Halaasana)

Plow Pose flows naturally out of Candle Pose, carrying the movement further by bringing the legs all the way back behind the head. It imitates the shape of the old-fashioned, hand-guided plows of yore, not the modern ones with engines!

Plow Pose is challenging but it feels great to finally gain the necessary flexibility to feel comfortable in it, and that builds confidence! Plow Pose helps to irrigate the brain and tones the thyroid even more than Candle Pose does. It strengthens the upper body, opens the chest, stretches the neck, shoulders and upper back muscles, stimulates circulation and energy flow through the entire body, improves digestion and elimination, relieves fatigue, soothes and energizes, and increases flexibility in the entire body. Talk about getting a lot of benefits from one pose!

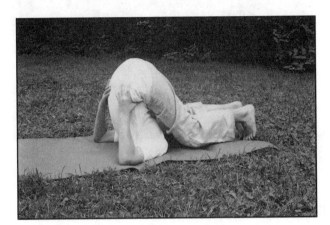

Plow Pose.

1. Begin in Candle Pose, then slowly lower your feet behind your head, keeping your legs straight and hands remaining on your back.

2. Rest for a few seconds with your feet on the floor behind you.

3. If you feel comfortable, slowly lower your knees so they rest on the ground on either side of your ears.

4. Hold this pose as long as you feel comfortable, then slowly straighten your knees and very, very slowly and gently, roll your body back down until you're lying flat.

➤ **For More Fun:** Before you roll out of Plow Pose, ask someone to put a light-weight object (like a Beanie Baby or other stuffed animal, or a small pillow) in between your toes or knees. Gently and slowly roll out of the pose, vertebra by vertebra, trying not to drop the object.

Fish Pose (Matsynasan)

Fish Pose is a great follow-up to Candle Pose and Plow Pose, because it arches the spine and neck, countering the previous poses and balancing the body. Fish Pose is challenging because it is not a position we would naturally get into. Once you've got the feel of it, however, it feels great, and you will feel great, too, knowing you've mastered this challenging yoga posture.

In addition to being an excellent counter pose to Candle Pose and Plow Pose, Fish Pose refreshes the body and the mind, and keeps the abdominal muscles healthy.

Fish Pose.

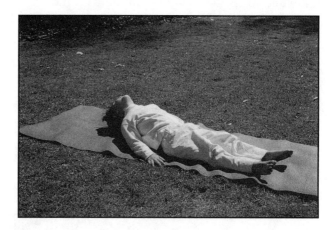

1. Lie flat on your back with your legs straight, arms down by your sides.

2. Press into your elbows and left your chest upward as you arch your back.

3. Rest gently and very lightly on the top of your head. Most of your weight should be on your elbows.

4. Hold this position for a few seconds, then slowly come out of it by bringing your chin into your chest and relaxing on your back.

➤ **For More Fun:** Purse your lips together like a fish. What sounds might a fish make underwater?

➤ **For Even More Fun:** Decide what color and kind of fish you are.

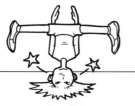

Ooops!

Headstand Pose can be hard on your neck if you put too much pressure on the head. Parents, show your child how to keep most of the weight centered over the forearms and elbows. To help your child feel the appropriate position, suggest resting the head so lightly on the ground that someone could slip a piece of paper under your child's head. Or use a folded blanket under the head for cushioning.

Headstand

Headstand is an impressive pose that kids just love. They feel great when they achieve it, although it is challenging and may take some time. It is a complete inversion with all the health benefits of inversions, increasing blood circulation to the brain, improving balance, and honing concentration. Headstand also promotes growth, strengthens the immune system, and builds energy. Adults should spot kids in Headstand, at least until the child is quite stable and confident in the pose.

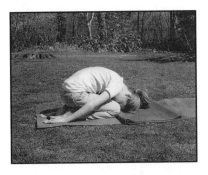 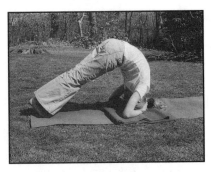 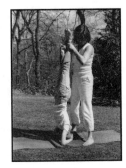

Start in Mouse Pose (left) and work your way to Headstand Pose (far right).

1. Begin by resting in Mouse Pose (see Chapter 12), near and facing a wall.

2. Interlace your fingers, making a basket, and place them very close to the top of your head so your hands, forearms, and elbows rest on the floor, forming an upside-down V around your head. For some, bringing the hands slightly back from the head in a tripod stance makes balancing easier.

3. Slowly roll forward onto the top of your head. Make sure you don't put a lot of pressure on your head. Most of your weight should be on your elbows and forearms.

4. Curl your toes under and straighten your legs, then take baby steps toward your face.

5. When you can't go any further, bend your knees, one at a time, and lift them up above your torso.

6. Slowly lift both your legs up toward the sky, using the wall for support.

7. Stay up for a short time, or as long as you feel comfortable, then slowly come back down into Mouse Pose and rest for a minute or two. All those mixed-up juices need some time to settle in!

➤ **For More Fun:** Once you are very comfortable in Headstand Pose, move out away from a wall and try it without support. Impressive!

➤ **For Even More Fun:** While inverted, open your legs to form a V shape, an inverted Tree Pose (see Chapter 11), or an inverted Pretzel Pose.

After a challenging workout like this, you may feel challenged, proud, or maybe a little frustrated. Parents, encourage your child to view challenging yoga poses as goals to reach at a gradual pace, step by step. Working toward a challenging pose builds self-discipline and self-control. And when your child finally gets it, he or she will enjoy a great boost of self-confidence, knowing the achievement came out of hard work, persistence, and dedication.

The Least You Need to Know

➤ Yoga poses that work both sides of the body at the same time synchronize body and mind.

➤ Mind–body poses improve mental and physical coordination.

➤ The Lotus Pose is a classic yoga pose that builds flexibility and self-esteem.

➤ Making progress toward, and eventually mastering, more challenging yoga poses helps kids feel great about themselves.

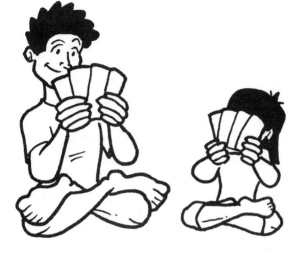

Chapter 18

Yogini Fun and Games

In This Chapter

➤ Yoga times two

➤ No-win, no-lose, all-fun yoga games

➤ Yoginis *en masse:* yoga fun in groups

➤ Inventing yoga games

Yoga is fun when done by one, but partner yoga is a great way for kids to bond with a parent, sibling, or friend. A group of yoginis playing yoga games also makes for spectacular fun!

In this chapter, we focus on fun partner and group yoga exercise and games. This is some serious yoga fun—so grab a friend or gather a group and get ready to play!

Two Can Be as Much Fun as One!

Traditionally, yoga is an individual activity designed to control the body to better facilitate meditation. But yoga has evolved! Why shouldn't kids do yoga with someone else? What better way to share a favorite activity?

We encourage all kids to practice yoga solo as well as with others. Solo yoga has many benefits including the development of concentration and the opportunity to focus inwardly on your own body, mind, and progress. But for a change of pace, to while away an afternoon, or when a kid and his or her buddy are just sitting around wondering what to do, partner yoga can be the perfect activity.

Partner Straddle Stretching

Many yoga poses increase flexibility, but a partner can further increase the flexibility-enhancing effects of a yoga pose with a little assistance. In Partner Stretching, two yoginis work together to maximize a straddle stretch. Partner Stretching teaches two yoginis to synchronize their movements, and gives their legs a nice, deep stretch.

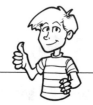

For Kids Only

While partner yoga can get giggly and even wild, it can also be quiet and meditative, depending on the mood of you and your partner. You can still get lots of benefits from partner yoga when you are feeling quiet and in the mood for a mellow, relaxing workout. A partner can help you stretch, concentrate, and focus.

1. Sit facing your partner with legs in a V shape or straddle position, feet touching your partner's feet so your legs form a diamond shape.

2. Stretch over your right leg as your partner stretches over his or her left leg. Try to touch your partner's fingertips on the side you are leaning toward.

3. Switch to the other side.

4. Now, lean toward the middle and hold hands with your partner if you can. If holding hands is easy, hold your forearms or elbows. Pull gently toward each other to really stretch those inner thighs.

Partner Straddle Stretching.

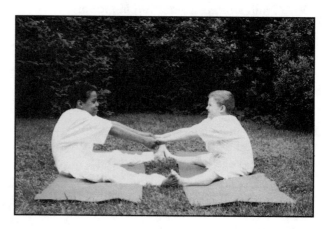

➤ **For More Fun:** If you or your partner needs an even deeper stretch, take turns gently pulling each other by the hands toward the middle. First pull your partner gently toward you, then let your partner pull you. Keep your feet together and relax into the stretch.

➤ **For Even More Fun:** Try to come up with other partner stretches in which both partners can feel a stretch simultaneously.

248

Mirror Me

The Mirror Me exercise is an excellent exercise for helping two people learn to pay attention to each other and become mentally attuned to each other. While we discourage the use of real mirrors in yoga, Mirror Me helps us to look further into ourselves while we also become more attuned to others. Mirror Me teaches kids about mirror effects (how a mirror works, how it shows things in reverse, etc.) and sportsmanship as it enhances balance, concentration, and arm strength.

1. Sit facing your partner, sitting on your heels with knees together in Japanese Sitting Pose (see Chapter 13) or in Pretzel Pose (see Chapter 17). Decide who will lead first.

2. Raise your hands and hold your palms up to your partner's palms, close but not touching, as if each of you was the other person's reflection in a mirror. Leave at least enough space for a piece of paper to fit easily between your palms.

3. Slowly move your hands in different ways, keeping them in the same plane, as if right up against the mirror. Move them up, down, side to side, around in circles, and so on, as your partner mirrors your movements. Don't move too fast!

4. After a few minutes, switch leaders.

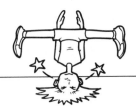

Ooops!

In partner stretching, remember to stay closely attuned to your partner's limits and comfort level. Don't yank on your partner or you could cause him or her to pull a muscle. Stretch together slowly and gently, and agree beforehand that if someone says stop, the stretch stops immediately. This not only helps preclude injury, but it teaches kids to connect.

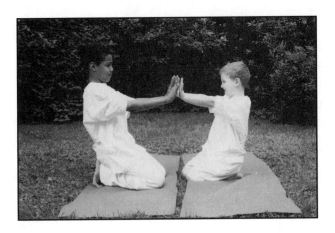

Mirror Me.

➤ **For More Fun:** Try playing a more intuitive version of this game. Instead of specifying who will lead and who will follow, take turns leading without telling each other who will do so. You may change leaders without even noticing! Concentrate on feeling the energy between your hands and letting the energy guide you.

➤ **For Even More Fun:** Make shapes with your hands—squares, diamonds, circles, hearts—as if drawing the shape on the mirror.

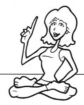

Yoga Stories

If you bring your palms up to someone else's palms without touching (or if you bring your own two palms together), then move your palms apart and together again, you can feel the energy between your hands. This energy, or chi, as the Chinese call it, forms the basis for the ancient Chinese art called Chi Kung (sometimes written as Quigong), which is the cultivation and manipulation of life-force energy (chi). Chi Kung movements come in different forms, including forms with such interesting names as Wild Goose Chi Kung and Five Animal Chi Kung. Chi Kung techniques also can be used as meditation exercises, martial art, or to enhance the practice of a religion, art, craft, performance, or self-discipline.

Assist Me

In this exercise, partners take turns helping each other get the maximum benefits out of specific poses. An extra body strategically placed can add an extra stretch or strengthening component to almost any yoga exercises.

While Assist Me can be used for many poses, for this example, let's use Downward Facing Dog. The stretch in Downward Facing Dog is achieved by reaching the hips back and up. A partner can help to increase this stretch. This pose works best with two partners of the same approximate size, including weight and height. Assist Me teaches kids about the dynamics of different yoga poses, encourages selflessness and teamwork, and facilitates a deeper stretch.

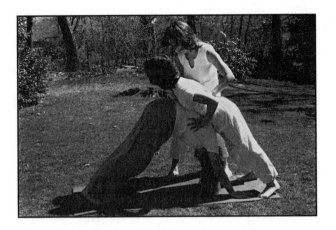

Jodi gives yoginis an assist.

1. One partner gets into Downward Facing Dog Pose (see Chapter 12).

2. The other partner stands on the side of the first partner's lowered head, then gently places his or her upper body on top of the back of the first partner and applies slight pressure. The idea here in this specific pose is to move up and back to help the first partner stretch his or her hips upward. The yogini in Downward Facing Dog should feel as if most of the weight is lifted off his or her hands.

3. Talk to your partner. Let him or her know how you are doing in the pose. Do you want more pressure? Do you need your partner to ease up a bit?

4. Let your partner know when you are ready to come out of the pose. Come out of the pose slowly, allow the partner who was doing the stretch to rest in Mouse Pose (see Chapter 12), then switch places.

➤ **For More Fun:** Experiment with all your favorite yoga poses. See how you and your partner can combine forces to enhance the stretch or strengthening power of each pose.

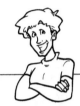

For Grownups, Too!

It may be tempting for parents to use Assist Me as a way to correct a child's form in a pose, but Assist Me isn't designed to fix incorrect form. Instead, its purpose is to enhance the power or stretch of a pose through the use of another body. It also gives a template for what the pose can be, and is beneficial for achieving proper alignment.

For the Whole Gang!

These poses are for a yogini gang. They are fun games to play in a group of any size, from 3 to 30. And remember, although we sometimes use the word "game" to describe the yoga activities in this book, yoga "games" have no winners or losers, no right or wrong. Keep the positive energy alive and be supportive of your fellow yoginis for maximum yoga fun!

Whisper in My Ear

This yoga game (created by Marsha Wenig of YogaKids) is a variation on the old standard circle game "Telephone." It uses creative combinations of yoga poses and silly instructions as the whispered message. Whisper in My Ear stimulates creativity, exercises receptive language skills, and enhances concentration and teamwork skills.

1. Sit in a big circle with your yogini group.

2. One person starts the message by whispering something in his or her neighbor's ear. The message can be something funny and mixed-up, like "Do Tree Pose and meow like a cat" or "Do Superperson Pose and sing 'Row Row Row Your Boat'" or "Do Downward Facing Dog Pose and croak like a frog." You get the picture!

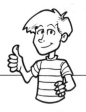

For Kids Only

Group yoga can stop being fun if people start laughing at each other, criticizing each other, or being otherwise unsupportive. There is a difference between laughing *at* each other and laughing *with* each other. Encouraging, supporting, even applauding your friends and siblings is extremely important for the success of group yoga. Appointing a leader to set a supportive tone can also help.

3. The yogini receiving the message whispers it to his or her neighbor until the message gets all the way around the circle to the person sitting next to the original message maker.

4. The final message recipient says the message out loud, then performs the yoga pose as heard—if he or she can still understand the message! Just like in the "Telephone" game, silly messages like these can easily get mixed up, and that's part of the fun!

5. Take turns being the first and last person to go.

➤ **For More Fun:** Have each person in the circle draw a picture of the mixed-up combo that was sent through the circle—a cat caught in a tree? A superperson riding in a rowboat? A dog-frog?

Yogini's Choice

This game gives each child a chance to play yoga teacher. It brings unity to a large group of yoginis, teaches listening skills, leadership skills, expressive language skills, and is a great confidence booster when the group is supportive of each yogini as he or she leads the group in their poses.

1. Each yogini in the group chooses a pose he or she would like to lead the group in doing. Choices can be known poses or made-up poses. If more than one person chooses the same pose, no problem! There isn't anything wrong with doing a yoga pose more than once.

2. One at a time, each yogini names the pose, describes the pose, and gives directions on how to do it.

3. The whole group listens, then follows the leader by doing the pose.

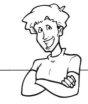

For Grownups, Too!

On nice days, you might direct your group of yoginis out into the yard or to a nearby park. Fresh air, sunshine, and a nice breeze make yoga games even more fun.

➤ **For More Fun:** Make a big circle when you do this exercise. Each leader stands in the middle when it is his or her turn to "teach" the pose.

➤ **For Even More Fun:** Make this a guessing game! Each leader gets in the center of the circle and does a yoga pose. The group has to guess the name of the pose. This also works for made-up poses, if the pose is imitating an animal or other known object. The group guesses what the pose is imitating.

Animal Enigma

This pose uses toy animals as props. Kids enjoy making yoga poses based on their favorite things! This is a fun game for a group of siblings or a small group of friends gathering informally after school. Fun props include Beanie Babies, stuffed animals, plastic animals, even photos of animals.

Animal Enigma helps kids with word retrieval skills, learning animal names and associated sounds, and of course, has all the benefits of each of the yoga poses involved.

1. Gather a bunch of stuffed animals, plastic animals, and animal figurines from around the house. Put them in a bag, pillowcase, or box.

2. Take turns choosing an animal from the bag and showing it to everyone. Then the whole group does the associated pose while making the sound of that animal.

3. Feel free to include animals without yoga poses. You can always invent one! If you have a favorite zebra toy, include it, and then the person who chooses the zebra can make up a Zebra Pose.

➤ **For More Fun:** Try to find animal noses from a party store or nature store. Pick a nose from a mystery bag, put it on, and then do the pose with the group.

➤ **For Even More Fun:** Play this game using animal categories: only birds, desert creatures, jungle animals, and so on.

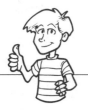

➤ **For Even *More* Fun:** Ask each person in the group to take turns gathering the items for the bag, or ask each person to bring from home one appropriate item.

For Kids Only

Hey kids, do you know where your grandparents are? Maybe they could use a good yoga workout, too! If you're looking for a yoga partner or another member or two for your yoga group, why not get grandma or grandpa into the game? They'll probably be more than willing to participate with a little encouragement, and family yoga is fun! Besides, yoga is good for them, too!

Synchronized Yoga

This game is fun with lots of yoginis—six or more work best. The idea is to do yoga poses in sync with each other. The poses look beautiful to an onlooker, like synchronized swimming! The group synchronizes by paying attention to each other, feeling the energy of the group, and watching to see that all the movements are together. Synchronized Yoga is wonderful group work, teaching kids teamwork, how to be attuned to others, group coordination, and of course, has all the benefits of the poses included.

For Synchronized Yoga, the group can decide ahead of time on a series of poses, or people can call out individual poses as you go. The following is only an example of one way to do synchronized yoga. You can synchronize any pose or poses. The point is to practice in unison.

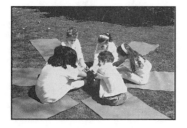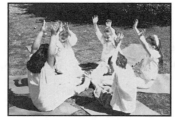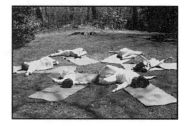

Synchronized Yoga.

1. Come into a circle with everyone's toes pointing to the center of the circle. Allow enough room for everyone to bend over without knocking heads.

2. Begin by doing Sandwich Pose (see Chapter 16). Really pay attention to the group and try to keep your movements in sync with everyone else's.

3. Next, move down into a Snake Pose (see Chapter 13), Downward Facing Dog Pose (see Chapter 12), Bridge Pose (see Chapter 16), or any other series you decide upon.

➤ **For More Fun:** Hold hands while doing yoga poses, or try Synchronized Yoga while each person faces the outside of the circle.

➤ **For Even More Fun:** Take turns coming out of the circle to watch how beautiful the group looks. See if you can get an aerial view (from above), maybe by standing on a sturdy chair.

➤ **For Even *More* Fun:** Try synchronized Yoga Sun Dance (see Chapter 15) or other vinyasa (flow series). Your group might look so good, you'll want to put on a performance for all your parents!

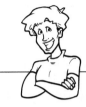

For Grownups, Too!

Encourage a group a yoginis to put their synchronized yoga routine to music (if they haven't already) and arrange for a performance in front of parents, neighbors, or even the school. What great publicity for a start-up yoga club, and even better, what a great boost for your child's confidence!

Yoga Games of Your Own Design

We've only scratched the surface of possibilities when it comes to partner and group yoga games. See if you can come up with your own yoga games and yoga in groups. Just remember, even though they can be highly energetic and/or challenging, yoga games aren't competitive. No winners, no losers. Just fun!

How do you make up a yoga game? Start with any pose and think of related poses. How might you string them together to create a game? Or, start with any regular game you like to play. (Volleyball? Ring Around the Rosy? Red Rover? Tag? Twister?) How could you incorporate yoga poses and take out the competitive aspect of your favorite games to "yoga-ize" them?

Yoga games can also take a quieter turn. Write stories with a group of friends based on yoga poses or the animals that inspire yoga poses. Make a group mural of each other doing yoga poses, or of animals doing yoga poses, or of the animals themselves.

Draw yoga pictures with sidewalk chalk on your driveway or make circles, lines, and other shapes to stand in while doing yoga poses (but be careful doing balance poses on cement). Tell stories in a circle, inventing ways in which you imagine how different yoga poses might have been invented thousands of years ago, or yesterday! You could even make up a yoga play.

Each child is a fountain of creativity, a beautiful rainbow of ideas, energy, and possibility. Yoga invention is just one way to encourage that fountain to flow and that rainbow to shine. Parents, step back and watch your child be a yoga artist. It's a beautiful sight.

The Least You Need to Know

➤ While traditionally a solitary activity, yoga works well with partners and even in groups.

➤ Partners can work together in yoga poses, helping to increase stretches and teaching each other to attune to the movements and energies of another person.

➤ Yoga games are lots of fun, but never competitive.

➤ Group yoga helps a group of people to work together, teaching teamwork skills.

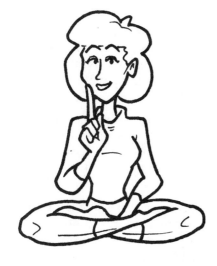

Chapter 19

Quiet Time

In This Chapter

➤ Quieting the body and mind

➤ Shavasana: yoga's deep relaxation

➤ Guidelines for practicing Shavasana

➤ Visual imagery exercises for relaxation

Wow! What a workout we've had. But it isn't over yet. It's time for Shavasana, a deep relaxation pose and the perfect way to end a yoga workout.

This is the time when we allow our bodies to absorb all of the benefits from the yoga practice we have been doing. It is also the time to quiet our bodies and listen to our internal selves. It is truly a time to do nothing, allowing our bodies and our minds to find quiet and stillness, something many people rarely take the opportunity to do.

How do you quiet your body and your mind? The answer is different for everyone. Some people thrive on high speed and find the idea of stillness challenging. On the other hand, some of us crave more quiet time and sink into relaxation with ease. Regardless of how you or your body feel about the idea, Shavasana is extremely beneficial for everyone.

Relaxation doesn't have to be hard or boring. In this chapter, we'll show you how to make relaxation comfortable and fun with lots of different relaxation and visualization exercises as we explore the ins and outs of yoga relaxation, contemplation, and stillness.

The Virtue of Stillness

What does it feel like to be alive? The question may seem silly, but try to answer it anyway. One of the keys to a full appreciation of life and being alive is taking the time to be quiet, be still, and just be. Stillness is a virtue because it allows us space to appreciate, savor, and make the most of our lives.

Without stillness, we couldn't appreciate movement, the vibrancy and action of motion. Without movement, we couldn't appreciate stillness. We need to balance our bodies, minds, and eternal energies, and bring the yin and yang in each of us into equilibrium. Movement and stillness work together to create a centered and whole person.

But when life gets busy, as kids' lives often do, stillness is sometimes the last thing families think about. Who has time to be still when we are busy in school, overwhelmed with homework, going to swimming, karate, soccer, ballet, playing with this friend, talking to that friend—the list goes on and on. Yet, allowing some time each day for stillness can have a magical effect on the mind and body, making life a little less stressful, more beautiful, and more meaningful, too.

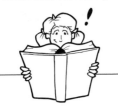

Learn About Yoga

Shavasana is the Sanskrit word for "dead pose" or "corpse pose." It is meant to bring the body into complete and total deep relaxation by lying in a prone position on the floor and centering the mind while relinquishing control of the body.

Parents who work with their young children in *Shavasana* for at least a few minutes each day can bring incredible peace to their children's lives and teach them valuable stress management skills. As your child relaxes, you guide him or her through any of the following visualizations, or make up your own. Children may also enjoy practicing Shavasana alone, and this is likewise beneficial and wonderful. Appendix B also contains books with additional visualizations to help promote deep relaxation.

Older kids might want to guide each other through Shavasana relaxation, or tape-record their own voices reading visualizations so they can relax on their own. And parents, don't forget to spend some time in Shavasana yourself! As we said, every person can benefit immensely from the regular practice of Shavasana.

Shavasana: Yoga's Peaceful Pose

Let's set up a structure to help establish the right environment, get really comfortable, and ease into total relaxation. The following scenario explains how to set the stage for the visual imagery exercises that you'll be practicing in a moment.

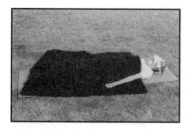
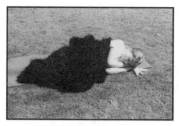
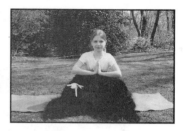

Rest in Shavasana (left). After deep relaxation, move into Pretzel Pose (far right).

➤ Dim the lights so your eyes can comfortably relax. Make sure your yoga space is as free from disruptions as possible. No ringing phones, beeping watches or toys, televisions, or people walking through the room, if possible. Shavasana is most beneficial if there are no distractions or interruptions.

➤ Put on some music that is soothing and relaxing, something with a slow tempo to help your body quiet and soften itself. Music without vocals is preferable, and music specific to a particular visualization is a nice touch (ocean sounds for a beach visualization, soft animal sounds for a safari or forest visualization, for example).

➤ Tuck yourself under a soft blanket. After doing many yoga poses, this is your body's opportunity to slow down and cool off, but you want to keep warm, because it's much easier to relax if you are warm and toasty!

➤ Place an eye pillow over your eyes to keep them relaxed and peacefully closed. You can purchase herbal eye pillows in animal shapes (see Appendix B), silk eye pillows, or simply use something as accessible as a soft scarf or clean sock draped over your eyes.

➤ Lie flat on your back and try to relax totally. Let your arms and legs drop to your sides. Don't try to hold them in any position. Just let them open up and relax. Keep your legs about 6 to 8 inches apart and rest your arms with your palms facing upwards, down by

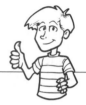

For Kids Only

When you work your body, you need to rest afterwards so your body has time to get stronger. Shavasana rests your body after a yoga workout, but it also rests your mind so it can work better, too.

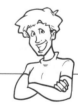

For Grownups, Too!

During Shavasana, you might want to massage your child's feet. Jodi does this for her students, sometimes with lotion, providing for wonderful sensory integration. Jodi's kids love this part! (Some kids don't care for it due to their extremely ticklish feet.)

your sides. Try to allow your body to become incredibly relaxed, almost as if you were melting into the floor.

Visual Imagery to Relax You

When the child is comfortably settled into the Shavasana Pose, a parent, friend, or sibling can read any of the following visual imagery exercises in a soft, soothing voice to help the child relax even further, easing away tension, balancing the body's energy, and relaxing the mind. Another option is to tape-record yourself and play the tape back.

Whenever the word "pause" appears in the following visualizations, the reader should pause for a few seconds, to allow the yogini in Shavasana to concentrate on the suggested feeling. Each one of the following visualizations also assumes the child is already resting in Shavasana as it begins.

Rainbow Relaxation

Turn your attention to your breath. Feel it moving in and out of your nose. Follow the sound and the feeling of your breath. [Pause] *Listen to your breath.* [Pause]

Now, assign your breath a color, to make it easier to follow. Notice the color moving all the way down into your belly, then back out through your nose. [Pause] *Watch your colored breath. Relax and breathe.* [Pause]

Imagine the color slowly leaving your breath. Return your breathing to normal. Now, imagine that high above your head is a beautiful waterfall. This is a special waterfall that will help to make you feel healthy and good. Another thing that makes this waterfall special is its color. This water is brightly colored. Imagine what color the water is. [Pause]

Now imagine the water streaming down over your head and body. It feels warm and comfortable, soothing and pleasant. Feel the water rushing and bubbling around you and through your body, moving through your head, your chest, your arms and out your fingertips, through your stomach, your hips, your legs, your feet, all the way down to and out of the ends of your toes.

Imagine the water is rushing through your body, taking with it anything stressful or unpleasant that happened to you today. Away it all goes, washed away by the rush of colored water. Tension, stress, fears, anything that happened today that bothered you, worried you, or made you feel bad. All are washed away with the rush of water. Feel the bad things wash away. [Pause] *Feel the beautiful water moving through you, clearing away everything negative and washing it out of your fingertips and toes.* [Pause]

Now that all the negativity is washed out of you, notice how healthy and calm and relaxed your body feels. Then, notice how the waterfall is slowing, the colored water becoming only a trickle, then a drip, and then disappearing. [Pause]

Now, imagine that above your body, a bright, vibrantly colored rainbow is forming. [Pause] *Watch it form.*

Notice all the colors. Red turning to orange turning to yellow turning to green turning to blue turning to purple. See the beautiful colors gleaming and shimmering above you. This is a special rainbow just for you, here to help you feel healthy and good. [Pause]

Now think of something positive that you experienced today. Think about that feeling as you feel the rainbow shining down on your body, enhancing the feeling and instilling your body with joy. The more the rainbow shines on you, the more delighted you feel. [Pause] *Feel the rainbow drenching you with happiness.*

You are like a glowing rainbow, filled with many different, beautiful colors. You are powerful and strong, amazing in your glory. Feel the empowerment of the rainbow within you. [Pause]

Now, slowly deepen your breath as you prepare to awaken your physical body. [Pause] *Then, slowly begin to move your toes.* [Pause] *Now your fingers.* [Pause] *Gently move your ankles and wrists.* [Pause]

Stretch your body as if you were a cat waking from a nap. [Pause] *Bring your knees into your chest and gently roll over to your side, making a pillow with your hands or with your eye pillow. Keep your eyes closed.* [Pause]

Slowly open your eyes half way as you use your hands to come up, sitting in Pretzel Pose.

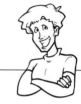

For Grownups, Too!

Visual imagery exercises can seem very real to kids, so make sure kids feel safe and comfortable. If you are describing a visit to the rainforest, assure your child that all the animals are guaranteed gentle and friendly. If you describe floating on a cloud, also describe the button your child can push to be returned immediately and safely to earth.

Cloud Floating Relaxation

Turn your attention to your breath. Feel it moving in and out of your nose. Follow the sound and the feeling of your breath. [Pause] *Listen to your breath.* [Pause]

Now, assign your breath a color, to make it easier to follow. Notice the color moving all the way down into your belly, then back out through your nose. [Pause] *Watch your colored breath. Relax and breathe.* [Pause]

Imagine the color slowly leaving your breath. Return your breathing to normal. Imagine that as you were breathing, a soft white cloud has drifted underneath you. [Pause]

Feel relaxed and comfortable as you nestle your body into the cloud. Feel the cloud beneath you. [Pause]

Now, imagine that this special cloud will take you to your favorite place in the entire world. Where will that be? It could be a place in your home, in your town or city, in your state or country, or even out of the country or out of the world. It can be a make-believe place or a real place. Tell yourself, inside, where the place is and think about the place. [Pause]

Slowly feel the cloud lift you off the ground and up, gently and slowly, into the air. Higher and higher you rise, into the sky. The cloud moves as quickly or as slowly as you would like it to move. You feel light and joyful as you ride on your soft, comfortable cloud. You look forward to arriving at your favorite place. You are enjoying the ride. [Pause]

Look around from your vantage point on the cloud. What do you see around you and above you in the sky? What do you see below you on the ground? You are almost there. [Pause]

At last you arrive. The cloud floats gently down into the middle of your favorite place. Imagine climbing off the cloud and knowing it will be waiting for you when you are ready to come back. But right now is the time to spend in your favorite place. Look around. Walk around. Be free. There are no limitations here. Just be! [Pause]

What will you do in your favorite place? Will you play with some of your favorite things? Explore? Eat some of your favorite foods? Listen to your favorite music? Spend some time here. [Long pause]

It is now about time to return to the present moment. Finish your visit and wander back to your cloud, waiting for you just where you left it. You feel content and happy after spending time in your favorite place. Feel that contentment in your heart, where you can hold onto it forever. [Pause]

Imagine climbing back onto the soft cloud and relaxing as it slowly rises and floats back through the sky, returning you to the present moment.

Now, slowly deepen your breath as you prepare to awaken your body. [Pause] *Then, slowly begin to move your toes.* [Pause] *Now your fingers.* [Pause] *Gently move your ankles and wrists.* [Pause]

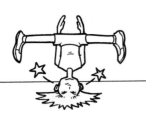

Ooops!

While some kids find relaxation challenging, kids who drink caffeinated beverages may find it more difficult. Caffeine is a stimulant and a diuretic, and it is not a healthy addition to the diet of any child. Caffeine isn't just in coffee, tea, and cola. It's also in some foods, such as chocolate and coffee ice cream, and even in some over-the-counter pain medication.

Stretch your body as if you were a cat waking from a nap. [Pause] *Bring your knees into your chest and gently roll over to your side, making a pillow with your hands or with your eye pillow. Keep your eyes closed.* [Pause]

Slowly open your eyes half way as you use your hands to come up, sitting in Pretzel Pose.

Rainforest Relaxation

Turn your attention to your breath. Feel it moving in and out of your nose. Follow the sound and the feeling of your breath. [Pause] *Listen to your breath.* [Pause]

Now, assign your breath a color, to make it easier to follow. Notice the color moving all the way down into your belly, then back out through your nose. [Pause] *Watch your colored breath. Relax and breathe.* [Pause] *Imagine the color slowly leaving your breath. Return your breathing to normal.*

Now, imagine you have just stepped into a lush, green, beautiful rainforest. You are the only human around, but you don't feel scared because you know it is a friendly place to visit. You look around at the trees and plants and flowers. You feel the moist rainforest air on your skin. You feel safe and happy. [Pause]

Imagine yourself slowly walking along the rainforest floor. The temperature is just right, perfectly comfortable. You can tell by the drops of water on the leaves and the dripping from the trees that it has just finished raining. It is the perfect weather for a walk. [Pause]

Imagine you are barefoot, walking on soft, velvety moss. You know you don't need to worry where you step because the ground is perfectly safe for your feet, soft and springy and comfortable. [Pause]

As you walk through the rainforest, listen to the rainforest sounds. What do you hear? Maybe you hear birds singing to each other in the trees, the sound of a distant waterfall, friendly animals scampering about, the drip of rainwater off leaves and flowers onto the rainforest floor. Listen carefully. What else do you hear? Try to hear even the faintest, most faraway sounds. [Pause]

Now, imagine all the colors of the rainforest you see around you as you walk. Notice all the exotic plants and flowers, the shapes and textures. Walk slowly and look carefully so you don't miss anything. [Pause]

Now look for animals. What animals do you see in the rainforest, peeking from behind trees and beneath leaves, flying overhead, or swimming in streams? [Pause]

What do you smell as you walk through the rainforest? Imagine the rainforest smell. Is it sweet? Clean? Musty? Wet? Does it remind you of anything else you've ever smelled? Think about whether you like the smell or not. Do you smell other smells, too? Flowers? Rain? [Pause]

Continue to explore the rainforest. Imagine you find some exotic fruit. Go ahead and taste it. It's fine to eat it. How does it taste? What is the texture? Is it sweet or sour, mild or strong? Does it taste familiar? [Pause]

Now, notice how things around you feel when you touch them. Touch a plant, a leaf, a flower. Nothing is dangerous here; everything is fine to touch. How do the leaves feel? Velvety? Slick? Wet? [Pause] *See if you can find an animal to touch. All the animals here are friendly and happy to play with you. What animals are you touching? The wing of a parrot? A monkey's tail? A scaly green lizard?* [Pause]

What else can you touch? Wet bark? Moss? Mud? Leaves on the rainforest floor? A stream? A boulder? Keep exploring and feeling the shapes and textures of everything around you.

Now, find a nice place to relax and recline in the rainforest. Maybe you will find a comfortable spot against a tree, or a bed of leaves, or a patch of soft grass. Imagine closing your eyes and settling in, safe and comfortable, to relax. Listen, smell, taste, and feel the rainforest all around you as you lie in complete, comfortable relaxation. [Pause]

Now, look inside yourself and notice how you feel about being in such a peaceful place. How do you like being immersed in nature, away from all other human beings? Think about it. [Pause]

Now, slowly deepen your breath as you prepare to awaken your body. [Pause] *Then, slowly begin to move your toes.* [Pause] *Now your fingers.* [Pause] *Gently move your ankles and wrists.* [Pause]

Stretch your body as if you were a cat waking from a nap. [Pause] *Bring your knees into your chest and gently roll over to your side, making a pillow with your hands or with your eye pillow. Keep your eyes closed.* [Pause]

Slowly open your eyes half way as you use your hands to come up, sitting in Pretzel Pose.

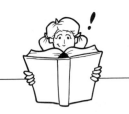

Learn About Yoga

Namaste is a Sanskrit word that means "I recognize and honor the divine light within you." It's a nice way to greet or say goodbye to someone, and an especially nice way to end a yoga practice when more than one yogini is involved.

After Visualization and Deep Relaxation

We like to end visualization and relaxation by chanting the word *Om*, which recognizes the unity of all our experiences, and by bowing to fellow yoginis, saying the word *Namaste* (pronounced *nah-mah-stay*), which means "I recognize and honor the divine light in you." Then it's time to give yourself a great big hug of thanks and self-affirmation!

It's also nice to talk about your relaxation experiences after they are over. How did it go? Where were you? What did you see, hear, and feel? You might like to describe the experience to a parent, friend, or the person who read the visual imagery exercise to you. Or you might like to draw a picture of it. But if you want to keep it to yourself, that's just fine, too.

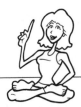

Yoga Stories

Getting in the habit of going to bed on time helps kids get the sleep they need, and Shavasana before bedtime makes a nice ritual to help ease kids into dreamland. The right amount of sleep is important for kids, from infancy through the teen years. Infants sleep, on average, 16 to 17 hours each day. By the time your child is in grade school, he or she needs about 10 hours of sleep each night, and some researchers believe teenagers need between 9 and 11 hours of sleep per night (much more than many of them get).

Moving from Shavasana into the Day

Once you have completed Shavasana, tune in to your body to identify the way you feel. More relaxed? More positive? Sleepy? Energized? Knowing how Shavasana makes a yogini feel can help determine what other times of day it might be appropriate, because while Shavasana is the perfect finish to a yoga routine, it can be practiced at any time of day. It can help kids fall asleep, relax before a test, get energized after a long day at school, or just give them a breather in the middle of a busy day.

The Least You Need to Know

➤ Shavasana is yoga's deep relaxation pose, traditionally practiced as the last pose in a yoga workout.

➤ Shavasana is best practiced in a dimly lit room with soft music and no distraction.

➤ The Shavasana Pose involves lying in a prone position, arms and legs apart, and eyes relaxed and closed.

➤ A parent, sibling, or friend can help the yogini relax in Shavasana by reading relaxing guided imagery visualizations such as the ones in this book.

Part 6

Especially for New Families

In this part, yoga is customized for all the unique and specific needs of new families. The postpartum period can be tough, both physically and emotionally, for new moms. Yoga can help ease the transition from pregnancy to motherhood through breathing exercises, deep relaxation, and certain poses of great benefit to a postpartum mom's adjustments. This time is challenging for new dads, too, and yoga is equally beneficial to help fathers handle their own physical and emotional needs.

Infant yoga can encourage healthy development and is a lovely, hands-on way for parents and newborns to bond. Toddler yoga is pure joy for toddlers and parents alike, as both explore the ever-expanding limits of a toddler's physical abilities and imagination.

Last of all, we'll give you some great ideas for using yoga to help siblings bond, with poses, games, and a whole new take on yoga's yamas and niyamas: the Yogini's 10 Steps for Sibling Synchronicity.

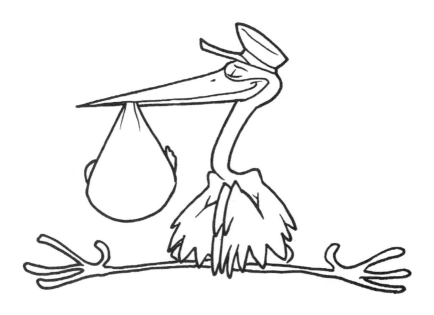

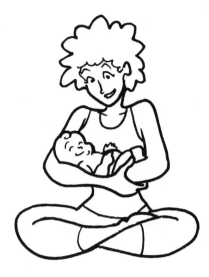

Chapter 20

Yoga for Postpartum Moms and Brand-New Dads

In This Chapter

➤ Your awesome new role as a parent

➤ Breathing exercises to calm new moms and dads

➤ Yoga poses for the postpartum period

➤ Yoga relaxation for new moms

➤ Yoga after Cesarean delivery

➤ Yoga breathing, poses, and relaxation for brand-new dads

Mom, Dad, this chapter is for you. While we've spent chapters talking about how important, fun, and beneficial yoga is for kids, we felt this is the place to stress how important yoga is for new parents, because nothing changes a family like the addition of a new baby.

For first-time parents, the change from childless couple to new parents can sometimes seem staggering, awesome, amazing, and a little overwhelming. Brand-new parents typically get very little sleep, often have a sudden decrease in income, are barraged with visitors, and are undergoing a sudden and dramatic shift in the family's focus from each other to that tiny little creature who is so beautiful and so entirely helpless! That's a lot to cope with.

But new parents can benefit immensely from a regular yoga practice.

While many of the yoga exercises and poses in this book are as good for parents as they are for kids, some work better than others for the individual needs of postpartum moms and brand-new dads, and those are the exercises and poses we will focus on in this chapter.

You've Got a New Baby!

Parenthood. It is a majestic calling. New parents often describe their stunned state of disbelief: me, a parent? How do I communicate with this little human being? How will I know what it wants? Will I do everything the right way?

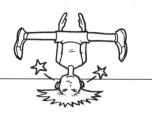

Ooops!

Even if you feel up to doing all your old and familiar yoga poses in the weeks after giving birth, use extra caution when attempting balance poses. Your center of gravity has changed since pregnancy and your body will have to learn to readjust, so take it slow until you feel comfortable with your recently altered body.

When life changes so dramatically, it is nice to have something that stays the same, something comforting, familiar, and really good for you. Something like yoga!

Parents may find a personal yoga practice incredibly rewarding during this transitional time. On top of all the external stresses, new moms are undergoing incredible hormonal changes that may catch them completely off guard. Yoga can help new moms maintain an emotional balance and can begin rebuilding strength and balance in that newly nonpregnant body.

New dads can also benefit from yoga, to help them relax or get energized, regain perspective, deal with the inevitable frustration of carving out a new role in the family, and to feel like an important part of the family circle.

Because the physical changes involved in childbirth and the postpartum period are so dramatic, let's start with yoga for new moms. Dads, you'll be next, so bear with us.

Yoga's Postpartum Poses for New Moms

Whether childbirth was easier than you thought it would be or a whole lot harder, that postpartum period of physical readjusting and roller coaster emotional changes can be pretty tough. Suddenly your center of balance has changed. You are probably sore in at least one place (depending on what kind of delivery you had), and maybe lots of places. You might be weepy, irritable, or sad one minute, then glowing with maternal feelings the next.

The first six weeks after childbirth are a challenge, and considering you probably aren't getting much sleep, you might wonder how you'll ever make it!

It gets easier. It really does! And yoga can help ease the transition. Making time for a daily yoga practice can do wonders for your emotional state and can help your body recover from pregnancy and childbirth more quickly.

We suggest that moms in the postpartum period take 20 minutes out of each day for some simple breathing exercises, targeted yoga poses, and deep relaxation. If you think you don't have 20 minutes, consider it an investment in your abilities to take better care of your infant. You've got time while your baby naps, or you can call on your family resources. Your partner, a parent, a mature older child, or a trusted babysitter could keep your infant entertained for 20 minutes. You need this, and your baby needs you to take care of yourself, too. Do it for the little one!

Breathing Exercises (Pranayama)

Pranayama is the Sanskrit word for breathing exercises. Keeping your body breathing efficiently will make you feel better, give you more energy, and even help you to relax when you finally have an hour or two to sleep. We described many breathing exercises for kids in Chapter 10. Any and all of these will work for postpartum moms and new dads, too.

Retraining your body to breathe deeply, expanding the abdomen with the inhale instead of the chest, feels great, will imbue you with energy you never knew you had, and will also help you to relax when you most need it.

The following exercises are especially good ones for postpartum moms to try (and new dads can benefit, too):

➤ **Belly Breathing** (described in Chapter 10) is a good way to begin getting your stomach muscles back in shape. For the last few months, you haven't had much room to breathe and those muscles have been stretched. Now you've got all that space again and your

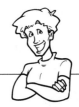

For Grownups, Too!

New moms sometimes find it incredibly difficult to spend time nurturing themselves. Doesn't motherhood mean giving all your energy to your child? Of course not! Moms who take care of themselves, stay healthy, listen to their bodies, eat well, exercise, and give themselves the relaxation time and personal space they need will be building the resources required to be a good mother.

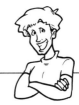

For Grownups, Too!

Depending on how you feel, lying flat on your back for deep breathing might be uncomfortable, especially if you've had a Cesarean delivery. Comfort is key to getting the most out of pranayama, so if it helps, prop yourself up on lots of pillows, on the floor, couch, or bed for your breathing exercises.

muscles need to remember where they are supposed to go! Lie down comfortably on your back and breathe into your belly, expanding and contracting your abdomen as you keep your chest and shoulders still.

➤ **Fly Like a Bird** (see Chapter 10) can help you gain control over your body and stay in a positive frame of mind about how you feel and look. Let yourself feel graceful and beautiful as you breathe while moving your "wings."

➤ **Alternate Nostril Breathing** (see Chapter 10) can help you to feel centered and focused when life has you frazzled and exhausted (which it will, at times). It is a good way to wind down after finally getting your baby to sleep, so you can focus on something else (like sleeping!).

➤ **Baby Breathing** is an exercise just for new parents. We don't mention it in Chapter 10 because it is a special one for parent-infant bonding, although a sibling could do this with a new baby as well. Baby Breathing is a lovely way to synchronize your energy with your infant's energy. When your baby is resting quietly in your arms or sleeping nearby, cuddle up close so your faces are near but not directly pointed toward each other. Cheek to cheek is nice, or when your baby is lying on your chest with his or her head nested under your chin. Listen for your baby's breathing. Then, in the same rhythm, let your breathing patterns synchronize (breathing through your nose). With each inhale your infant makes, you *exhale* gently. With each exhale your infant makes, you *inhale* gently. Imagine the air between you is infused with love that your baby breathes out and you breathe in, that you breathe out and your baby breathes in. Ah, this is what it's all about!

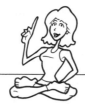

Yoga Stories

Those postpartum weeks are full of surprises. Beyond the notorious mood swings, you might also find you keep forgetting things, losing things, tripping over things, dropping things, and suddenly having no idea why you came into a room or what you were about to say. Don't worry, you aren't losing your mind. You are just experiencing some dramatic hormonal swings as your body adjusts to not being pregnant anymore. Take a little extra care of yourself during this time. Sleep whenever you can, eat fresh, healthy foods, drink lots of water, and take a few minutes to yourself each day to relax and breath.

Yoga Poses for Postpartum Moms (Asanas)

Sometimes moms need a real energy boost, and asanas are a great way to get one. When you are feeling blue, out of sorts, or just plain tired, gentle asanas can be a real pick-me-up to get you through the rest of the day (or night!).

About two weeks after the birth (about four weeks after a Cesarean delivery), you can start doing many asanas, but take it easy and start slowly. If you notice an increase in *lochia* or if you start to bleed, that's a sign you're doing too much. Take it back a notch.

Following are some of the poses we find helpful for new moms in the postpartum period. Each of these poses was described and discussed in earlier chapters (as referenced) for children, but they are all appropriate for adults, too.

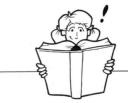

Learn About Yoga

Lochia is the fluid and blood you will pass for a week or two after giving birth. Your body is getting rid of all that excess fluid gradually. The amount and color of lochia are helpful indicators that can tell you if you are doing too much. Lochia should taper off gradually and turn browner; if it suddenly turns bright red or increases in amount, slow down now! If the flow increases dramatically, call your doctor.

➤ **Pretzel Pose** and **Lotus Pose** (see Chapter 17) are great ways to sit, energize and stretch your hips, and regain your confidence and sense of self. Start with Pretzel and work up to Lotus Pose.

➤ **Mouse Pose** (see Chapter 12), also aptly called Child's Pose, is a wonderful way to take care of yourself and "mother" yourself for a few minutes.

➤ **Snake poses** (see Chapter 13) are wonderful for reenergizing and activating the stomach muscles and strengthening the arms (you'll need it—you've got a bundle of joy to carry around!). Nursing a baby or cradling your infant tends to round the back and slump the chest forward, and snake poses help to strengthen and tone the back muscles. Start with Baby Snake Pose and work your way up as you're ready.

➤ **Cat Pose** and **Cow Pose** (see Chapter 12) are great for easing lower back discomfort that so often accompanies that shift in balance from pregnant to no longer pregnant.

➤ **Camel Pose** (see Chapter 13) is a lovely way to open up the front of your body and let your emotions out as you give your back and spine a nice arch, to counteract the forward-bending effect of carrying and leaning over a baby all day.

➤ **Bear Walk** (see Chapter 14) lets you loosen up, have a little fun, and take some of the weight off your feet. Plus, babies think it's funny to see mommy walking around like that!

➤ **Mountain Pose** (see Chapter 11) can help you feel grounded and strong.

➤ **Tree Pose** (see Chapter 11) is a great way to regain balance. Try it holding on to the back of a chair or a wall until your body can remember how it feels to stand on one foot without all that extra weight in front!

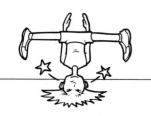

Ooops!

Lots of new moms get the postpartum blues, consisting of mood swings, fits of weepiness and/or irritability, and occasional feelings of anxiety. Some moms get a more serious form of postpartum depression, however. If you feel unable to cope with the demands of parenting or can't seem to stop extremely negative or irrational feelings, see your doctor immediately. Postpartum depression is very treatable and more common than you may think.

➤ **Warrior Poses I, II, and III** (see Chapter 16) are power poses that can imbue new moms (who sometimes feel a little fragile and unsteady) with a sense of confidence, authority, vigor, courage, and energy. Nothing beats a series of warrior poses for energizing a new mom, both physically and mentally.

➤ **The Yoga Sun Dance** (see Chapter 15) or Sun Salutation, as it is also known, is a great exercise for new moms. It helps you to feel bonded with nature and part of the processes of the natural world, connecting you with the sun and the Earth. Depending on how you feel, you might want to modify parts of the Yoga Sun Dance so they feel more comfortable. For example, if you've had a Cesarean delivery, you might not want to raise your arms all the way up over your heads. Raise them out to the sides instead. When coming down into Downward Facing Dog, you might prefer to stand on your hands and knees instead of your hands and feet. Just listen to your body and make adjustments to keep yourself comfortable.

Deep Relaxation (Shavasana)

If we could pick just one single yoga pose that would most benefit new moms, it would be Shavasana (see Chapter 19). This valuable, calming, energizing, centering, balancing exercise gives each body what it needs at the moment. Committing to just 10 minutes a day for Shavasana, with or without accompanying spoken visualizations, can be the nicest, best, and most productive thing a new mom can do for herself and her new baby during the postpartum weeks.

The visualizations we provided in the last chapter were kid oriented. The following visualization is nice for postpartum moms, to help them relax and feel great. Have a partner or older child read this to you while you relax, or record yourself reading it on a cassette tape and play it back. Feel free to make this visualization longer, shorter, or different in any way. Or make up your own.

Lie back comfortably, close your eyes, and relax. [Pause] Breathe gently and deeply, and imagine that with every inhale, you take in love, peace, and serenity. [Pause] With every exhale, you let go of stress, negativity, and confusion. Breathe in peace, breathe out stress. Imagine your breath filling your body with light. [Pause]

Now feel your body against the Earth. Imagine the Earth is cradling you in its arms. Imagine the Earth speaking to you: "You, too, are now a mother. We are a family of creators, you and I. See the beauty of our creation." [Pause]

Now, imagine the Earth lifting you gently up and handing you to the sun. You feel your body growing lighter and lighter as the sun wraps you in light and lifts you. [Pause] You feel warm and safe, utterly cared for. The light within you seems to buoy you up and you float, weightless, gently, slowly into the sky. You look below and see miles of rolling green hills, fields of flowers, sparkling lakes and rivers flowing into green oceans. You feel safe and comfortable, still cradled by the warm sun. Take a minute to look at the lovely Earth below you. [Long pause]

Now, you slowly begin to sink back down as the sun brings you back to Earth. You come down and down, getting closer to the green, the blue, and the other bright colors. [Pause] You come back down into your own home and you look down to find your baby cradled and sleeping in your arms. You hear the Earth's voice again: "What you have made is equally beautiful, just as miraculous, and vaster than all the Earth." You know it is true. [Pause]

Now, imagine placing your sleeping baby gently into its crib, covering it with a blanket, watching for a moment, then slowly, slowly, prepare to come out of the deep relaxation and awaken your body. [Pause] Slowly wiggle your toes and your fingers. Stretch your arms and legs in any way that feels comfortable. Gently roll to your side and curl up into the fetal pose, the pose that your baby was in when inside your belly. Rest here for a moment. [Pause] Now, slowly, open your eyes, and slowly, slowly use your hands in front of you to come to a sitting position. Thank yourself for your practice.

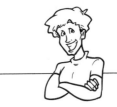

For Grownups, Too!

The visualization in this chapter has to do with creation and your new infant. Sometimes you might want to focus on things other than motherhood for your visualizations. Try adapting the visualizations in Chapter 19 according to your own interests.

When You've Had a Cesarean Delivery

We certainly don't mean to imply, by this separate section, that the previous advice and postpartum poses don't apply to those of you who had a Cesarean delivery. Listen to your body and proceed as you feel ready.

However, if you've had a Cesarean delivery, the thought of yoga might make you cringe. It hurts to move! How are you supposed to do yoga? The hours and days after a Cesarean can be extremely frustrating. Doctors tell you not to lift your baby, not to let your older children jump on you, and all you want to do is scoop up everybody and give them a reassuring hug! Well-meaning family and friends might try to do everything for you and this can be frustrating, too (although sometimes it can be a great relief to let people help you).

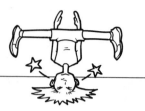

Ooops!

After a Cesarean delivery, wait three or four weeks before trying yoga poses beyond the most basic (such as Mountain Pose and Shavasana). To protect your incision, avoid any poses that really stretch your abdomen. Also, if lying flat on your back is painful, again, use lots of pillows to prop yourself up and make yourself comfy.

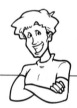

For Grownups, Too!

If the weather permits, one of the nicest ways to recover after a Cesarean delivery is to take a walk outside in the fresh air and sunshine. No need to walk fast. A slow, leisurely pace is all it takes. Your body will benefit from the exercise and your soul will be nourished by the contact with nature.

But here is a very true and very important fact about recovering from a Cesarean delivery: The sooner you move, the sooner you will stop hurting. It's true! As much as it hurts to try to sit up that very first time, if you try it the very next day after your delivery (with help), you will recover much, much faster.

Of course, you shouldn't tax yourself beyond your limits. You have had surgery, and too much bending, stretching, or shaking could damage the incision or put too much stress on your recovering body. We aren't suggesting you do a headstand. But we are suggesting you practice sitting up and, most important, walking as soon as you can. We know. It hurts! But you can do it. (Again, we stress, let someone help you with sitting up and walking, especially at first.)

You can do a few yoga poses right away, even the day of your Cesarean:

➤ **Balloon Breathing** (see Chapter 10) is great to do after a general anesthetic or an epidural (the anesthetic that numbs you from the waist down so you can be awake during a delivery). It is important to begin breathing deeply right away. Begin Balloon Breathing right away to practice filling your lungs completely and emptying them fully, and also to help reactivate those abdominal muscles.

➤ **Butterfly Pose** (see Chapter 11) is a nice hip stretch that very gently and only peripherally engages your abdominal muscles.

➤ **Japanese Sitting Pose** (see Chapter 13) is a pose where you sit on your heels with your feet and knees close together. This is a nice position to help get your leg muscles stimulated while talking to your baby.

➤ **Mountain Pose** (see Chapter 11) is appropriate for when you are ready to stand. Sustained for short periods, it's a stabilizing and confidence-building pose to try.

➤ **Warrior II Pose** (see Chapter 16) gives you an incredible sense of power and confidence, and it raises your arms and moves your body just enough to begin activating your body without putting excess strain on your incision, which the other warrior poses might do.

➤ **Shavasana** (see Chapter 19) is a wonderful pose to do right after a Cesarean (or any birth). You will probably be much more comfortable if, rather than trying to lie flat, you prop your upper body on a load of pillows (or crank up the top end of that hospital bed if you had a hospital birth).

Although many of the visualizations in this book are wonderful and beneficial for any postpartum mom, the following visualization is specifically designed for moms who have experienced a Cesarean. It is designed to help the body heal. Have someone read it to you as you relax in Shavasana, or read it on a cassette tape and play it back as you rest:

Imagine a light shining over your body. [Pause] First it is white, then it turns into a color, any color you would like. Choose the color and see the light as it changes. [Pause]

Now feel the light shining down over your entire body. As the light shines on you, it sends healing energy and peace into your body. [Pause] Feel the light as it covers you and surrounds you with healing energy. [Pause]

Now that the colored light has infused your body, imagine your body glowing from within with the beautiful light. Feel the healing and peace within you. [Pause] Imagine your body mending and adjusting, coming back into balance. [Pause] Breathe and meditate for a few minutes on the healing power of the light within you. [Pause]

Now slowly, slowly, prepare to come out of the deep relaxation and awaken your body. [Pause] Slowly wiggle your toes and your fingers. Stretch your arms and legs in any way that feels comfortable. Gently roll to your side and curl up into the fetal pose, the pose that your baby was in when inside your belly. Rest here for a moment. [Pause] Now, slowly open your eyes and slowly, slowly use your hands in front of you to come to a sitting position. Thank yourself for your practice and recognize how your body feels after this deep relaxation.

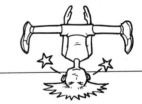

Ooops!

Even months after your incision is healed, you might occasionally feel a twinge in the area. However, if you experience an area of bright redness or discharge on or around your incision, see your doctor immediately. You might have an infection.

Hey, Dad!

This is a time when dads sometimes feel a little left out. Although they may participate in the birth, they are, by biological necessity, mostly observers. While they can bond with their newborn, they may believe they should step back and allow the new mother to take her primary role.

Mothers are the primary focus of a child's attention for the first few years, but primary doesn't mean *only*. Dads who are involved from the beginning develop strong, lasting, valuable relationships with their children, and a great way to get involved is by doing yoga—with your new baby and on your own, too.

Whether or not you've ever done yoga before, now is a good time to start, because yoga is an excellent way to manage stress, diffuse anxiety, and even channel anger.

Sometimes new dads get angry. We aren't suggesting you are angry at your partner or new baby, but new fathers do sometimes experience frustration and anger as they attempt to adjust to a new role, deal with changing family dynamics, and handle the awesome responsibility of being, in many cases, the sole financial provider for the family, at least for awhile.

On top of these feelings, new dads are often extremely tired because they are up at night helping with feeding the baby. Dads are often expected to participate actively in infant care but at the same time, aren't supposed to miss a beat when it comes to their jobs. That's a lot to handle.

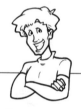

For Grownups, Too!

New parents can gain a lot from a regular meditation practice. New parenting is taxing and meditation helps to balance the whole self by stilling the mind for awhile each day. After Shavasana, try five minutes of quiet, alert sitting in Pretzel Pose or Lotus Pose. Notice, observe, breathe, be, but don't think, solve, try, or do.

Yoga is a great way to help new dads feel more in control of their feelings. The following poses we find particularly helpful for new dads, although any yoga pose, including the many we mentioned in earlier chapters, is appropriate. These poses help channel excess energy, keep dads calm and centered, and even provide an energy boost for dads who are ready to fall asleep on their feet.

➤ **Warrior Poses I, II, and III** (see Chapter 16) are great for helping dads regain a sense of balance, control, strength, and power. They boost confidence and balance the emotions, streamlining energy so it can be channeled more productively.

➤ **Camel Pose** (see Chapter 13) opens the front of the body and helps dads to get in touch with their emotions while stretching overworked backs and necks. This pose feels good after a long night.

➤ **Tarzan Holler** (see Chapter 14) lets you let loose some of that excess energy. You may feel like a little kid doing this one, but that can be great! (Just don't do it when the baby is asleep, or the baby won't be asleep for long!)

➤ **Handstand** (see Chapter 16) is the perfect pose for dads who feel their worlds are turning upside-down. Go with the flow and turn upside-down yourself! Do Handstand against a wall for stability. Handstand builds arm strength, reestablishes focus and concentration, and encourages confidence.

➤ **Baby Lift** is a nice way for dads to bond with their infants. Do this exercise when your infant is awake, alert, and ready to play. But not right after a meal! (Keep a spit-up rag handy in any case.) Lie on your back and place your infant on your chest. Place your hands securely around your baby and lift him or her over you (not over your face, but over your spit-up-rag-clad chest). Lift your baby up, down, up, down, up, down. Maintain eye contact and smile, talk, coo, sing, or otherwise engage your baby's attention. Continue until either baby or your arms tire.

Baby Lift.

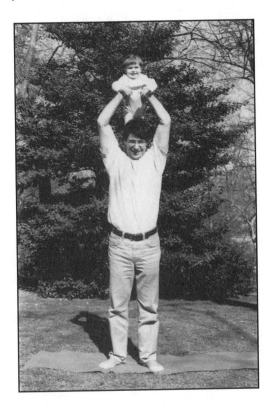

➤ **Shavasana** (see Chapter 19) benefits anyone and everyone, new dads included. Not only do you need a good rest but the centering and calming benefits of deep relaxation will help you feel confident, calm, and secure in your new role as dad. Spend 10 minutes a day in Shavasana and enjoy newfound self-control, concentration, and peace of mind. New dads can also appropriately adapt any of the visualizations in Chapter 19.

While everyone can benefit from yoga, it can change the lives of new parents for the better in so many ways that we can't help but recommend it with the greatest enthusiasm. But wouldn't it be fun to include your new infant in your yoga routine? You can! Read on. The next chapter will show you how.

The Least You Need to Know

➤ The awesome responsibility and associated stresses of new parenthood can be managed and greatly eased by a regular yoga practice.

➤ Yoga breathing, poses, and relaxation help new moms feel emotionally balanced as they regain their physical strength and balance.

➤ Yoga can speed up recovery for moms who delivered by Cesarean.

➤ Yoga can help new dads feel energized and confident as family dynamics and roles change with the arrival of a newborn.

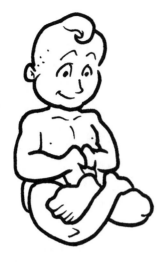

Chapter 21

Yoga with Infants and Toddlers

> **In This Chapter**
>
> ➤ Your infant is a natural yogini!
>
> ➤ How to bond with your baby through yoga
>
> ➤ Toddler playtime is learning time, too
>
> ➤ The imagination explosion of toddler yoga

People are often incredulous when they first hear that infants can do yoga. "How can a baby do yoga?" they ask, eyebrows raised.

Yoga is easy for babies! We're not saying your eight-week-old infant is suddenly going to assume the Lotus position all by him- or herself. But yoga poses are based on natural human movements, and those are just the movements infants and toddlers spend their days exploring.

The first two years of life mark an explosion of brain growth. This chapter explores yoga activities for infants and toddlers, to help take full advantage of this developmentally active time. Yoga can quickly become an essential and much anticipated family time, a lovely way to introduce a new baby to the world, to get to know your child, and to channel your toddler's energy.

Getting to Know You

A new infant can seem at once incredibly foreign and as familiar as the palm of your hand. How do you get to know this little person? You can't have a conversation, exactly. But you can bond and communicate in other ways.

While infants naturally assume certain yoga-like poses, infant yoga involves a parent/child (or teacher/child) interaction. This interaction is like a conversation, but it uses touch and movement instead of words. Yoga between parents and infants is an incredible, nurturing, bonding experience that provides infants (and parents!) with exactly what they crave: touch, warmth, and closeness.

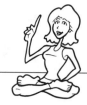

Yoga Stories

Infant yoga is great for any baby, but is extremely beneficial for kids with special needs. For example, infants with Down's syndrome or cerebral palsy can benefit immensely from an early intervention yoga program. These children often experience delays in developing motor coordination, and yoga practice seems to stimulate muscles, organs, and glands in a way that assists and promotes development. Performing yoga with your baby is helpful in bringing development closer to what is considered "typically" age appropriate. For more information on the effects of early intervention yoga on children with special needs, refer to the seminal work on the subject, Sonia Sumar's *Yoga for the Special Child* (see Appendix B).

In addition to establishing a physical bond with your child, infant yoga is also highly beneficial for the child's burgeoning development. Moving an infant in certain ways and into certain positions helps to stimulate and activate muscle development, bone strength, joint mobility, and the development of the arches of the feet, the five senses, and the very first communication skills—eye contact, cooing, gesturing, reaching, repeating. All of these influences help establish the synaptic connections that grow a baby's brain to its fullest potential. What a wonderful gift to give to your child!

Infant yoga can also help to alleviate a number of physical discomforts for infants, including colic, constipation, and gas. It helps to strengthen and maintain the nervous system, improves motor coordination, and even increases lung capacity.

The following sequences of infant yoga poses are adapted from Sonia Sumar's book *Yoga for the Special Child*. Yoga with babies is best practiced on a soft, safe, firm surface, such as a carpeted floor, covered with a soft baby blanket. If you have a hard floor, considered using a mat covered with a blanket. And remember, babies are people, too! If they don't feel like doing yoga or act resistant, try again later. Respect your yogini's reactions and always tell him or her what you are doing, such as, "Good morning, yogini! Shall we do some foot circles?"

Baby Breather

We believe that if a parent exposes an infant to specific breathing exercises, such as Breath of Fire (see Chapter 10), eventually the baby will join in. Obviously, a baby must be ready, developmentally, to do specific breathing exercises, but when the time is right, the yogini will already be familiar with what the technique sounds and looks like. Practicing breathing exercises around a baby is cleansing and rejuvenating for the parent doing the exercise, and a productive stimulus for the baby. Any breathing exercise in this book will work.

Footsies

Time to play a little footsy with your baby! The feet are less sensitive than other parts of your baby's body, so they are a good place to warm up and prepare your yogini for more stimulating yoga poses. Footsies increases joint elasticity in the feet and ankles, and strengthens the tendons, nerves, and muscles of the feet. It also helps develop your yogini's arches.

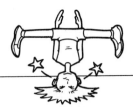

Ooops!

Sensory stimulation is great for babies, but babies can easily get overstimulated, too. Signs that your baby is suffering from sensory overload include a refusal to look you in the eye, suddenly falling asleep, crying for no apparent reason, or staring blankly. Suspect sensory overload if you have been on the go all day with no down time for your baby to relax.

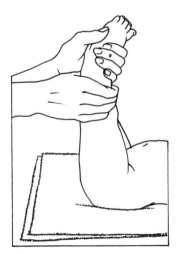

Footsies.

(Drawing by Wendy Frost)

1. Place your baby on his or her back and sit at your baby's feet. Take one of your baby's feet in your hand.

2. Hold your yogini lightly by the ankle with one hand and with the other hand, hold your baby's toes.

3. Move your baby's foot in circles, first one way, then the other way. A few circles should be enough unless your yogini is gurgling for more!

4. Now hold your baby's leg just above the ankle and with the other hand, again grasp your baby's toes.

5. Gently flex and point your baby's foot a few times.

6. Now give the soles of your yogini's foot a gentle massage with your fingertips and thumb, working from toes to heel. Don't forget to massage the inside arch.

7. Repeat with your baby's other foot.

Knees, Please!

Knees, Please! is a relaxing movement for babies that increases mobility of the knees and hips, and stimulates the abdominal organs. It can even help to relieve colic and gas, and relax your baby before naptime or bedtime.

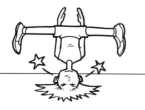

Ooops!

When manipulating your yogini's feet, legs, and hips, always keep his or her spine in alignment by keeping the raised leg vertical, rather than bending it to one side, and by keeping both hips flat on the floor.

1. As your baby lies on his or her back, place one hand on top of your baby's thigh and the other below the knee. Raise your baby's leg off the ground, flexing the knee as it rises. The other leg should stay straight and flat on the floor.

2. Gently move your baby's raised knee toward his chest, bending the knee and stopping just at the point when you feel resistance. Don't force your baby's leg beyond this point!

3. Return the leg back to the floor, and repeat a few times, then repeat with the other leg.

4. Now raise both knees toward your baby's chest, repeating a few times.

Get Hip, Baby!

Babies' hips may seem much more flexible than adult hips. Babies can lift their legs and bat effortlessly at their toes! But hip exercises are still great for babies as their muscles and bones grow. Hip exercises tone the organs of the abdomen as well as increase hip and knee mobility.

1. Coming out of the knee exercises, return both of baby's legs to the floor, then place one hand on top of your baby's thigh and the other below the knee.

2. Raise your baby's leg and make gentle, slow circles with his or her knee. First move the leg out to the side as you bend the knee. Use your other hand to keep the other leg flat on the floor.

3. Now move your baby's knee in an arc-like motion toward the center of your baby's body, then extend the leg straight out and back down to the floor where it started.

4. Repeat several times, then repeat with the other leg.

Yogini's Sleep Pose

Rock a bye baby ... while this comfy pose may not exactly induce instant sleep in a yogini baby, it is excellent for increasing flexibility of the hips, knees, and back. It may also help to relieve colic.

1. From the hip exercise, take hold of your baby's ankles and raise the legs off the floor until they are at a right angle to the floor.

2. Gently bend your baby's legs and hold the soles of the feet together, making a diamond shape with the legs.

3. Holding this position with one hand, use the other hand to gently lift the baby's head toward the feet. The feet should come above the chest, toward or touching the head.

4. Don't force your baby into the position if he or she doesn't want to do it, but for many babies, this position is easy, relaxing, and interesting. You want to bring the feet above the chest area and head to meet.

Up in Arms

This arm exercise activates your baby's upper body, developing strength, coordination, and lung capacity. Your baby can see her arms more easily than her legs, so these exercises also promote visual-motor (eye-hand) coordination and body awareness.

1. Place your baby on his or her back and take a hand in each of your hands.

2. Gently stretch your baby's arms out to each side, straight out from the shoulders.

3. Press your thumb into each palm to stimulate a grasping response.

4. Now raise one arm, bringing it perpendicular to the floor, above your baby's chest. Lower it and stretch the arm arms to each side again.

5. Repeat several times, then repeat with the other arm.

6. Now raise both arms straight up at the same time, bringing your baby's hands together above his or her chest.

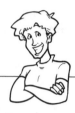

For Grownups, Too!

Few things feel more wonderful to new parents than being the recipient of an infant's smile. Social smiling is smiling in response to external stimuli such as the sight of a mother's face, certain noises, or the appearance of a toy. Spending lots of time making eye contact with and talking to your yogini will get you lots of smiles!

7. Stretch your baby's arms out to the sides again, then lower.

8. Now raise your baby's arm straight up and over so it is reaching over your baby's head. Lower that arm as you bring the other arm over your baby's head. Repeat, slowly alternating arms back and forth in a scissors-like motion.

Tummy Time

This series of exercises are performed with your yogini lying on his tummy. Some babies love this position. Others prefer to be on their backs where they can see what is going on around them. If your baby resists, try these poses again another day.

These tummy poses strengthen your baby's lower back, buttocks, abdominal and leg muscles, tone the abdominal organs, and increase the mobility of the hip and knee joints.

1. Place your baby on his or her tummy with both legs outstretched and both arms next to his or her body.

2. Place one hand on your baby's lower back. Place your other hand under one knee, securing it from bending.

3. Slowly raise one leg off the floor, keeping your other hand in place to secure your baby's hips against the floor. Stop at the point of resistance, then return the leg to the floor.

4. Repeat several times, then repeat with the other leg.

5. Try lifting both legs at the same time with one hand. Keep your other hand in place on baby's lower back.

6. Now hold baby's calf with one hand and lift baby's lower leg only, bending it at the knee. Lower the leg back to the floor.

7. Lift and lower the leg several times, then repeat with the other leg.

8. Lift both lower legs at the same time. Remember, never move past the point of resistance.

9. Try a modified Cobra Pose (we call this Baby Snake Pose in Chapter 13). Kneel behind and over the baby. Make a cooing sound or other attractive sound, to get your baby's attention. This will prompt the baby to press into his or her hands and come into Cobra Pose!

Upside-Down Baby!

Inversions are as good for babies as they are for big kids (and grownups!). Although babies don't feel the effects of gravity as much as kids who walk around all day do, inversions nevertheless redirect blood and fluid flow in their bodies, flooding their brains and upper-body organs and glands with oxygen and other nutrients. Inversions are great for your baby's nervous system, sensory organs, and even memory. Inversions also help your baby's digestion and elimination systems work more smoothly.

Prepare young babies for the more dramatic inversions older kids practice with this gentle, well supported inversion.

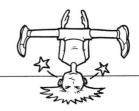

Ooops!

Babies are very flexible but also fragile. Never manipulate a yogini's body beyond where it naturally wants to go, and always pay attention to your baby's reaction to what you do.

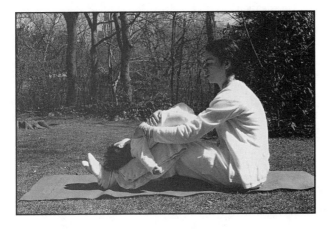

Upside-Down Baby Pose.

1. Sit with your legs outstretched and together. Cover your legs with a soft blanket or towel.

2. Place your baby on your legs, on his or her back, with your baby's feet on your thighs and baby's head resting just above your ankles. Your baby's spine should be centered between your legs.

3. Hold baby's thighs with one forearm, and baby's upper body with your other forearm.

4. Slowly raise your knees to form an inverted V with your legs. Don't increase the angle of your legs beyond 45 degrees from the floor.

5. Hold for about 10 seconds at first. Work up to two minutes (if your baby is uncomfortable, end the pose).

6. Slowly lower your legs to the floor, then lift your baby off your legs, allowing your baby to rest on his or her back for a few minutes. This rest time allows your baby's blood pressure to equalize after the inversion.

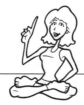

Yoga Stories

Many studies have been conducted to determine how infants see the world around them. Infants prefer to look at striped patches rather than solid patches, may be partially color-blind (although this is difficult to determine), and prefer to look at a picture of a normally constructed face as opposed to a picture of a rearranged face. Four-month-olds can perceive a partially covered object as a whole object, six-month-olds have depth perception, and spatial perception continues to develop throughout childhood. Parents can use all these cues to make infant yoga more fun and effective, such as using striped toys and pictures or partially covered objects and pictures to get a baby's attention or to help direct a baby into different poses.

Baby Relaxation

It's a lot of work being a baby. That constant movement, exploration, discovery, and growth take a lot of energy. After a nice workout of infant yoga, your baby can benefit immensely from deep relaxation similar to the Shavasana Pose (see Chapter 19) practiced by bigger kids and adults.

How do you get a baby to lie still and relax? By minimizing sensory input and by giving him or her a nice infant massage. Deep relaxation releases tension from your baby's body, gives your baby's mind and body a rest from the stimulation of the day, and balances your yogini's internal energies.

1. Place your baby on a blanket, on his or her back. Dim the lights, put on some soft, gentle, relaxing music, and minimize the possibility of distractions (unplug phones, ask other family members to keep voices down, and so on). Cover your baby with a soft blanket if you think he or she might get cold.

2. Sit at your baby's feet and spread your baby's legs about six inches apart.

3. Take one of your baby's feet in each hand and gently massage the soles with your thumbs. Work your way around to the top of each foot.

4. If your baby seems to be enjoying the massage, keep rubbing your baby's feet, or massage baby's legs, arms, shoulders, and scalp, too. Or, if baby seems to want to be left alone, let your baby rest.

5. Allow your yogini to relax for as long as he or she likes. Five to ten minutes is an ideal time, but if your baby falls asleep for an hour, that's fine! If your baby squirms upright and wants to play after two minutes, that's fine, too. Let your baby set the time limit.

6. After about 10 minutes, if your baby is awake but still relaxing, gently rouse your baby by singing softly, talking to him or her, chanting, or resuming the foot massage.

7. When your baby is awake and ready to play, give him or her lots of hugs, kisses, and affirmation. Assure your baby that he or she is a natural yogini! And of course, tell your baby how much you love him or her.

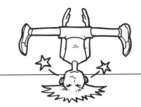

Ooops!

Sometimes infants resist yoga, squirming against your movements or crying. Resistance doesn't necessarily mean your baby doesn't like yoga. Your baby could be crying for a number of reasons: hunger, fatigue, colic, or gas, for example. Play with the timing of your yoga sessions. You can also move babies into yoga positions while they are sleeping, but wait until the end of naptime.

Toddler Land: Learning Through Play

Once your tiny, helpless little infant manages to tip upright and start toddling across the room, the world changes—your baby's world, and your world, too! Suddenly your baby isn't a baby anymore. Your baby surprises you each day with his or her new skills, astute and original questions, and resourcefulness. And the energy ... oh my goodness, the energy!

Anyone with a toddler knows that toddlers don't learn by sitting and studying for long periods of time. Toddlers learn through play. That's why toddlers love yoga! Yoga is learning play, and a regular yoga practice provides moving, growing, curious toddlers with a great outlet for their energies and explorations.

Toddlers may be small, but with a few adjustments here and there, they can do lots of yoga poses older kids can do. Toddlers love to pretend, test their limits, try new things, and move, move, move.

*Jodi assists a toddler yo-
gini with headstand fun.*

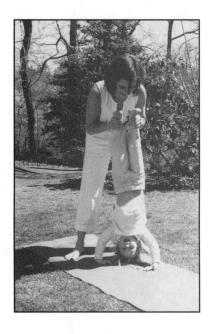

Toddler yoga practice may not be a peaceful or calm affair, but it is certainly fun! A
playful attitude is best. Be prepared to answer questions, change the plan, keep up
the pace, go with the flow, and learn as much from your toddler as your toddler
learns from you.

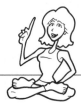

Yoga Stories

Back in the early 1930s, psychologists developed six categories of play based on observations of nursery school children. **Unoccupied play** refers to random behavior, standing,
looking around, and movements without a goal. **Solitary play** refers to play independent
of and without interest in others. **Onlooker play** involves watching others with interest,
talking to but not engaged with them. **Parallel play** refers to playing alone but with similar toys or in a similar manner to children nearby. **Associative play** involves social
interaction but little organization. **Cooperative play** involves group identity and organized activity. Yoga with kids can be solitary, parallel, associative, or cooperative, depending
on many factors.

Imagine This!

Toddlers have brilliant and surprising imaginations, even before they are competent talkers. Yoga poses that allow them to pretend and envision different scenarios are often a great success. The following yoga exercises are perfect for toddlers, individually or in a group.

A Trip to the Zoo

Little ones love a trip to the zoo, real or pretend! For this exercise, pretend you and your toddler are visiting all the different animals in a zoo. Help and encourage each other in the game. As you cue your toddler, he or she will probably cue you. Ask, "What do you see?" "What should we do now?" "Where are you going?" "What's that over there?" Every animal pose in this exercise has its various benefits. Overall, this exercise also helps stimulate creative and mental flexibility.

1. Time to go to the zoo! Pretend to get in the car. Sit, turn the key, rev up the engine, grab the steering wheel, and go! (See Driving My Car Pose in Chapter 15.) Talk about the scenery you see on the way to the zoo. You can even use a big cardboard box, bed, carpet square, or blanket as the "car."

2. We're here! Get out of the car and ask your yogini what he or she would like to see first. The lions? Let's do Lion's Breath (see Chapter 10). Roar!

3. Next, you might visit the bears and do Bear Walk (see Chapter 14).

4. Proceed through the zoo, visiting all the different animals. If you know a pose for that animal, try it. If you don't, make one up. You might see turtles, giraffes, seals, fish, snakes, butterflies … the list goes on. (See Part 4 for lots of animal poses.)

5. When your zoo trip is over, spend some time in Shavasana. Depending on your toddler's mood, he or she may not spend much time relaxing, but encourage taking a rest after that long, tiring trip by doing Shavasana Pose (see Chapter 19). For a visualization during Shavasana, talk your yogini through a descriptive ride on one of the animals. An elephant? An eagle? An antelope?

➤ **For More Fun:** Incorporate music, complete with animal sounds, or make all the animal sounds yourself.

➤ **For Even More Fun:** Incorporate animal puppets, stuffed animals, and/or animal masks in your visit to the zoo.

For Grownups, Too!

Toddlers are notorious for resisting naptime and bedtime, but a tired toddler who has had sufficient exercise during the day (and, interestingly, sufficient naptime) is more likely to take a nap or go to bed without a fight. Yoga promotes more regular sleep patterns and more restful sleep.

A Trip to the Park

Whether you take your toddler to the park every day or not, an imaginary park has so many more possibilities than the real thing, and it doesn't matter what the weather is doing outside. A Trip to the Park also includes benefits from all the poses it might include, as well as stimulating creativity and mental flexibility.

1. What a beautiful, sunshine-y day outside. Let's skip to the park! (Even if your toddler doesn't yet know how to skip, she can pretend.) As you skip, sing "Skip to my Lou."

2. Here we are! Smell the fresh air, the green grass, and the beautiful flowers. Notice the sun and the lovely weather. Smell the flowers while doing Breath of Fire (see Chapter 10). Use an imaginary flower, or even a pinwheel!

3. Take a look around you. Is this park filled with tall green trees? Try Tree Pose (see Chapter 11). Toddlers find it challenging to stand on one foot, but they have a lot of fun trying! It's fine if they want to do it against a wall or even against you!

4. What else do you see in this park? A sprinkler to run through? Pretend to run through the spray. Yikes, you got wet!

5. Over there you might find a nice pond full of fish. Pretend to be a fish swimming in the water.

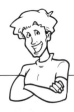

For Grownups, Too!

Everyone talks about those "terrible twos." We think the "twos" are pretty terrific! Two-year-olds are just coming into their own, learning new skills and independence. But some kids between the ages of 12 months and 4 or 5 years can be prone to temper tantrums. Yoga can help! A regular yoga practice gives young kids a sense of self-control and an outlet for excess energy, both tantrum tamers.

6. Do you see swans floating on the pond, or pigeons near the popcorn stand? Try some bird poses (see Chapter 12).

7. Look at the butterflies fluttering over the flowers. Do Butterfly Pose (see Chapter 11).

8. Are you getting hungry? Pretend to make a sandwich (see Chapter 16), then have a picnic lunch at your very own table (toddlers or mom or dad can oblige by doing Table Pose, Chapter 16).

9. Don't drop that sandwich or the ants might come marching two by two! Try "The Ants Go Marching" (see Chapter 15).

10. Phew, what a fun and exciting day in the park! Time for a nice rest in a big, green, grassy field. Rest in Shavasana (see Chapter 19)—for as long as you can convince your toddler to do it. For a visualization, describe a ride on a rainbow. Suggest your child use the rainbow as a slide!

➤ **For More Fun:** Spread out a picnic blanket to really set the mood.

➤ **For Even More Fun:** When the weather permits, go to the real park and do your yoga poses there!

Toddler Trip

This is a toddler's-choice trip. Let your toddler think about where he or she would like to visit. Now that your toddler has some experience with yoga, follow your yogini's lead.

Where would you like to go today? Maybe you'll go to the land of the dinosaurs, or never-never land, or the ocean. Maybe you'll enter the setting of a favorite book or video, go on a hunt for pixies and gnomes, or travel on a rocket into outer space. You never know what that little brain will invent!

To add to the fun, help your toddler into an appropriate costume and wear a costume yourself. Set the stage. Use props. You might even want to videotape your trip to create a precious memento.

The Least You Need to Know

➤ Parent–infant yoga is a great way to bond with a new baby.

➤ Infants receive physical and mental developmental benefits from a regular yoga practice.

➤ Yoga helps toddlers expend their energy, develop coordination, and channel their active imaginations.

➤ Toddler play is easily transformed into yoga play, especially with the parent along to cue the toddler, suggest direction, and of course, play along!

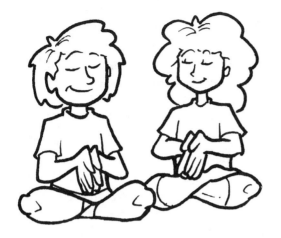

Chapter 22

Hey, Kids: Do Yoga with Your Little Brother or Sister

In This Chapter

➤ A new baby? Hooray! But can they play?

➤ Give older siblings the attention they need with yoga

➤ Teaching baby brother or sister yoga through observation

➤ Yoga bonding between siblings

➤ Yoga poses for siblings

For families who are welcoming child number two, three, four, or more, yoga is not only an excellent way to bond with the newborn, but the perfect introduction between new siblings.

We've already mentioned, throughout this book, many ways in which poses can be adapted to include more than one child, and more specifically, a younger sibling. In this chapter, we will offer some more ideas, and explore the ways in which siblings can bond and form a deeper, more meaningful relationship through the use of yoga.

There's a Baby in the House!

Bringing home a baby is a huge transition for new parents, but it may be an even bigger transition for a new sibling, especially if the child is making the adjustment from being an only child to being the big brother or sister.

Suddenly, parents are busier, distracted, tired, and overwhelmed. The new baby is downright demanding. New siblings may suddenly be expected to be patient, quiet, understanding, gentle. "Shhh, the baby is sleeping. Just a minute, I have to change the baby. Could you please wait while I see why the baby is crying? Be gentle!"

Of course, new parents don't mean to expect anything unreasonable of a new sibling, but even under the best of circumstances, major life changes can be stressful. Whether big brother or sister is 2 or 12, things change with a baby in the house. What's a stressed-out new sibling to do? Think about the following points:

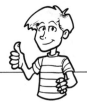

For Kids Only

It's easy to feel left out when your parents seem to spend so much time with the new baby, but just remember, they need you more than ever! Remind your parents that you would like to be involved and ask how you can help with the baby.

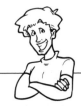

For Grownups, Too!

No matter how busy everyone gets, don't forget to touch base with your older child or children at least once every day. Ask them how they're doing, and if there is anything you can do to help them out. Really listen to what they say.

➤ Remember that your parents love you just as much as they always did. You haven't been re-placed. Your family is just growing!

➤ Remember that change is hard on everyone—you, your parents, and the new baby. But stick-ing together makes change easier on everyone.

➤ Remember that the baby will look up to you, admire you, and want to be like you. Think of ways in which you can start setting a great ex-ample for your new little sibling.

➤ Remember that babies are delicate, but they also love to play. Have fun making funny faces, telling stories, and singing to your new sibling.

➤ Remember that it is your baby, too! Your par-ents have the responsibility for seeing that the new baby is properly cared for, but when it comes to love, your bond with the baby can be just as strong as theirs.

➤ Recognize that it's okay to feel negative about the baby sometimes. It doesn't mean you don't love the baby!

➤ Keep up that yoga practice! It can help you relax, energize you when you are tired, make you feel calmer, and it is a great thing for you to teach your new sibling when he or she is old enough to learn. Doing yoga for a baby can be great entertainment and babies learn from watching and listening to your yogic breathing and poses. (It won't be long before the baby will be a yogini and joining in!)

How Yoga Helps When You Bring a New Baby Home

With all the household chaos surrounding your family's new little (but noisy!) bundle of joy, yoga can be an oasis of serenity. New babies take up lots of parents' time and energy, but older children also experience some profound needs at this time.

While some siblings don't seem to be jealous of the new baby at all, they may feel as if they are getting less time from their parents. It's probably true! While parents can involve their older children actively in many aspects of baby care, spending a sacred time together without the baby is an important way to maintain emotional contact and feed their children's need for reassurance, love, and attention.

A daily yoga practice, during baby's naptime or with one parent while the other watches the baby, is a wonderful way for parents and their first children to keep in touch. Set aside a period of time—just 20 minutes can accomplish a lot—to be together, breathing, yoga-cizing, imagining, relaxing, and being peaceful together.

This is not the time to talk about the baby (unless the child wants to), or chores, or responsibilities, or school, or anything else to do with outside commitments. This is your time together. Savor it. Be fully present during this time. It will do wonders for both of you. End your yoga sessions with a big hug!

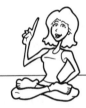

Yoga Stories

Research supports the notion that sibling interaction may be even more influential on children than parental interaction, especially the influence of older siblings on younger siblings. Observations of sibling interactions at a young age (approximately 19 months and 4½ years) revealed the tendency of younger siblings to watch and imitate older siblings. Siblings may be a stronger socializing influence than parents in adolescence, as well, especially when it comes to dealing with peers, physical appearance, identity issues, school difficulties, and the discussion of "taboo" subjects such as sex and drugs. Studies show that parents often focus on the apparently negative aspects of sibling interaction, such as rivalry and competitiveness, but that most sibling relationships also include many neutral and positive exchanges.

For teenagers, parents should encourage the maintenance of individual yoga practice in addition to family yoga time. Individual yoga can be a great stress-management tool for kids undergoing any transition. It can also give kids energy when they need it (if the baby is keeping parents up at night, the baby may be keeping others up, too), and can relax them when they are feeling stressed, left out, or overwhelmed.

When a yogini is fed by the physical, mental, and spiritual nourishment of a regular yoga practice, he or she gains greater self-control, a sense of personal responsibility, becomes more self-sufficient and self-possessed, and learns about priorities: love, caring, kindness, and good health. Sounds like the makings of a pretty stellar role model!

Yoga Unions: Forging the Sibling Bond

Older siblings can start teaching the new baby about yoga from the first day the baby comes home! Set the baby up in an infant seat to watch the older child do animal poses, nature poses, movement poses, and other fun yoga games. Babies love to hear sound and watch movement and fun.

The older the baby gets, the more likely he or she will strive to imitate big brother or big sister. Children who are exposed to yoga at an early age will feel comfortable and at ease with a yoga practice when they are able to move around on their own.

As They Grow

When babies become more mobile, pushing their heads and chests off the floor, rolling over, scooting, sliding, and eventually crawling, they will probably try to do many of the yoga poses their older siblings do. Letting them try is an excellent way to encourage blooming development.

Depending on their ages and stages of development, babies may be able to push up into Mother Snake Pose, bend down into Downward Facing Dog, stand in Mountain Pose, breathe like a bunny, imitate chanting, and make certain animal sounds as they crawl or scoot. Babies may find other ways to express their budding yogini status.

The more different kinds of movements, positions, sights, and sounds babies are exposed to, the more those little brains will work to take it all in, internalize it, and then express it through imitation. This is how babies learn, so make the most of it through plenty of daily yoga interaction!

The Yogini's Ten Steps for Sibling Synchronicity

As we've mentioned before, yoga is more than poses. It is also a spiritual journey and a way of life. Remember the yoga values (yamas) and habits (niyamas) we talked about in Chapter 4? In addition to being individually helpful, these values and habits can be excellent ways to teach cooperation, sharing, mutual respect, empathy, and other relationship-enhancing qualities to siblings.

Let's review them now. We've renamed them the "Yogini's 10 Steps for Sibling Synchronicity" and slightly revised them to have a family focus.

Step 1: Live in Peace

Fighting isn't any fun. Who wants to fight? Sometimes siblings make each other angry, but making an effort to solve arguments peacefully will help siblings cherish and value each other. While toddlers may be too young to understand the reasoning behind nonviolent interaction, children as young as three or four can begin to understand that a sibling is a human being and deserves respect and gentle treatment, and that working out problems by talking instead of reacting physically has better results for everyone.

Step 2: Tell the Truth

Siblings who begin life as truthful companions will build allies in each other. If children make it a rule and a habit to tell each other the truth, later in life they will know they can trust each other, confide in each other, and depend on each other.

Step 3: Let Go of the Toy

One way to practice respect for each other is for siblings to stop taking things from each other. While babies may not mind if a sibling takes away a toy, toddlers tend to feel that anything in their possession, or even within the range of their eyesight, is theirs, theirs, theirs. Teaching older children to refrain from grabbing things out of a sibling's hand will soon set an example for a younger sibling.

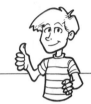

For Kids Only

Are you feeling frustrated that the new baby can't do anything fun, like play games or talk? Instead of focusing on what your new sibling will be able to do *someday*, focus on what he or she can do *now*. Each stage of development is fascinating. What is fascinating about your sibling today? Your new baby brother or sister will never be this age again.

Step 4: Practice Self-Control

This is a tough one for young children. Kids' tempers sometimes run high, and it is easy to lose control. Whether losing control for a child means grabbing away toys, hitting, or throwing a tantrum, self-control is an important and valuable lesson for kids to learn at an early age. They may not always be successful in their efforts, but if kids understand when self-control is warranted, they can begin to practice.

Step 5: Share and Share Alike

Sharing is also hard for lots of kids. Among toddlers, one is likely to hear lots of "Mine! Mine! Mine!" Older kids can quickly learn the importance and value of sharing, however. Another, even more important lesson is learning to live with less. How many toys does a child need? How many outfits? In what ways could a child be happier, more imaginative, and less limited, with fewer possessions? Siblings who learn to live with less and share what they have will be more interested in playing with each other and developing a friendship than in who gets to hold what toy.

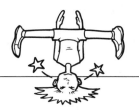

Ooops!

Germs get passed around easily with babies and kids in the house. Sick yoginis can't have nearly as much fun, so wipe off toys and other kid-contact surfaces frequently, and get in the habit of washing your hands before every meal. If kids scrub their hands while singing the whole ABC song, the soap and water will have more time to wash away those germs and bacteria!

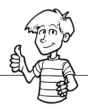

For Kids Only

Babies love music. If your little brother or sister is upset, bored, or frustrated, try singing a little song or playing some music and dancing. You might just be able to sing or dance those baby cares away! How about singing the song "Don't Worry, Be Happy" (see Appendix B)?

Step 6: Clean It Up

Messy, messy, messy. Does that describe your room? While some kids tend to be naturally neat (and others have neatness forced upon them), when siblings share a room, failing to keep things clean can be a source of frustration, irritation, and dissension. Parents should cultivate in their children an attitude that everyone is responsible for cleaning up his or her own mess, and that everyone should also make an effort to help other people clean up their messes, too. A clean, neat environment helps everyone who lives in it feel more organized, calmer, and happier. Sibling harmony through clutter control!

Step 7: Don't Worry, Be Happy!

Kids can be worriers, just like adults, but siblings who make an effort to remind each other to practice contentment and who cultivate a positive attitude, will help each other with stress management as well as gain a deep inner feeling of satisfaction. Worries can seem inconsequential if put into perspective by a trusted sibling. Even young children can be taught to help each other cheer up. Never underestimate the power of a sibling to modulate a child's mood. Also, parents should look at their own tendencies to worry. Constant worrying and fretting can present kids with an undesirable model.

Step 8: Work Together

Self-discipline is hard for lots of kids (and lots of adults!), but having a sibling to help and encourage self-discipline can go a long way toward teaching a child how to put self-discipline into practice. A younger sibling can help an older sibling practice the piano by joining the practice as page-turner and cheerleader. The older sibling might reciprocate by helping the younger sibling pick up that puzzle or by helping out with a difficult math assignment.

Step 9: Study Together

Siblings who spend time together, not just playing but learning, may learn even more than they would on their own. Whether kids do homework together, work on a special school project together, or simply read books and mold clay together, their joint efforts can teach each of them more about the world.

Step 10: Believe in Magic

We aren't suggesting kids should literally believe in magic, but we are suggesting that they engage on their spiritual journeys together. If kids talk about philosophical questions, work out ethical dilemmas, seek out universal truths, and try to uncover the mysteries of the universe together, they can go further, understand more, and come up with more fascinating questions if they do it together. Embarking on a spiritual journey together—even if children come to very different answers and conclusions—will help kids forge a relationship that can last a lifetime.

Loving Responsibility

Yoga values and habits promote not only harmony but a sense of responsibility toward oneself and toward others. Yoga practice builds family harmony in many ways: It teaches parents and siblings to accept the responsibility of living in a family, to care and love each other, to support each other, and to move through life together.

While bonding between siblings will largely happen on its own, parents have their own responsibility to oversee the process, keep rivalry under control, rechannel aggression and dissension, and promote an environment of loving kindness. If every family member, from the most senior grandparent to the youngest infant, lives and loves in an environment that promotes loving responsibility for others, your family will surely thrive.

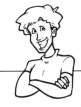

For Grownups, Too!

Set up a plain table instead of a formal desk in your child's room or playroom to create a work surface for two. Put a chair on either side and your kids can study or work on other projects together.

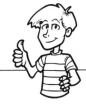

For Kids Only

Babies love hugs and kisses ... most of the time! Remember to show your new baby brother or sister lots of affection, but don't be offended if he or she cries or pushes you away. Sometimes babies get too much stimulation and they need some time alone. It isn't you—there's just too much going on.

Yoga Poses Yogini Brothers and Sisters Can Do Together

Let's play yoga! Younger siblings are delighted to have the attention, engagement, and guidance (well, not always the guidance) of an older sibling. Following are some yoga pose ideas to add to the other poses in this book that already include options for sibling involvement.

Puppy Play with Downward Facing Dog

Every puppy loves to have a bigger dog to play with! In this pose, the traditional Downward Facing Dog Pose gets an added element of movement and fun.

Puppy Play with Downward Facing Dog Pose.

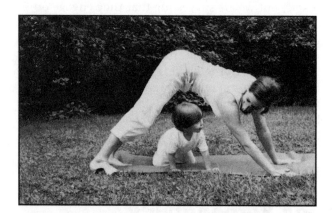

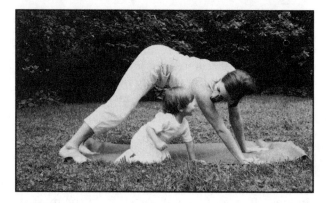

1. The older sibling does Downward Facing Dog Pose (see Chapter 12).
2. The younger sibling also gets into Downward Facing Dog, then crawls and scampers around the older "dog." Go under the bigger dog, around, between the feet, and in figure eights. Don't forget to bark like a puppy!

3. The older sibling can pretend he or she is the puppy's mother or father dog. Bark like a parent dog. See if you can get that puppy to calm down. No? If you can't beat 'em, join 'em! Romp around the room on all fours with your "puppy."

The Cobra Family

In this exercise, siblings assume whichever level of snake pose they are able to get into. The result is a family of cobras ready to slither around the room together.

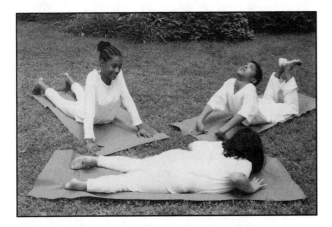

Cobra Family Pose.

1. Each sibling lies on the floor face down, forehead on the floor, palms on the floor on either side of the chest.

2. Rise up into Baby Snake Pose, Mother Snake Pose, or Father Snake Pose (all in Chapter 13), according to your abilities or inclinations.

3. Everybody hiss! Get those tongues out! Have a conversation in Cobra: "Nice-s-s-s-s-s day, is-s-s-s-s-s-s-n't it, s-s-s-s-s-s-s-son?" "Yes-s-s-s-s-s-s! Let's-s-s-s-s-s-s go for a s-s-s-s-s-s-s-slither!"

4. Slither around the room. What games would cobras play? Where would they go to look for food? What would they talk about?

Family Picnic

We described this variation of Table Pose in Chapter 16, but it bears repeating here. In this exercise, the older sibling (or a parent) acts as a picnic table. And then, the ants come marching in ....

Family Picnic Pose.

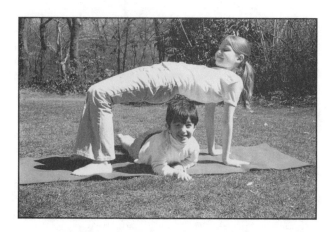

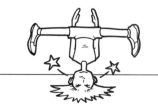

Ooops!

We encourage parents to always supervise sibling yoga interactions. Older siblings sometimes overestimate what they can do, how much they can hold, or how long their patience will last. They might also overestimate what their younger siblings can do.

1. The older sibling or a parent assumes Table Pose (see Chapter 16). Pretend you are a picnic table. Where are you? In the park? In a forest? In the backyard?

2. Younger siblings pretend to be ants. Get down on hands and knees. Do you smell something? Sandwiches? Pie? Go investigate!

3. Younger siblings march around the picnic table as in the Ants Go Marching exercise (see Chapter 15), and might even try to climb aboard looking for tasty crumbs. Yum yum!

4. A younger sibling can be a picnic blanket lying flat on the floor, while an older sibling gets a turn as the ant. Is that a cookie crumb? Nibble nibble that tummy!

Club Sandwich

What sandwich isn't improved by an additional layer? In this variation of Sandwich Pose, a younger sibling gets to be a part of the sandwich. This pose is like a big hug!

1. The older sibling sits on the floor with legs outstretched in a narrow V.

2. The younger sibling sits on the floor between the older sibling's legs, with his or her back to the older sibling and legs outstretched.

3. The older sibling raises his or her arms, then bends over forward, folding the body over into a sitting Sandwich Pose, folding the younger sibling (gently!) into the sandwich.

4. The younger sibling stretches fingers toward toes and enjoys the sandwich squeeze!

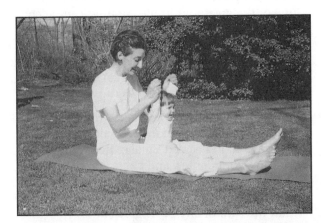

Club Sandwich Pose.

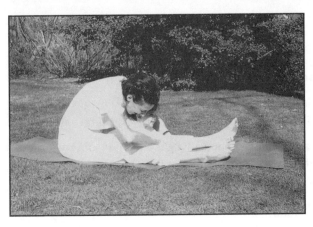

Foot Massage Fun

Older kids usually have an easier time relaxing into Shavasana than do younger kids, and they will enjoy the relaxation even more if their younger siblings give them a nice, relaxing foot massage! Young kids love to rub feet, especially if they get to use a special lotion.

1. The older sibling lies back into Shavasana (see Chapter 19).

2. The younger sibling sits at the older sibling's feet and rubs them, with or without lotion. Encourage the younger sibling to spend as much time as possible, rubbing the entire tops and soles of the feet, including each toe.

3. If younger siblings would like a foot massage, too, older siblings can return the favor. This is a good way to begin to teach younger children how to relax in Shavasana. (Unless their feet are too ticklish!)

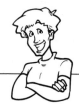

For Grownups, Too!

Massage is a great way to help kids relax each other for Shavasana. Show your kids how to give each other foot, leg, arm, back, and even head massages. The touching is good for them and will help them relax as well as trust each other. (No tickling allowed!)

It Takes a Family

Having a good relationship with a sibling or siblings is one of the great joys in life. Siblings can be cherished, trusted, supportive friends throughout a lifetime. And while sibling harmony sometimes seems to "just happen," it usually takes the involvement of every family member acting with love, mutual respect, and caring toward each other to set an example.

But what a wonderful project for the family! While we don't choose who our families will be, that doesn't mean we can't decide to make them our friends, companions, confidantes, and cherished ones. Working on every different family relationship with purpose and love will make the entire family stronger and greater than the sum of any of its parts.

The Least You Need to Know

➤ Yoga can help kids adjust to the presence of a new baby by giving them a stress management tool and by giving them special alone time with parents.

➤ Babies love to watch older siblings practice yoga, and their observation sets the groundwork for future yoga accomplishment.

➤ The yoga yamas and niyamas (values and habits) can be applied to sibling relationships for greater harmony.

➤ Siblings doing yoga together forge a strong bond and a positive relationship.

➤ Many yoga poses can be adapted to accommodate the participation of a younger sibling.

Part 7

Yoga All Day Long!

In this last part, yoga moves beyond exercises and techniques to become a part of your whole day. We'll talk about the yoga way to eat (hint: it's a lot more than "good for you"!), and the ways in which yoga is good medicine. Yoga can be a part of an overall health plan that addresses specific problems in kids (colic, asthma, constipation, backache), in conjunction with therapies administered by qualified health professionals.

We'll go into more detail about the ways in which yoga therapy targets the unique challenges of kids with special needs, we'll talk about yoga for teens, and we'll help parents surprise and delight their children with a yoga kids party! From decorations and favors to recipes and theme-party ideas, we'll take you through the easier-than-you-think process from start to finish.

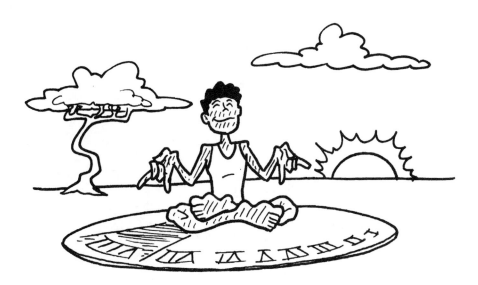

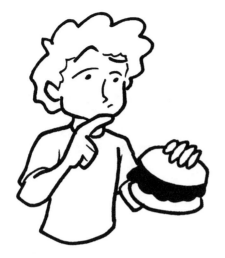

Chapter 23

Eating for Strong Minds and Bodies

In This Chapter

➤ What are you eating—and what could you be eating to feel better?

➤ Food, yoga-style

➤ What about vegetarianism?

➤ Eating beyond the dinner plate

➤ The revival of the family meal

➤ Yoga snacks for healthy kids

We've explained in other chapters some of the ways that yoga is about more than exercise, but did you know that yoga even has a particular way of eating?

Eating yoga-style isn't weird or unpleasant, or even difficult in the least. The yoga style of eating is based on common sense and, even though the theories were derived thousands of years ago, is perfectly in line with all the scientific knowledge about nutrition we have today.

What you eat is an essential part of who you are; but before we talk about eating in the yoga style, let's look at how Americans tend to eat, how your family tends to eat, and what kids are eating when parents aren't around to watch!

Food, American-Style

Americans tend to know a lot about nutrition. We are bombarded with the information from all kinds of sources: television, magazines, books, the Internet. However, knowing how to eat well and actually eating well are two different things.

Many Americans enjoy fast food, red meat, processed convenience food, sugar, white-flour products, and lots of other foods processed way beyond anything they looked like when they were alive. It's a long way from a field of wheat to a perfectly round, snow-white, soft hamburger bun; a long way from a chicken to a shaped and processed chicken nugget.

Even though you can probably name at least one known health consequence for eating too much fat, sugar, and processed foods, you probably don't avoid these things entirely. Should you? Maybe not. Moderation is usually the most sensible course for any dietary plan, but many children in America don't practice moderation when it comes to less-than-ideal dietary choices. Parents, do you know what your children are eating?

What Do Kids in America Eat?

Ask any child what he or she sees friends eating in the cafeteria or after school and you probably won't be given long lists of fresh vegetables and fruits.

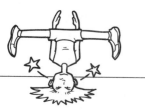

Ooops!

As much as parents would like to encourage their kids to eat healthy foods, making food a source of tension may contribute to future eating disorders. Parents can offer a wide variety of healthy foods and make junk food mostly unavailable at home, but shouldn't force their kids to eat. Kids may be more willing to eat healthy foods if they feel it is their own choice, not something forced upon them.

Data compiled by the USDA/ARS Children's Nutrition Research Center (based on the U.S. Department of Agriculture's 1996 Continuing Survey of Food Intakes by Individuals), reveals that children aren't getting enough of the healthy foods they require (as compared to the recommendations in the USDA Food Guide Pyramid).

According to the survey, kids of all ages consumed more dietary fat, including saturated fat, and much more added sugar than they require for good health. Many choices in the "breads and grains" category included calorie-dense but nutrient-poor refined carbohydrate sources such as cakes, cookies, and donuts. Very few kids consume whole-grain foods, an important source of fiber, certain vitamins, and minerals.

Nutritionists recommend one serving each per day of dark, leafy green vegetables and deep yellow or orange vegetables. However, fewer than one in three children under the age of 11 eat the recommended minimum servings of fruit and vegetables each day, and among adolescents, the vegetables of choice are rarely dark and leafy or deep yellow. French fries, potato chips, and tomatoes (eaten in salsas, pizzas, and spaghetti sauces) are the most commonly chosen vegetables.

While about half the children under five get enough fruit, most of it is in the form of fruit juice, which has no fiber. Fewer than a fourth of children over the age of five get enough fruit, and when it comes to beverages, over the past 20 years, soda consumption has risen 16 percent while milk consumption has fallen 16 percent.

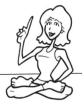

Yoga Stories

Although some kids are lactose intolerant, milk is sometimes unfairly blamed for stomach discomfort in children. Many children drink large amounts of juice each day, and juice contains sorbitol, a naturally occurring form of sugar that can cause stomach cramps, gas, and even mild diarrhea. Prune juice is a laxative because of high sorbitol content, but apple, pear, peach, and cherry juices also have high levels of sorbitol. Parents, if you think your child is allergic to milk, consider limiting juice consumption first. Nutritionists typically suggest that young children drink no more than four to eight ounces of juice each day. If your child is thirsty for juice more often, stick to this amount but double the volume of liquid by adding clean, purified water.

How can parents reverse these trends for their kids? Of course, they can't always control what their child will eat, especially when he or she is at school or at other people's houses. However, making healthy foods available at home and eating the same food themselves is the best way for parents to set an example that kids will probably follow eventually.

What Is Your Family Eating?

Eating right is often a challenge for parents, but healthy eating at home is an important way to set a good example for kids.

Conscious eating is the first step toward good nutrition, so we would like to suggest that the whole family spend three days writing down everything they eat—every single thing, whether a meal or a snack or food eaten while preparing food. Sometimes, just knowing you'll be writing it down will keep you from making an unhealthy food choice. However, be honest. If you eat it, write it down, then sit down with your family and take a good, hard look at how you eat.

What Could Your Family Be Eating?

Take a look at your dinner plate tonight, and your lists of foods from the past three days. Is your diet mostly filled with whole grains like whole-wheat bread, brown rice, whole-grain pasta, and whole-grain cereals? Do you eat fresh salad greens, raw or steamed vegetables, and fresh fruit every day? Does meat take up only a small portion of your plate?

Most nutritionists agree that to get sufficient vitamins, minerals, fiber, and protein, most adults should center their diets on whole grains, fruits, vegetables, legumes, nuts, and seeds. Protein from animal sources need only be an occasional addition to the diet, or used to flavor grain or vegetable dishes. High-fat, high-sugar foods should be eaten only occasionally.

If that sounds exhausting and, as a parent, you tend to prefer grabbing a can of diet soda and a bag of chips to eat in the car while driving the kids home from soccer practice, we would like to encourage you. Healthy eating doesn't have to be difficult. Who has the time or patience to measure foods, count calories, or keep track of fat grams? Not us! Yet, we agree that healthy eating is important, even vital, for healthy living in the true spirit of yoga. So, we like to use yoga's philosophy of eating. We think you'll find it to be easy, sensible, nutritionally excellent, and delicious.

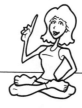

Yoga Stories

According to the USDA/ARS Children's Nutrition Research Center at Baylor College of Medicine in Houston, Texas, almost two-thirds of all children eat almost 30 percent of their daily calories away from home. That means parents can't control everything their kids eat. However, teaching children about nutrition will best prepare them to make their own decisions. The USDA encourages parents to teach children to "count to five" every day to ensure the consumption of five daily servings of fruits and vegetables. This alone can vastly improve children's diets because fruits and vegetables are concentrated sources of vitamins, minerals, fiber, and phytochemicals, those nonnutritive substances in plants thought to have immune-boosting and disease-fighting properties.

Food, Prepared Yoga-Style

What is the yoga philosophy of food? In brief, eating in the yoga style involves three main considerations:

➤ Eat mostly fresh foods that look pretty much the way they looked when picked or pulled from the ground or taken from the animal (like milk), or that have most of the food still intact (like whole grains as opposed to refined grains and other minimally processed plant foods).

➤ If it is highly preserved, artificially colored, or has been around for a long time, avoid it most of the time.

➤ If it is stimulating (like coffee, tea, or chocolate), high in saturated fat, or has lots of added sugar, avoid it most of the time.

Isn't that simple? Each of these points has a basis for it that has nothing to do with nutrients, fiber, calories, fat grams, or any of the other typical considerations of Western nutritional science. Instead, the point of eating in the yoga style is to eat mostly food that is *sattvic,* and minimize foods that are *rajasic* or *tamasic.*

Is Your Food Sattvic, Rajasic, or Tamasic?

Every food has a certain energy or quality to it that has an effect on the body. Some foods are balancing, promoting clarity, lightness, and balance in the body. These foods are sattvic, and include fresh, whole plant foods that are minimally processed so they look pretty much the way they did when harvested, whole-grain foods, nuts and seeds, dried beans and peas, honey (a yoga favorite!), and dairy products like milk and butter. Eating primarily sattvic foods makes you feel great, balanced and energetic, centered and serene.

Some foods tend to be rajasic. These foods are the spicy, sour, or pungent foods, including stimulants and anything else that seems agitating. Examples of rajasic foods include meat, eggs, strong spices like pepper, coffee, tea, and cola. Rajasic foods tend to make people feel agitated, anxious, and overly stimulated.

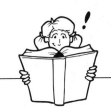

Learn About Yoga

Sattvic, rajasic, and tamasic are Sanskrit words used to describe the quality and effect of a food, or anything else, on the body and mind. **Sattvic** influences promote balance, lightness, and clarity. **Rajasic** influences promote agitation, movement, and increased activity. **Tamasic** influences promote laziness, heaviness, and inactivity.

Tamasic foods are on the opposite end of the spectrum from rajasic foods. Tamasic foods are the foods that are overly processed, preserved, stale, or addictive, including alcohol and tobacco (not a food, but tamasic nevertheless). Coffee, tea, and cola are both addictive and stimulating, so they have both rajasic and tamasic qualities—a double whammy! Too much tamasic foods make people feel lazy, sap energy, dull ambition, and drain away joy.

Do You Have to Be Vegetarian?

Lots of people who do yoga are vegetarian. Lots aren't. We would like to state up front that vegetarianism is by no means a requirement for yoginis.

However (isn't there always a however?), many people who practice yoga eventually choose to become vegetarians. Why? We can't answer that question for every yogi and yogini, but we will say that yoga tends to transform the individual in such a way that internal awareness increases and values become externalized. If a practicing yogini begins to think seriously about the meaning of nonviolence or respect for all living things, he or she may decide to experiment with a meat-free diet.

Parents of kids who decide to try a vegetarian lifestyle are often thrown for a loop if they aren't accustomed to eating vegetarian. If you were raised in an environment that encouraged meat eating and taught that a daily hearty serving of meat was necessary for healthy growth (as many of us were), the transition to vegetarianism (or living with a vegetarian yogini) can be tough. But just to put your mind at ease, here are a few points to consider:

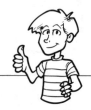

For Kids Only

Lots of teenagers try vegetarianism, if only for a little while. If you decide to try giving up meat, we hope you will spend some time thinking about why you have made that choice, noticing how it makes you feel, and thinking about the implications of your dietary choices. Vegetarianism can be a wonderful way to explore your beliefs about nonviolence, kindness, and respect for life.

➤ A diet that includes dairy products and eggs but no meat (called a lacto-ovo vegetarian diet) is a safe and healthy alternative for kids, as long as they include lots of fresh, healthy whole grains, fruits, vegetables, protein, and a good calcium sources such as milk, tofu, sesame seeds, and leafy green vegetables.

➤ Well-planned vegetarian diets tend to be higher in fiber and phytonutrients (nonnutritive plant substances with protective health benefits) and lower in saturated fat than the typical American diet.

➤ Vegetarians typically enjoy lower rates of cardiovascular disease, Type-2 diabetes, hypertension, and weight problems.

If a yogini is interested in eating vegetarian, parents should have a discussion about what vegetarianism means to the child. What kind of vegetarianism is the child planning? Semi-vegetarians may choose to eat fish or poultry and eliminate only red meat. Lacto-ovo vegetarians eat dairy products and eggs but no red meat, fish, or poultry. Lacto vegetarians also eliminate eggs, and vegans, or strict vegetarians, avoid all animal products.

Lacto-ovo vegetarianism is a safe and healthy alternative for teens, as long as they eat a wide variety of healthy foods, center their diets on whole grains, fruits, and vegetables (and not just vegetarian junk food), get plenty of exercise (like yoga!), and make a point to learn about and practice good nutrition.

Vegetarianism can be a great adventure for kids seeking alternatives, but again, it isn't a requirement for yoga. It is simply a choice that many come to on their own.

Developing Good Eating Habits

Changing from a junk-food-loving family to a family of healthy eaters overnight isn't easy. Changing any dietary pattern too drastically or quickly usually results in failure. Families can work together to plan healthy meals and encourage each other to stick to healthy eating habits. Many parents find their kids are even better at healthy eating than they are! Following are some tips to help your family get on the right nutritional track:

➤ Don't buy junk food. Boxes of snack cakes, candy bars, and chips are easy to grab and eat after school or in the evenings. If they aren't there to begin with, hungry yoginis (and their parents) will have to grab an apple, a handful of baby carrots, a carton of yogurt, or a peanut butter sandwich on whole-wheat bread instead.

➤ Forget the soda and sugary drinks and stock your refrigerator with easy-to-grab, individually sized bottles of spring water, low-fat milk, and 100 percent juice (calcium fortified is best).

➤ Hate making salad? Those salad-in-a-bag salads often contain a healthy mix of different greens, and they are extra easy to prepare. Just grab a handful of greens, throw it in a bowl, drizzle on a little olive oil (a healthy source of fat), and enjoy!

➤ Got the munchies? Stir up a big bowl of dried fruit (raisins, apricots, dates, bananas), whole-grain cereal, almonds or walnuts, and whole-wheat crackers, then store in snack-sized bags for easy access.

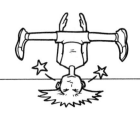

Ooops!

Kids on a strict vegetarian or vegan diet are at greater risk for nutritional deficiencies than kids whose diets include milk and eggs. Vegan kids may lack sufficient calcium, iron, and zinc (to counter this, consume lots of fresh vegetables, especially leafy greens, and calcium-fortified tofu or soymilk), and they need a source of vitamin B12 (available in fortified cereals and multivitamin supplements).

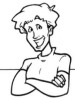

For Grownups, Too!

Packaged salad mix may seem like an extravagance, but no matter how little you pay for a head of lettuce, it's a waste if you end up throwing it away because you didn't want to bother washing and chopping. Also, many of the highly nutritious greens in salad mixes aren't conveniently available in other forms.

➤ Keep a bowl of washed, fresh fruit on the counter or kitchen table.

➤ Visit local farmers' markets in season. Yoginis can pick out new kinds of fruits and vegetables and then wash, clean, chop, and (if necessary) cook them together—a culinary adventure!

➤ Even if the whole family isn't vegetarian, parents should plan at least two or three vegetarian meals each week. Try veggie pizzas; tostados or burritos filled with beans, cheese, tomatoes, lettuce, and olives; vegetable/tofu stir fry; pasta with different combinations of sautéed or sauced veggies. Use your imagination or find vegetarian cookbooks in the library and experiment.

Healthy eating just takes a little practice, and the increased energy and life you will feel from eating a healthy diet full of fresh whole foods will more than make up for any extra effort you might take in breaking old habits and trying new recipes.

Practice Mindful Eating as a Family

Now you know what to eat. But do you know *how* to eat? Yes, we're sure you are perfectly coordinated with your utensils, but that isn't what we mean. We are talking about mindfulness.

Have you ever sat down to a fantastic meal but been so distracted that you didn't even notice what you were gulping down? Have you ever enjoyed a supposedly "decadent" meal so much that you couldn't quite believe it was bad for you?

Just as the mind is an integral part of the body, it is also an integral part of the eating experience. We would encourage yoginis to savor every bite of whatever they choose to eat. Eating a piece of cake with guilt and shame will turn that food into a negative force in your body. Eating a piece of cake with joy and appreciation, noticing and reveling in every moment of the experience, can transform that cake into a positive energy inside your body.

Mindful eating means paying attention to eating. It means not watching TV, reading a magazine, or doing anything else when you eat, but really, truly eating. Any food can nourish and support the body if eaten mindfully (and in moderation). Any food can fail to nourish the body if eaten with negativity.

Let every bite of your wisely chosen diet count, and you will have mastered the final step to true nourishment, yoga-style.

The Sacred Ritual of the Family Meal

We also encourage families to resurrect the tradition of the family meal, even though families are busier than ever and everyone's activities seem to happen at a different time than everyone else's. Families with a sacred mealtime, which they hold as a priority, have the benefit of a bonding, grounding time together every day when they can relish the food they share and the company they share it with.

Even if everyone can't be there all the time, we suggest that families get together and decide to make the family meal a priority. Children will cherish such a tradition someday, and parents will cherish it, too, because it allows them to keep in contact with their busy little yoginis no matter what else is going on in their lives.

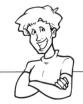

The Zen of Who You Are, What You Eat, and What You Do

To focus on food in a manner that is truly worthy of a yoga lifestyle, we must, last of all, talk about the importance of eating for the whole self. Eating isn't just fuel. What you eat is energy you take into yourself that becomes a part of you. What you eat is who you are, just as what you do, say, and think becomes a part of who you are.

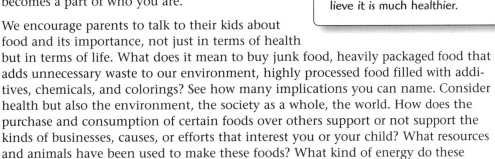

For Grownups, Too!

Once available only in health food stores, organic produce and other organic foods are now widely available. While standards vary and the industry isn't yet regulated, in general, organic food is grown without pesticides and chemical fertilizers. Organic food typically costs a little more, but it tastes better, and we believe it is much healthier.

We encourage parents to talk to their kids about food and its importance, not just in terms of health but in terms of life. What does it mean to buy junk food, heavily packaged food that adds unnecessary waste to our environment, highly processed food filled with additives, chemicals, and colorings? See how many implications you can name. Consider health but also the environment, the society as a whole, the world. How does the purchase and consumption of certain foods over others support or not support the kinds of businesses, causes, or efforts that interest you or your child? What resources and animals have been used to make these foods? What kind of energy do these foods impart to the body, considering their history? Do you know where your food comes from?

Awareness of what you eat and its implications beyond the borders of your dinner plate is the first step toward eating with a conscience, being mindful of bringing life, rather than eventual disease, to your whole self.

The energy in food is a function of that food's whole existence, from seed or embryo to salad or omelet or cheeseburger. The nutritional composition of the food is only part of the story, and this is something we hope you and your child will consider when making your dietary choices. Eat to live, to live well, and to promote life.

Good Snacks

Let's end with some delicious and healthy snacks, perfect for hungry yoginis after a vigorous yoga workout. These are some of our favorite recipes. Feel free to adapt them in any way you like. Happy snacking!

➤ **Bugs on a Rug:** Spread peanut or almond butter on whole-wheat toast, then dot with raisins, currants, dates, and snipped dried apricots.

➤ **Dip It!:** Mix a half-cup plain yogurt and a half-cup low-fat cottage cheese in a blender and blend until smooth (or, don't blend if you don't mind it lumpy). Use this dip for veggie sticks (carrots, celery, other root vegetables), toasted tortilla strips, or pita bread triangles.

➤ **Beanie Greenies:** Take a leaf of lettuce or other greens and put a spoonful of white or pinto beans, a few chopped tomatoes, and some shredded cheese in the middle. Roll it up and eat it like a burrito.

➤ **Tomato Kisses:** Cut cherry tomatoes in half, scoop out the seeds, and fill with a dollop of cream cheese, cottage cheese, or plain yogurt.

➤ **Nuts to You:** Toss banana slices and whole almonds or walnut pieces (or both) with a little honey, top with milk, and enjoy.

➤ **Yogurt Surprise:** Invent ways to add tastes to plain yogurt. Stir in chopped or dried fruit, seasonal berries, homemade granola, honey and sesame seeds, maple syrup and chopped pecans, or a dollop of orange marmalade. Much nicer, more fun, and less sugary than sweetened yogurt.

The Least You Need to Know

➤ American kids tend to eat more fat and sugar and fewer fruits and vegetables than they should for optimum health.

➤ Families can work together to improve their eating habits.

➤ Kids with nutritional know-how will be more likely to make smart nutritional choices.

➤ Eating yoga-style means focusing on sattvic foods (foods that add balance and clarity) and eating fewer rajasic (anxiety-provoking) and tamasic (fatigue-provoking) foods.

➤ Eating mindfully and with a social conscious can improve your whole eating experience.

➤ Make the family dinner a sacred ritual and enjoy renewed contact and communication with parents and siblings.

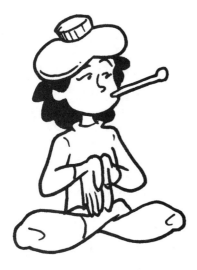

Chapter 24

Yoga to Make Kids Feel Better

In This Chapter

➤ Yoga, the natural remedy

➤ Other natural healing methods

➤ Allopathic vs. natural vs. complementary medicine

➤ Yoga for what ails kids

On top of all its other benefits, yoga is a natural healer. But yoga isn't like a pill or a cough syrup, or even like an operation or a splint. Yoga itself doesn't fix health problems. Instead, it helps the body to help itself, and our bodies are our best allies when it comes to good health. Bodies know how to fix themselves. Sometimes they just need a little help.

Yoga is just one of many natural approaches to health that focuses on balancing and centering the entire body, mind, and spirit for greater health and healing. In this chapter, we'll talk about how yoga addresses specific health concerns, as well as give you an introduction to the natural health movement.

Yoga Is a Great Natural Remedy

The natural health movement is booming. Why? Because people are feeling the need to return to their roots, to a more natural way of addressing health that doesn't rely on chemicals and manmade drugs. People are also tiring of the expense and the lack

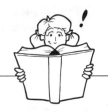

of results they sometimes experience with *allopathic* (standard Western) *medicine. Natural medicine* doesn't try to fix a disorder directly. Instead, in various ways, natural medicine empowers the body to heal itself by maximizing its healing energy.

And while natural remedies aren't always free, their cost may be so much less than with standard medicine that people don't mind. People like the idea of helping their bodies to help themselves. Natural healing returns the power of healing to the individual, and many people prefer this less invasive form of care for themselves and for their children.

Yoga, Plus Other Great Health Alternatives

Yoga is a wonderful natural remedy. It aligns the body so energy can flow unimpeded to every part. It massages, stimulates, activates, or releases tight or blocked organs and glands. It sends blood from the feet to the head and back again, nourishing every inch of you. It lets yoginis take action toward healing themselves.

Yoga strengthens and nourishes the spine—the body's command central where messages are alternately delivered and received—for better head-to-toe communication. And, last but not least, it eases, clears, and centers the mind for a better focus on healing, positive energy, and good health.

Yoga isn't the only natural remedy available. It is, on the contrary, one of hundreds, but most natural healing methods employ the same philosophy and techniques as yoga. They align or otherwise guide the body and its energies to maximize the natural healing process. They don't fix symptoms. They work from the inside out, fixing the whole self for greater healing capacity.

Some of the integrative healing techniques becoming more and more popular today include ...

➤ **Acupuncture** and acupressure, techniques for activating energy points for better energy flow throughout the body. While acupuncture uses needles (not a favorite with kids), the needles are so fine that acupuncture is relatively painless.

➤ **Homeopathy,** a technique that uses diluted plant and other substances to balance the body in a symptom-specific way.

➤ **Massage therapy** in all its variations (such as cranial-sacral therapy, which reorients the bones of the skull, and reflexology, which works on pressure points in the feet and hands), to release muscle and tissue tension, and increase mobility.

➤ **Chiropractic or osteopathic care**, to align the skeleton for freer energy movement.

➤ **Reiki** and other forms of energy manipulation, to balance the body's energies toward healing.

➤ **Animal, music, art, dance, play, and yoga therapy**, which can all be excellent for children's needs by helping them to get balanced and focused in ways they can easily understand and enjoy.

➤ **Naturopathy**, a healing method that employs the best of many different therapies.

These are only a few examples of the types of alternative care available, and further investigation into the natural healing movement will uncover many more.

Knowing When to Call the Doctor

If there is so much natural healing going on, is visiting the "regular" doctor ever necessary? Certainly.

Natural healing has certain strengths. It is excellent for chronic pain, allergies, degenerative conditions, and problems allopathic doctors can't diagnose or for which there is no "standard" cure.

But nothing can beat allopathic medicine when it comes to addressing acute conditions. Serious health problems requiring immediate attention, such as heart attacks, broken bones, accidents, acute infections, and trauma, are best handled by a conventional medical doctor.

Perhaps the best approach is to embrace *integrative medicine*. Integrative medicine uses and integrates both allopathic and natural medicine for a more complete and truly holistic approach.

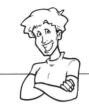

For Grownups, Too!

If you decide to seek a natural healer for your child, ask around for recommendations and check the credentials of the natural health practitioner. Specifically, talk about his or her experience working with children. You will feel safer and more confident working with a children's chiropractor or homeopath accustomed to preparing remedies for children.

Learn About Yoga

Integrative medicine uses the best of both worlds, depending on the ailment, integrating traditional, holistic, and conventional techniques. It is truly holistic, as it incorporates both allopathic and natural medicines.

We recommend parents seek out an allopathic family doctor or pediatrician to oversee their child's health care, but choose one who is open to alternative methods of care when warranted for chronic injuries, pain, allergies, asthma, digestive problems, or other ailments that typically respond well to a more natural approach.

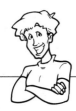

For Grownups, Too!

Not all allopathic physicians are open to natural healing methods. If natural healing interests you and you have a choice of physicians, talk with several before choosing. How would each doctor feel about you seeking alternative care for certain conditions? Would he or she be willing or able to advise you? Find a doctor whose beliefs in integrative medicine coincide with your own, if possible.

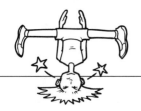

Ooops!

Parents, before you assume your baby has colic, check for other reasons for prolonged crying. Are you sure your baby isn't hungry? Tired? Scared? Wet? Could your baby be sitting on something uncomfortable, wearing something uncomfortable, or suffering some other discomfort, such as from a diaper pin, car seat buckle, or even a hair wrapped around a finger or toe?

Yoga for What Ails Kids

Let's look at some of the ways specific yoga poses, movements, and exercises can address health problems many kids experience. Once again, yoga isn't designed to immediately relieve pain (although it sometimes does), miraculously cure asthma or allergies, or solve health problems caused by genetic or environmental factors.

However, yoga does help the body to help itself, aligning, strengthening, toning, opening, massaging, stretching, and releasing in ways that can help kids feel much better and, ultimately and under the right circumstances, heal.

Yoga to Relieve Baby's Colic

When a baby has colic, he or she cries inconsolably for long periods of time. Nobody is sure exactly why, although many people will tell you colic is caused by this or that, from intestinal gas to sensory overstimulation.

Whatever the cause of colic, colicky babies often pull their knees up or strain as if they are experiencing gas. Any yoga pose that bends the legs at the hips and brings the knees to the chest (either one at a time or both together), and any kind of hip rotation (as in the Get Hip, Baby! exercise in Chapter 21) can ease the discomfort that seems to be associated with colic. Baby Relaxation (Chapter 21) is also good for colicky babies, especially when practiced in a quiet room free of distractions, with lights dimmed and soothing music playing in the background.

Yoga for Kids' Asthma and Breathing Problems

Yoga breathing exercises promote long, deep breaths instead of the short, fast breaths that can aggravate asthma. Using the breath to help with breathing problems trains the body to breathe in the most efficient and productive way it can. During any yoga pose, try to remain conscious of what the breath is doing. Any yoga posture that opens and expands the chest is excellent for aiding asthma and other respiratory problems. Some yoga poses that work well include ...

- ➤ Tree Pose (Chapter 11)
- ➤ Snake Poses (Chapter 13)
- ➤ Cow Pose (Chapter 12)
- ➤ Flamingo Pose (Chapter 12)
- ➤ Swan Pose (Chapter 12)
- ➤ Camel Pose (Chapter 13)
- ➤ Crocodile Pose (Chapter 14)
- ➤ Hero Pose (Chapter 16)
- ➤ Superperson Pose (Chapter 16)

- ➤ Warrior poses (Chapter 16)
- ➤ Table Pose (Chapter 16)
- ➤ Slide Pose (Chapter 16)
- ➤ Twister Pose (Chapter 16)
- ➤ Bridge Pose (Chapter 16)
- ➤ Wheel Pose (Chapter 16)
- ➤ Fish Pose (Chapter 17)
- ➤ Shavasana (Chapter 19)

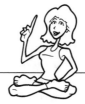

Yoga Stories

Many children suffer from allergic rhinitis aggravated by pollen, pollutants, mold, pet dander, or dust. Symptoms include sneezing, watery eyes, and itchy, runny nasal passages. One version of a common yoga cleansing ritual, called neti, washes the irritated sinuses with clean water, a process that can help soothe an attack of allergic rhinitis. Mix about a teaspoon of salt into a pint of lukewarm water, then using a bulb syringe or even a neti pot (a small pot with a long spout made for this purpose), squirt or pour the salted water gently in each nostril, then blow it out. Then, rub a little sesame oil, olive oil, or mineral oil inside each nostril to keep nasal tissue lubricated.

Yoga for Kids' Upset Stomachs, Gas, Constipation, and Diarrhea

Yoga is an excellent remedy for upset stomachs, including those caused by constipation, gas, and diarrhea. You know yoga is working if you pass gas while doing it! The following poses are excellent for stomach ailments of any sort. They are also good for promoting digestion and helping with other gastrointestinal problems:

- ➤ All breathing exercises (Chapter 10)
- ➤ Frog Pose (Chapter 11)
- ➤ Star Pose (Chapter 11)
- ➤ Cat and Cow Poses together (Chapter 12)
- ➤ Mouse Pose (Chapter 12)
- ➤ Deer Pose (Chapter 14)

- ➤ *T. rex* Pose (Chapter 14)
- ➤ Yoga Sun Dance (Chapter 15)
- ➤ Flopping Rag Doll (Chapter 15)
- ➤ Bow Pose (Chapter 16)
- ➤ Twister Pose (Chapter 16)
- ➤ Sandwich Pose (Chapter 16)
- ➤ Shavasana (Chapter 19)

Yoga to Ease Kids' Aching Backs

People tend to associate back pain with grownups, but kids can suffer, too. Chronic back pain can be eased and even cured by doing yoga on a regular basis. However, knowing what to do for back pain can be tricky. Back pain could be caused by a pulled muscle, tight muscles due to stress, radiating abdominal pain, or something more serious like a slipped disk or scoliosis. Any serious or extreme back pain should be addressed by a doctor.

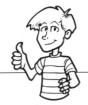

For Kids Only

Slouching and slumping over in your chair may feel more comfortable at the moment, but it holds your spine in a crooked shape and doesn't give your lungs enough room to breathe deeply. The eventual effects of slumped posture aren't worth the temporary lazy feeling of semicomfort. Get in the habit of sitting up straight and you'll feel better in the long run.

Those Backpacks Are Heavy!

Carrying around a heavy backpack all day is enough to give anyone a backache. Part of the problem is that a heavy, book-laden backpack worn over one shoulder pulls your whole body to one side, throwing your back out of balance. Try to carry your pack on both shoulders, not just one. That way, you at least balance the weight—and remember, yoga is all about balance!

Or, if you really can't make yourself wear your backpack on both shoulders, alternate between shoulders, or even wear your backpack as a front pack occasionally. When you are standing in one place for awhile, take your backpack off and put it down. Give yourself a rest.

Keeping the Spine Healthy

Doing yoga will keep your entire back elongated, flexible, and in alignment. Certain poses target the back more than others, however. Some good poses for keeping your spine in top condition include:

➤ Mountain Pose (Chapter 11)

➤ Cat and Cow Poses together (Chapter 12)

➤ Downward Facing Dog Pose (Chapter 12)

➤ Mouse Pose (Chapter 12)

➤ Swan Pose (Chapter 12)

➤ Snake poses (Chapter 13)

➤ Camel Pose (Chapter 13)

➤ Deer Pose (Chapter 14)

➤ Alligator Pose (Chapter 14)

➤ Yoga Sun Dance (Chapter 15)

➤ Hero Pose (Chapter 16)

➤ Superperson Pose (Chapter 16)

➤ Warrior poses (Chapter 16)

➤ Twister Pose (Chapter 16)

➤ Bow Pose (Chapter 16)

➤ Sandwich Pose (Chapter 16)

➤ Bridge Pose (Chapter 16)

➤ Wheel Pose (Chapter 16)

➤ Shavasana (Chapter 19)

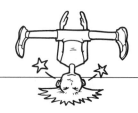

Ooops!

Whenever picking up or putting down anything, heavy or not (a backpack, a little brother, a musical instrument, or even bending down to pick up a ball or a piece of paper you dropped), remember to use your knees and legs to bend down, rather than locking your knees and doing all the work with your back.

Recovering from Sprains, Strains, and Breaks

While some people advise against any physical activity when recovering from *sprains, strains,* and breaks, we have found that gentle, targeted yoga poses promote healing and make the recovery period more comfortable.

Even if the injured area is still tender, there are poses you can do. Just listen to your body and don't do things that hurt a lot. The kind of mild, gentle pain that feels like stiff muscles stretching and becoming active again is good. Sharp, severe pain or pain that makes you very uncomfortable is probably not good. Listen to your body and go at your own pace.

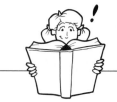

Learn About Yoga

A **strain** is a tearing of muscles or tendons (bands of tissue that connect muscle to bone). A **sprain** is an injury to a joint resulting from stretched or torn ligaments (bands of tissue that connect bone to bone and support joints).

Different poses are good for different injuries. Experiment and see what feels rehabilitative. For example, if you have sprained a wrist, try Downward Facing Dog. Ease into the pose gently and just put as much weight on your wrist as feels manageable. This

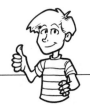

pose actually helps strengthen a healing wrist. If the pain becomes sharp or severe, of course, stop.

We don't want to give you the impression that yoga is meant to "harden you" or teach you to ignore pain. On the contrary, yoga teaches you to listen to pain, feel it, distinguish different types of pain from each other, and learn from it for better healing.

Yoga to Help Kids Concentrate and Increase Mental Alertness

When you feel like your concentration is ailing, yoga is also helpful. Just as the physical body sometimes gets out of sorts, our mental processes can get frazzled and in need of some gentle rehabilitation. Poses effective for helping with concentration and increasing mental alertness include …

For Kids Only

It may take you awhile to differentiate between a good stretch that might hurt a little bit and serious pain that is bad for your body. When you feel pain during yoga, ask yourself, is this good pain or bad pain? After you have experience with yoga stretching, you'll better understand and be able to feel the difference.

➤ All breathing exercises (Chapter 10)

➤ Eye exercises (Chapter 17)

➤ Chanting (Chapter 10)

➤ Yoga Sun Dance (Chapter 15)

➤ Mountain Pose (Chapter 11)

➤ Tree Pose (Chapter 11)

➤ Flamingo Pose (Chapter 12)

➤ Eagle Pose (Chapter 12)

➤ Crow Pose (Chapter 12)

➤ Headstand (Chapter 17)

➤ Wise Owl Pose (Chapter 13)

➤ Roller Coaster Spin (Chapter 15)

➤ Volcano Blast (Chapter 15)

➤ Hero Pose (Chapter 16)

➤ Toe-Ups (Chapter 17)

➤ Windmill (Chapter 17)

➤ Crossovers (Chapter 17)

➤ Mirror Me (Chapter 18)

➤ Synchronized Yoga (Chapter 18)

➤ Shavasana (Chapter 19)

Teaching kids how to help their bodies heal themselves through yoga is an incredibly powerful way for kids to understand how much health and healing is in their own hands. People who take their own healing seriously enough to take control of it, learn about it, and direct it tend to feel less helpless, more able to bear pain, and better able to maintain a positive attitude. That's healing power!

The Least You Need to Know

➤ Yoga, and other natural healing methods, can be less expensive and, in some cases, more effective than conventional or allopathic healing methods.

➤ Sometimes conventional medicine is best, especially for acute conditions, trauma, and other emergency health problems.

➤ Certain yoga poses can help kids with colic, asthma, breathing problems, stomach and digestive problems, and back pain, and can even help in recovering from sprains, strains, and breaks.

➤ Yoga heals the overworked brain as well as it heals the body.

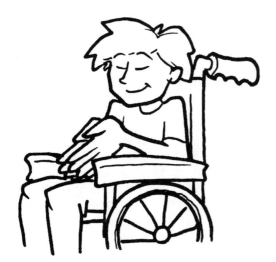

Chapter 25

Yoga for Kids with Special Needs

In This Chapter

➤ Everybody has special needs

➤ Your child can excel at yoga

➤ Yoga and learning challenges

➤ Yoga and physical challenges

➤ Accentuate the positive!

Everyone has special needs. Everyone needs individual attention, has a unique approach to learning, and his or her own personal challenges. For this reason, we don't want this chapter to seem exclusive from the others. Kids with special needs, such as physical or learning challenges, are just like any other kids.

Certain challenges can be specifically addressed through yoga. We address those challenges in this chapter to show parents and teachers how much yoga can help kids rise to meet their personal challenges with confidence and success.

We do recommend that children with moderate and severe disabilities learn yoga under the guidance of a certified yoga instructor experienced in working with children with special needs. See Appendix B for finding certified children's yoga therapists. Because it is a parent's job to locate a qualified instructor, we have addressed this chapter primarily to parents. We do not, in any way, intend to exclude kids from reading this chapter themselves, and we hope they will do so.

Every Kid Can Excel at Yoga

We've said it before and we'll say it again: Yoga is not competitive! There is no being "good" or "bad" at yoga, which is why anyone at all can do it: infants, toddlers, kids, teens, adults, seniors, people with hearing loss, those who are blind, those with paralysis or other physical disabilities, people with emotional ailments, and people with medical illnesses.

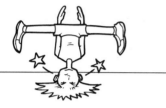

Ooops!

Parents, we encourage you not to correct your child's form. Your child with special needs will do some of the yoga poses quite different from what you might expect, and that's perfectly fine. Keep yoga positive, fun, and affirmative for your child.

We all go at our own pace. No matter how long you can hold a pose or how close to the ground you can get your heels in Downward Facing Dog, what the next person is doing doesn't matter. The only wrong way to do yoga is to do it unsafely. Each person sets his or her own standards, goals, and progress, and each individual's progression is a success.

Designing a Yoga Practice for Each Unique Child

When designing a yoga practice for your child, the first and most important thing to do is determine which benefits of yoga are most important for your child. Yoga has millions of benefits. What does your child need from a yoga practice? What do you expect from a yoga practice for your child?

Flip through this book and make some notes. Which poses target areas that are relevant to your child's needs? Of course, you won't want to limit yourself solely to poses that address a certain challenge. Yoga is about balance and each child needs to move and develop the whole self. However, knowing your particular focus can help shape and focus your yoga plan.

For example, perhaps your child has attention deficit disorder (ADD). Look for specific poses to help your child with focus and concentration, but you will also want to include other poses. Those that help with fine and gross motor coordination, interrelational skills, strength building, and flexibility help your child find and maintain a good balance.

No matter who you are or what your child's individual needs are, we would like to suggest one ultimate goal: fun! Providing your child with a yoga plan and yoga poses that he or she will find irresistibly fun will make yoga a positive and, ultimately, a more effective experience. Forcing your child into doing poses just because they are "good for you" could turn your child off to yoga, and then no one will benefit.

Even children with severe impairments who benefit from a more therapeutic yoga approach should enjoy their yoga therapy. Keep it easygoing! Kids with learning and physical challenges often have a slew of therapies—speech therapy, physical therapy, occupational therapy, tutoring, and the list goes on. Let yoga therapy be fun!

To help you focus and form a plan, we've provided space (headed "Challenge") for you to write down some of the challenges you would like a yoga practice to address for your child. There's space (headed "Beneficial Poses") to list the poses you find in this book that would be beneficial, according to our descriptions, in helping with the child's challenge. And there's also space (headed "Complementary Poses") to list poses that complement or balance your listed beneficial poses by working on other areas. We suggest you also write down the benefits next to all the poses you select. Once you've got it all written down, you'll have a basic focus for your child's daily yoga practice.

CHALLENGE: _____

BENEFICIAL POSES:

_____

_____

COMPLEMENTARY POSES:

_____

_____

CHALLENGE: _____

BENEFICIAL POSES:

_____

_____

COMPLEMENTARY POSES:

_____

_____

CHALLENGE: _____

BENEFICIAL POSES:

_____

_____

COMPLEMENTARY POSES:

_____

_____

CHALLENGE: _____

BENEFICIAL POSES:

_____

_____

COMPLEMENTARY POSES:

_____

_____

Yoga for Kids Who Learn Differently

While some kids have physical challenges to contend with, such as injuries, illness, or developmental issues, other kids have less tangible challenges. For kids affected by attention deficit hyperactivity disorder (ADHD), dyslexia, and other learning challenges, school and other activities requiring concentration and standard learning modes can become frustrating. Grades, relationships, success in extracurricular activities, and even self-esteem may suffer.

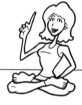

Yoga Stories

Recent studies in the news have suggested that many of America's children may be over-medicated. Many children are on medication for attention deficit hyperactivity disorder (ADHD) when perhaps they shouldn't be, and many parents (especially those who practice yoga) whose children are on medication for ADHD would prefer their children find a more natural form of relief without side effects. Some children with ADHD respond so well to yoga that they are able to stop taking medications that assist with concentration, such as Ritalin (according to many anecdotal claims). This is an excellent goal for a yoga practice. However, please don't make any decisions about stopping medications without consulting with your pediatrician or child psychiatrist/specialist.

Yoga is an excellent therapy for kids who learn differently. Here's how.

ADHD (Attention Deficit Hyperactivity Disorder)

Attention deficit hyperactivity disorder (*ADHD*), sometimes called attention deficit disorder (ADD), is a condition characterized by an inability to sustain attention for a length of time considered appropriate for the child's age, excessive talking and interrupting, a tendency to shift from one uncompleted activity to another, and difficulty in remaining seated, listening to directions, following instructions, and waiting for his or her turn. While some kids outgrow ADD, in other cases, the condition persists into adulthood.

Other symptoms characterize this disorder as well, and we don't intend to offer any tools of self-diagnosis in this book. Diagnosis is for your doctor or pediatrician.

Children who experience difficulty in paying attention, following directions, or who become easily overstimulated, may benefit initially from private or at-home yoga lessons. Once your child is familiar with yoga and experienced in some of the basics, including breathing exercises, eye exercises, asanas, and Shavasana, he or she might try a group class. (See Chapter 9, which describes how to find the right teacher.)

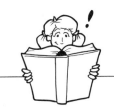

Learn About Yoga

Attention deficit hyperactivity disorder (**ADHD**), also known as attention deficit disorder (ADD), is a condition characterized by an attention span shorter than would be expected for the child's age, and sometimes hyperactive or impulsive behavior considered inappropriate for the child's age. ADHD is currently considered to manifest itself in three forms: children who are primarily inattentive, children who are primarily hyperactive or impulsive, and children who are both.

Learning Disabilities

According to the National Institutes of Health in Bethesda, Maryland, a learning disability is generally characterized by a two-year delay in grade level in reading, spelling, or math. More generally, a learning disability is any condition that interferes with a child's ability to learn. Even if your child isn't delayed two grade levels, however, certain learning disabilities such as *dyslexia, developmental writing disorder* (*DWD*), or *developmental arithmetic disorder* (*DAD*) can make school seem exceptionally difficult.

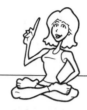

Yoga Stories

Some facts on attention deficit hyperactivity disorder (ADHD):

➤ ADHD affects 3 to 10 percent of all school-aged boys, and is 3 to 10 times more common in boys than in girls, although researchers aren't sure why.

➤ Up to 60 percent of hyperactive children continue to have related problems into adulthood, and there is no way to determine which children will outgrow the condition and which won't.

➤ Hyperactivity is the most common reason why children are referred to mental health centers in the United States.

➤ ADHD is not a learning disability. However, about 40 percent of children affected by ADHD have learning disabilities, and approximately 15 to 20 percent of learning-disabled children have ADHD. So, while there is some crossover, many children with ADHD don't have difficulties in school and some are in gifted and talented programs.

Children with learning disabilities often have difficulties utilizing both brain hemispheres. They also struggle with language, including expressive and receptive language. Sometimes they experience delays in social skills.

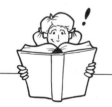

Learn About Yoga

Dyslexia, also called developmental reading disorder (DRD), is a reading disability resulting from an inability to correctly or completely process graphic symbols.

Yoga can certainly help to benefit kids with learning challenges, especially if the yoga practice is fun and playful, incorporating the multiple intelligences theory of Professor Howard Gardner we described in Chapter 8. Children with learning differences should include yoga poses and exercises that work across the body's midline, such as Windmill, Crossovers, and Bicycle Pose (all in Chapter 17).

Yoga can also teach body awareness skills. Encourage children to play creative yoga games such as Mirror Me, Assist Me, and Synchronized Yoga (all in Chapter 18). Children with learning disabilities should practice yoga in a setting that will help them to feel confident, whether that means yoga at home, in privacy, or with a group of peers.

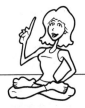

Yoga Stories

In the United States, it is estimated that 5 to 10 percent of children between the ages of 5 and 17 have at least one learning disability. Children with learning disabilities are not less intelligent than other children. They simply process information differently or are experiencing developmental delays in certain areas. Learning disabilities include disorders that keep a child from correctly reading or writing words, correctly speaking or hearing words, or correctly interpreting math symbols. Injuries, diseases, vision or hearing loss, lack of early experiences, or congenital conditions can cause learning disabilities.

Yoga for Kids Who Have Physical Challenges

Whether your child is physically delayed, in a wheelchair, has some paralysis, is immobile, or is missing certain limbs, your child can do yoga, too. If your child requires assistance getting into certain poses, bear in mind that lots of children require assistance and there is nothing wrong with that. Remember our Assist Me exercise in Chapter 18? As we've said before, each person is unique and each child's version of a pose, as long as it is safe, is correct and fine for that child. It doesn't have to look like the picture in a book.

Too Loose: Hypermobility and Down's Syndrome

Some children are hypermobile, or very flexible. Children with Down's syndrome are susceptible to this condition. Extremely flexible kids can certainly benefit from a yoga practice. Just because they are particularly flexible in certain areas of the body doesn't mean they should ignore poses that target that area. Actually, doing poses for a certain area where flexibility is already present is actually beneficial because such targeted yoga will help to strengthen a hypermobile area.

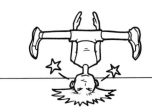

Ooops!

Many times in yoga books or other books, we see models doing yoga poses perfectly. A "perfect" model is not necessarily a good model, since few people do a pose exactly the same and no one is perfect (whatever "perfect" means!). Rather than comparing a child's pose to a picture in a book, go by how the pose feels and works for the individual.

Children with moderate to severe cases of Down's syndrome will benefit from working one-on-one with a certified yoga instructor. Most of this work will be hands-on and interactive until the child is able to perform the yoga poses independently. The focus of yoga therapy for children with Down's syndrome is to strengthen the muscles, enabling more yoga poses and greater overall physical control. (See Appendix B for information on Sonia Sumar's book, *Yoga for the Special Child,* and on finding a certified yoga teacher.) Some relevant poses might include Bridge Pose (see Chapter 16), Butterfly Pose (see Chapter 11), and Mother Snake Pose (see Chapter 13).

Too Tight: Stiffness and Cerebral Palsy

Yoga helps to loosen stiffness and joints by keeping the body mobile and by working the limits of flexibility for each individual. Children with l palsy will benefit from working one-on-one with a certified yoga instructor (again, see the Appendix B for information on Sonia Sumar's book and for a list of certified yoga instructors). Cat and Cow Poses (see Chapter 12), Mother Snake Pose (see Chapter 13), Twister Pose (see Chapter 16), and yoga breathing exercises would all be appropriate inclusions in your yoga plan.

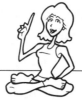

Yoga Stories

Parents can try to help their children understand that yoga is about working with the individual body's natural tendencies and movements, no matter how large or small. Whatever challenges your child has, encourage your child to listen to his or her body to reveal what yoga can do. If your child discovers movements that seem like yoga movements or positions that feel like yoga poses, encourage your child to name them and use them. Be sure to help your child understand that yoga is about him or her, not about the limits of the poses in this book.

Paralysis, Immobility, and Yoga

Kids with joint stiffness or soreness, paralysis, or other types of immobility can also benefit from a yoga practice. Children who are in wheelchairs or even bed-bound can certainly do many yoga poses, with the assistance of either a parent, sibling, or teacher. Remember, yoga is all about what the individual can do and about nudging personal limits without pushing, but never about competition.

For some kids, even the slightest movement is a huge accomplishment, and that's wonderful. A certified yoga instructor specializing in working with physically challenged kids can provide specific exercises and poses that can benefit your child. Some relevant poses are breathing exercises …

➤ Mouse Pose (Chapter 12)

➤ Butterfly Pose (Chapter 11)

➤ Cactus Pose (Chapter 13)

➤ Yoga Dancing (Chapter 15)

➤ Sailboat Pose (Chapter 15)

➤ X Pose (Chapter 16)

Too Little Tone: Hypocerebratonicity and Weak Muscles

Many kids are hypotonic, meaning their muscles are underdeveloped. These kids may be quite flexible but lack a balanced level of muscle strength. Yoga poses that work as a focus for hypotonic kids are those that emphasize gross motor movements, such as Bear Walk, Giraffe Walk, *T. Rex* Walk (all in Chapter 14), and the Yoga Sun Dance (see Chapter 15).

Helping Kids Believe They Can Achieve Their Goals

Just as important as teaching yoga poses to kids with challenges is maintaining a positive energy about the practice of yoga. Yoginis can feel your energy, even if they can't or don't always express what they feel. If you believe your yogini can achieve his or her yoga goals, your child will believe it, too. So believe it! Because your child can do it.

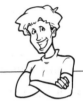

For Grownups, Too!

If you feel unsure about how to help your child do yoga, take a yoga class with your child and consider yourself in training! Have the certified instructor show you poses you and your child can do together at home. Also look through this book to find appropriate poses. Your shared yoga practice can turn into a bonding experience that will help your relationship grow and develop.

The Least You Need to Know

➤ Everyone has special needs and a yoga class should be designed to recognize the special needs of each unique individual.

➤ Parents can help their kids with learning or physical challenges by designing a unique yoga practice that addresses particular needs and a balanced approach.

➤ Some learning challenges that yoga can benefit include dyslexia, developmental writing disorder (DWD), and developmental arithmetic disorder (DAD). Attention deficit hyperactivity disorder (ADHD), which can result in learning challenges, can also be helped with yoga therapy.

➤ Physical challenges that respond well to yoga therapy include the hypermobility associated with Down's syndrome, cerebral palsy, joint problems, paralysis and immobility, and hypotonicity.

➤ If you believe your child can accomplish yoga goals, your child will believe it, too.

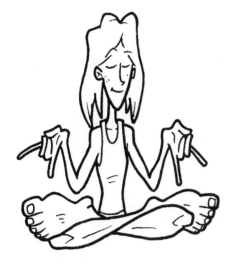

Chapter 26

Yoga for Teens

In This Chapter

➤ Teens and yoga for greater independence

➤ Boys can do yoga, too!

➤ How yoga helps girls become women

➤ What's in store for the next generation?

Wait a minute ... how did that little child turn into a teenager? Wasn't it just yesterday she was toddling around, holding onto the furniture for balance? Wasn't it just yesterday that he was struggling to pronounce the words "mama" or "dada"?

Guess what, mom and dad? Your son or daughter is almost a grownup. "Wait!" you may protest. "My daughter is only 15! She isn't an adult! She doesn't even do her own laundry!" Teens do still depend on the adults in their lives for many things, but we can't deny that very soon, they will be adults themselves.

As parents, how can we help our kids make that final step into grownup land? Should we push? Nudge? Hold on as tight as we can to prolong the inevitable? Close our eyes, hold our breaths, and hope for the best? What's a parent to do?

Yoga, anyone? Yoga can help teens find their way, developing their confidence, self-control, even a sense of right and wrong. It can also help parents to get through the teen years, to relax, breathe, and focus instead of worrying every second their son is away with the family car, driving it (gulp) *all by himself!*

Independence Day

Babies need adults. They can't do much on their own. Toddlers don't think they need adults, but clearly, they do. Preschoolers and grade-schoolers are moving out into the world, but rely on the safety and security of an adult in control.

But teens? Hey, it's independence day! Teens are practically adults themselves, and while they may not always make smart decisions (then again, adults don't always

make smart decisions, either), they are fast developing into capable, mature, self-possessed young adults with the ability to carve their own paths through life.

While some teens mature faster than others and teens may often feel less than sure of themselves out there in the world, one thing *is* for sure: Adulthood is imminent. This is a scary time for parents, as they slowly loosen their grasp and let their children go their own way.

Adolescence is a natural time for teens to search for different ways of thinking, alternative exercises, and brand-new philosophies, and it's a time for them to explore the world and strive to find their places in it. Many of us first discovered yoga in our teens for these reasons. Even if parents are already into yoga, teens can make yoga their own by developing a personal practice tailored to uniquely adolescent needs. Yoga can provide both family time and the alone-time teens sometimes need to explore who they are and where they are going in life.

For Kids Only

Sometimes it's really hard for parents to let go, even when you want them to let you become an adult. Try to be patient with them. They still think of you as a little kid. The best way to show them you are growing up is to behave like an adult: trustworthy, responsible, mature, and passionate about your pursuits, whatever they are (yoga, school, friends, basketball, music, and so on).

*Yogini teens practice
Warrior I.*

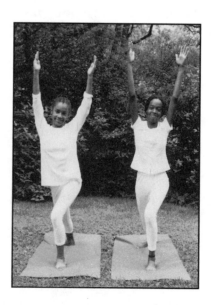

Yoga is great for teens in all the ways it is great for anyone: building self-confidence, strength, flexibility, coordination, concentration, focus, and self-control. Yoga gives teens a context from which to develop a personal philosophy, a physical fitness plan, or a meditation practice. Yoga can be anything a teen wants it to be. It can give a structure and a purpose to a teen's burgeoning independence.

Welcoming Teens into the Adult Community

Our society doesn't have a law that specifically says when a child becomes an adult. We can drive at 16 or 17. We can vote at 18. We can drink at 21. But that doesn't necessarily mean that any of those ages signal adulthood.

A child becomes an adult when he or she acts like an adult. As a parent, you can respect and support your teen's attempts to become an adult. The teen years aren't always as easy as we may remember them. It can be tough out there, but with your love and your teen's personal effort, nothing can stop him or her from success (whatever that means for the individual).

When adults welcome teens into the adult community, teens feel a part of that community. When communication develops between the young and the old, and everyone in between, fear and misunderstanding are replaced with love, empathy, and hope. Parents, unite with your yoginis and we can all look forward to the future.

What Yoga Teaches Young Men

Yoga for boys? Some people question the notion of teenage boys doing yoga. While lots of parents are happy to bring their preschool-aged sons to a yoga class, people say older boys wouldn't enjoy yoga … or would they?

Actually, many pre-adolescent and adolescent boys take yoga classes. Boys are naturally less flexible than girls, so yoga is extremely beneficial for balance in male athletes. In fact, more and more male celebrities and sports figures are doing yoga to build a better balance in their minds and bodies. Some popular male yogis you may know are Sting, Ricky Martin, Jerry Seinfeld, and Kareem Abdul-Jabbar.

Because yoga teaches noncompetitiveness and non-violence, it can help boys to control the sense of competition and aggression that contemporary society sometimes nurtures in its young men. It also

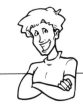

For Grownups, Too!

Boys in our culture are often pigeonholed into male stereotypes: good athlete, potential good provider, strong, able to suppress emotional displays, and so on. These stereotypes limit boys and can stunt their emotional growth. Try to let your son be whoever he is. Let him decide. Encourage him to look beyond societal stereotypes to his inner self.

teaches boys (and men) to respect all life and see things with a broader and more compassionate perspective. That isn't "girl-y." That's maturity.

And even though many yoginis are girls in this country, in India, yoga has traditionally been mostly a practice for males. Yogis in other countries recognized long ago the many benefits of yoga for the male body, mind, and spirit. Tune up your male energy with a daily yoga workout and watch your confidence, strength, and athletic abilities soar!

Getting Strong

Boys may think yoga is all stretching, but many yoga exercises and poses use the body's own weight, often coupled with challenging balances, to build muscle strength.

Many sports build muscle and increase strength in boys, but overlook stretching and flexibility. Yoga balances this disparity with plenty of stretching to balance its strength-building aspects. For maximum physical potential, boys need both.

Boys to Men

Many other countries and cultures, especially ancient ones, have rituals for boys entering manhood. Our culture largely overlooks this tradition. Bar Mitzvahs or less formal marker events, such as father-son camping trips, can serve as "manhood" rituals. Parents, if your family hasn't found a symbolic and celebratory way to recognize your son's transition into the adult world, we hope you will create one.

Boys need to know that this important and often confusing time of transition is recognized, normal, natural, and a cause for joy. Sure, adolescent boys sometimes feel confused, nervous, insecure, even scared. It happens to everyone. Hormone levels in adolescent boys are changing and causing these intense feelings.

But these hormonal changes signal one of the most significant rites of passage in a boy's life. Parents, let it be known your son has become a man! You might even consider throwing a yoga party to celebrate (see the next chapter). Be sure to include lots of warrior poses (see Chapter 16), which build strength and confidence in growing boys.

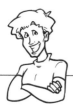

For Grownups, Too!

Many ancient cultures took their young boys on some form of a quest as a rite of passage into manhood. Trips into nature with father and son (or another trusted male adult) can create significant, lifelong memories for a young boy. Go out into nature and have an adventure (your adventure needn't include hunting!). Talk about what it means to be a man.

Boys Growing Up Yoga Style

How do you convince a boy that he can benefit from yoga? Do yoga together! Dads, this is a great way to spend time with your son and set an example by showing him that "real men" do yoga. Embarking on a yoga plan together will help both of you get into better balance. If you and your son play sports together, make a plan to evaluate your performances before and after instituting a daily yoga practice. Many parents coach their children's sports teams. What a great opportunity to integrate yoga exercises as warm-ups!

For even more direction and a great role model, seek out a male yoga teacher from whom to take classes. A practiced male yogi can tell you even more about the flexibility, range of motion, endurance, and other qualities yoga promotes in men.

What Yoga Teaches Young Women

As they face the many changes in adolescence and struggle to find their own place in the world, girls can learn a lot from yoga. Yoga is an excellent way to boost self-confidence, something not always easy to maintain in the face of puberty and its associated hormonal changes.

But being a teenaged girl isn't all about hormones. As young women today prepare to make their own way in life, they face many personal and societal challenges. Although every woman is different, yoga can help young women build the confidence they need to become responsible for themselves, develop a strong sense of self, nurture and respect their bodies, and form strong, healthy, equitable relationships.

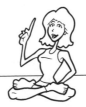

Yoga Stories

Girls in our society today are afflicted with an epidemic of eating disorders, often starving themselves (a sign of a condition called anorexia nervosa), eating excessive amounts of food (a sign of binge eating disorder), or bingeing and then purging by vomiting or using laxatives (a condition called bulimia). While the causes may be complicated, many believe eating disorders are partially a response to beliefs that happiness or confidence comes from body size and shape. Eating disorders are much more common in girls than in boys, and they are very difficult to control without professional help. Kids, if you suspect you have an eating disorder, please seek professional help immediately. Every year, several thousand women die from eating disorders or their complications.

Entering the Cycle

Girls begin menstruation at different ages, but usually between 9 and 15 years of age. This is a difficult time for girls because they aren't used to this monthly process and may be unprepared for the associated discomfort and the "technical" aspects of dealing with the menstrual flow. We hope you will talk to your daughter openly about what to expect and how to handle the details.

Those "hormonal" days can make everyday obligations, such as school and after-school jobs, more difficult than usual, but a regular yoga practice can greatly reduce the uncomfortable symptoms associated with menstruation. Breathing exercises, deep relaxation, and exercises that stretch and massage the abdomen and back are great for girls experiencing menstruation-related discomfort such as cramps, bloating, or lower backache. Some great poses for relief include Bridge Pose (see Chapter 16), Cat and Cow Poses (see Chapter 12), and deep relaxation (Shavasana; see Chapter 19).

Yoga can also help girls stay in touch with their womanhood. Menstruation is a very real and exciting sign that a girl has become a woman. A monthly mother-daughter celebration seems in order! Give your daughter a backrub, enjoy a quiet cup of tea together, and do some mother-daughter partner yoga. How about a few rounds of the Yoga Sun Dance (see Chapter 15)? What better way to nurture your blossoming daughter?

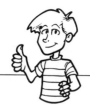

For Kids Only

Feeling insecure today? You aren't alone. Teenaged girls sometimes have a hard time feeling confident. The trick is to know how to handle these temporary feelings (we know they don't *seem* temporary). Be kind to yourself and your body. Express your feelings. Tell yourself you are beautiful, inside and out. Get involved with something you love. These are positive responses that can make you feel great!

Girls to Women

The signs of womanhood are obvious in a teenaged girl. Her body changes, she begins to menstruate, and she feels different: emotional, confused, super-confident one moment and timid the next. Hormones are the culprit, not a girl's "inner self" or personality.

These hormonal changes are exciting for young girls and their parents. They signal the entrance into womanhood and that is a significant time in a girl's life. Parents can help their daughters make this important transition by keeping communication open and by celebrating this rite of passage. We aren't saying you should throw a party when your daughter starts her period. How embarrassing! But celebrating your daughter's journey into the adult world? We can think of no better reason for a celebration.

Sweet sixteen parties, Bat Mitzvahs, and debutante "coming out" parties all contain the spirit of this celebration. Parents, if your daughter isn't celebrating any of these particular rituals, we hope your family will create its own. The next chapter gives you lots of ideas for yoga parties to honor your teenage daughter's coming of age.

Girls Growing Up Yoga Style

Mothers who do yoga with their daughters set a great example for how to treat the body, respect the self, and build health and vibrant energy for life as an adult and, potentially, pregnancy, childbirth, and motherhood. Although daughters don't always choose to emulate their mothers, mothers have a significant influence on who a girl becomes. Moms, be the best woman, mother, and yogi you can be, and your daughter will eventually be inspired to be the most she can be, too.

Next Generation Yoginis

Yoga has been around for thousands of years. Each generation that practices yoga helps to continue that auspicious tradition. A generation of yoginis ready to take on the world is an exciting prospect.

Teens involved in a regular yoga practice as well as other activities that interest and inspire them will already be exercising their bodies and their passions. Teens who understand that they *are* the future will be better prepared to take on the weight of the world with lightness and joy, serenity and love. There is no one else to do the job. The job has already begun. And, parents, we think your yogini will be a wonderful member of the next generation.

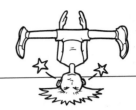

Ooops!

Hormonal changes and increased responsibility can make life tough for teens. Frustration, irritability, anger, and sadness are common. The best medicine is movement! Vigorous yoga poses and a brisk walk in the fresh air are great mood enhancers. If teens can't control their sadness or anger or have thoughts of suicide, they may be suffering from a more serious form of depression. See a doctor immediately. Depression is highly treatable.

The Least You Need to Know

➤ Teens struggling to become adults can gain strength, self-confidence, values, and maturity from a regular yoga practice.

➤ Yoga isn't just for girls. Boys benefit immensely from yoga, becoming more physically balanced and gaining better self-control.

➤ Yoga is an excellent way for girls to handle the hormonal changes associated with puberty and to build the self-confidence so important for girls to be successful.

➤ Raising kids in a yoga tradition with respect, support, and lots of love will create a next generation of world citizens in whom we can all take pride.

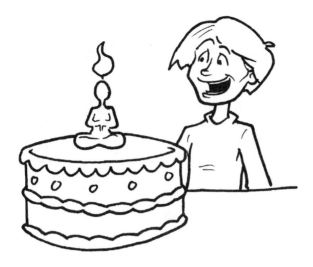

Chapter 27

Surprise: A Yoga Kids Party!

In This Chapter

➤ How to make yoga into a party

➤ Safety first

➤ Yoga party basics: invitations, decorations, food, and favors

➤ Theme-based yoga poses and games

➤ Are grownups invited?

If you think yoga is fun, wait until you've hosted or attended a yoga party! Yoga can provide the perfect theme for a budding yogini's next birthday party. Or, celebrate other marker events with a yoga party: the first day of any season, New Year's Day, Valentine's Day, May Day, Independence Day, Thanksgiving, New Year's Day, half-birthdays, a child's coming of age, or just because you feel like having a party!

This chapter will tell you everything you need to know to organize, set up, and host a yoga party. A yoga party can be for a child of any age, so some of the ideas in this chapter will be geared for younger children, some for older. Pick and choose the ideas that suit you.

Are you getting in a party mood? Then let's party on!

Yoginis Unite!

Even if your only experience so far with yoga is to have flipped through the pages of this book, you can hold or attend a yoga party. All it takes is some creativity and a little team spirit.

Yoginis coming together to experiment with yoga for the first time can have just as much fun as yoginis who have been doing yoga for a couple of years. A group of toddlers can have a blast at a yoga party, and so can a group of teens. Even a group of new mothers could collect for a new-baby shower or a first birthday and do yoga together with their infants.

A Kid Party Every Parent Can Love

Most parents have probably already attended and hosted their fair share of kid birthday parties. If you're one of them, you know the drill: Hang the streamers and balloons, order the cake and matching cupcakes, buy the requisite bags of chips, cartons of dip, plates of sandwich fixings, cartons of ice cream. Decorate the table with birthday paper plates and coordinated plastic ware. Buy the matching centerpiece. Spend hours dividing treats and toys into party favor bags and tying with ribbons.

But imagine a party where the focus is on the child's creativity and imagination, a party that is economical, ecological, and educational. A yoga party makes kids the center of the action, and that's not only fun for kids, it's easier on parents.

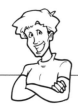

For Grownups, Too!

The easiest, and often the most fun, place to have a yoga party is outside in a yard or park. Weather permitting, outdoor parties require few decorations because nature provides the beauty. The fresh air is great for kids and you will typically have a much larger space for yoga play.

What Parents Need to Know About Kids' Parties

If you think throwing a party for kids is complicated or expensive, think again! The only thing really necessary for a great kid party is plenty of fun things to do, a good space to do them in, and some tasty food (the less "junky," the better—healthy food that tastes great will keep kids feeling great). Props, decorations, favors, all that other party stuff can be creatively acquired, hand-made from things you already have around the house, or recycled from past parties.

To assess what you really need for your own yoga party, sit down with your child and make a list of what things are really important to your yogini. Then, go over your list one more time and see if you can cross off anything. The simpler the preparations are, the more energy you can pour into the party itself.

Keeping Kids Safe

Any child's birthday party should be well supervised by several adults. Ask a few parents to stick around and join the fun. A large group of small children can be hard for one or two adults to supervise. Make sure the party is in an area where small children can't wander into the street or another yard, or into an unsafe part of the house such as steep basement stairs.

If the kids are young, parents could attend with their children and do the yoga poses and games, too. Parental involvement keeps each kid safer, and the parents can have a lot of fun, too!

If the kids are older, supervision is equally important, although parents may be more or less involved in the party, depending on the child's party plan. Parents should be nearby, just in case.

What You'll Need for a Karma-Licious Yoga Party

Now let's get down to details. A yoga party works best with a specific theme. For young kids and older kids alike, animal and nature themes are appropriate, such as a Rainforest Gala, a Desert Soirée, a Trip to the Zoo, a Day at the Beach, or a Bird Bash. For example, young kids could celebrate at a Bird Bash by dressing up like different birds before each pose, picking costumes from a box of scarves, masks, beaks, hoods, wigs, boas, and capes provided by the host.

Older kids could hold a Rainforest Gala by doing yoga poses to appropriate music and talking about steps they could take to help preserve rainforest environments all over the world. They could even make rain sticks (sticks that, when turned over, make the sound of rain) from recycled wrapping paper or paper towel tubes filled with twigs, leaves, sand, and gravel, and sealed on each end with a circle of cloth and a few sturdy rubber bands.

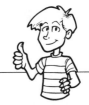

For Kids Only

Kids sometimes have a hard time figuring out whom to invite to a party. Base your guest list on a specific group and invite everyone in that group to avoid hurt feelings: your yoga class, school class, girl scout troop, kids in your neighborhood, etc. Even if you are tempted to leave certain people out, think how they would feel. Be a kind, empathetic yogini and include the whole group.

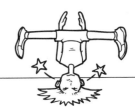

Ooops!

Outside parties are great, but be sure kids are well supervised, away from traffic, and in a fenced area, or have several people in charge of safety. Kids should be instructed to stay with the group, avoid strangers, and look out for hazards, such as sharp objects on the ground and stinging insects. And don't forget the sunscreen!

Yogini Party Invitations

How do you invite your friends to a yoga party? Very gleefully! Make your own invitations cut into animal shapes, foot shapes, a circus tent, a cactus for a desert theme, a big feather for a bird theme, or whatever else is appropriate. A child may like to decorate invitations with drawings, paintings, or stickers. For the computer literate, design an invitation using a card-making computer program. Or, think of your own clever idea. Your invitation could look something like this:

Come to our yoga party!

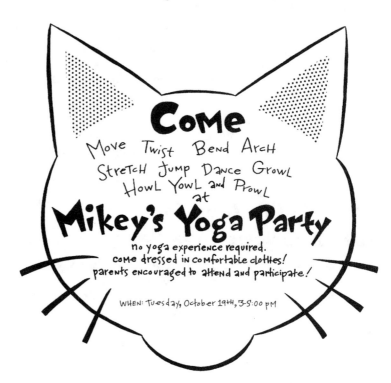

Yogini Party Decorations

Decorations for a yoga party can be simple or fancy. Outside parties don't need much. Keep in mind that yoga respects the natural world. Your party can be both economical and ecological.

Use a sheet or blanket on a picnic table instead of a throw-away paper table cover. For a centerpiece, find pieces of the natural world that are easily borrowed—pretty rocks, fallen leaves, pine branches, pinecones, and acorns. Don't pick flowers unless they are plentiful or planted specifically for cutting. Let the flowers around you serve as decoration as they grow!

350

Children can participate in the decorating by making nature collages, leaf rubbings, and collecting decorations from nature.

Many natural decorations can also be brought inside. An inside yoga space can also be adorned with crystals, wind chimes, and draped sheets, scarves, ribbons, and beads. Use what you have in a new way. Opening the windows and turning on appropriate music are decorations in themselves.

For younger kids especially, parents should really emphasize the theme, whatever it may be. You don't necessarily need to spend money. Collect all your child's stuffed animals and fill a room or a yard with them. Make construction-paper cutouts of circus shapes, desert shapes, feet, and so on, and have your child decorate them. You could make a piñata of a tree, an elephant, a beach ball, or a cloud, for example. Hang decorations everywhere, or glue them to skewers or Popsicle sticks and "plant" them in the ground.

Theme-related books piled in corners, posters hung on the wall, mobiles, animal puppets, and any actual pets you happen to have can all add life and fun to a room, backyard, or other party area. (Don't let pets loose in areas where they might escape or get injured, please.)

Yogini Party Food

Much of your decor, whether inside or out, can come from creatively designed yoga party food, a sure way to make the table attractive. We like yoga party food that is fun, healthy, delicious, and that sustains body and mind. Parents, enjoy the following recipes, or adapt your own favorites.

Yogini Finger Food

Make sandwiches spread with a variety of healthy fillings or toppings, such as peanut or almond butter, cheese, hummus, tomato, or avocado on whole-grain bread. Cut the sandwiches into animal shapes using cookie cutters.

Yoginis love to dip! For a delicious savory dip, beat together one cup of plain yogurt or sour cream with eight ounces of cream cheese, then add various herbs, ketchup, pesto, or mashed avocado to accompany whole-grain baked chips, baby carrots, celery sticks, strips of baked white or sweet potato, pita bread triangles, or strips of toast.

Sweet dips are delicious, too! Serve a sweet dip made from 1 cup of plain yogurt, ¼ cup honey, and a dash of cinnamon with apple slices, banana wheels, or other chunks of fruit on plastic toothpicks (keep toothpicks out of reach of young children).

Let kids create their own fruit-and-veggie animals! Serve big bowls of fruits and veggies cut into random shapes: circles, triangles, rectangles, squares, crescents, and other shapes. Give each child a white paper plate and let him or her build their own edible works of animal art. Don't forget to take pictures!

Not every party needs a cake. For a sweet treat, make peanut butter or molasses cookies and cut them into animal shapes with cookie cutters. Bake, decorate, and pile the cookies on a platter. Or, use animal-shaped cookies (homemade or store-bought animal crackers) as the decoration on top of cupcakes or around the sides of a larger cake (an animal parade!).

For a truly yoga-licious yet nutrient-dense party cake, try the following yummy recipe for Yogini Party Cake. It is moist, delicious, sweetened with honey, and can be customized to include whatever yummy ingredients your child favors.

Yogini Party Cake

3 large eggs
½ cup canola oil
1 cup unsweetened (natural) applesauce *or* unsweetened pumpkin puree
1 cup finely shredded carrots
1 8-ounce can crushed pineapple with juice
2 cups honey, divided (save 1 cup for after baking)
1 cup whole-wheat flour
1 cup white flour
1½ teaspoons baking powder

1½ teaspoons baking soda
1 teaspoon cinnamon
1 teaspoon ginger
2 cups total of any of the following, or a combination equaling 2 cups:
- finely or coarsely chopped almonds, walnuts, or pecans
- raisins (dark or yellow), dried cherries, dried blueberries, or currents
- chopped dried apricots or dates
- grated coconut
- finely chopped fresh apples, peaches, or apricots

In a large mixing bowl, combine the eggs, oil, applesauce or pumpkin, carrots, pineapple and 1 cup of honey. Beat until well combined.

In another bowl, add flours, baking powder, baking soda, cinnamon, and ginger. Stir with a fork until well combined, then add to the wet ingredients.

Fold in the two cups of fruit, nuts, or whatever combination you choose.

Pour into a greased 13 × 9-inch cake pan and bake at 350 degrees for about 35 minutes, or until a wooden toothpick comes out clean.

After you take the cake out of the oven, heat the remaining cup of honey on the stovetop or in the microwave (about 30 to 45 seconds) until it has a watery consistency. Using the wooden toothpick or a skewer, poke holes all over the top of the warm cake, then pour the warm honey evenly over the top. Pour slowly, allowing it to sink into the holes.

Serve warm, at room temperature, or cold, plain or with a dollop of vanilla- or honey-flavored yogurt.

You can also frost this cake. Cool completely, then frost with eight ounces of cream cheese softened with just enough honey or thawed apple juice concentrate to make it spreadable (add just a little at a time).

Serves approximately 24 party guests.

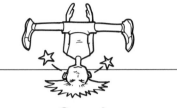

Ooops!

Don't forget that children under one year of age aren't usually supposed to eat eggs or honey. Until you have your pediatrician's or doctor's okay, don't serve cake to the babies.

Yogini Party Favors

Everyone likes to have a favor to take home as a memento after a great party, and if people have brought gifts, favors are an extra-nice way to say thanks!

Appropriate favors for a yoga party vary widely, depending on the age of the guests. Here are some fun, age-appropriate ideas:

➤ For toddlers: animal, bird, clown, or other appropriate figurines and a box of animal crackers

➤ For preschoolers: a "treasure" or two, such as an inexpensive, small crystal or other colorful rock, perhaps in a box wrapped with shiny foil; and a pinwheel to practice breathing exercises

➤ For grade-schoolers: a small potted bulb flower or other plant for them to nurture, or a potted pinwheel

➤ For teens: a crystal or other small stone on a chain or leather tie, a beaded bracelet, or some other "wearable" form of nature

➤ For any age: a tie-dyed or otherwise hand-decorated T-shirt; a nicely decorated, printed list of all the yoga poses and games featured at the party; a copy of this book for each guest!

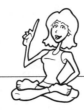

Yoga Stories

Colors symbolize many things, including each of the seven chakras, different types of energy, different personality types, and even the different months of the year. Kids love getting something personalized, so when offering colored stones as party favors, consider coordinating them to the color of each child's birthstone (you can ask for birth dates along with RSVPs). Birthstone colors are as follows: January is dark red (garnet); February is purple (amethyst); March is light blue (aquamarine); April is transparent (diamond); May is green (emerald); June is white (pearl); July is bright red (ruby); August is light green (peridot); September is blue (sapphire); October is multicolored (opal); November is yellow (topaz); December is blue-green (turquoise).

Yogini Party Fun

Now for the party itself. What do you do at a yoga party? Yoga, of course! After a brief gathering and social period, assemble guests into a group. You might like to begin with something vigorous like Yoga Dancing or the Yoga Sun Dance to get everyone warmed up and engaged.

Then head straight for your theme destination! Remember to get there, yoga-style (Driving My Car Pose, Boat Pose, Camel Pose, for example), then do your theme-related poses—circus, desert, beach, park, rainforest, and so on. Use appropriate music, props, costumes—whatever adds a festive atmosphere.

Remember, yoga is movement, so whatever you do at your destination, even if it doesn't seem much like anything you've read in this book, it is yoga. Don't worry if you don't cover all the yoga poses you had planned. Stay flexible and let the kids lead the action (within reason!). Kids come up with some great ideas about where they will "go" next or what they will "see" on their journey.

Somewhere along your yoga trip, don't forget to light the "Candle." Have everyone do Candle Pose (see Chapter 17), then sing "Happy Birthday" (or just

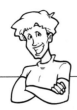

For Grownups, Too!

One of the challenges of organizing yoga poses for a group with varied experience and fitness levels is to make sure everyone feels comfortable doing poses their own way. Everyone's version is the right version, even if everyone does the poses differently. Remember, the point is fun, not "winning" or being "right." Celebrate difference!

"Happy Day" if it isn't a birthday party) while in the pose! Then, have everyone blow out their flames (in other words, their feet).

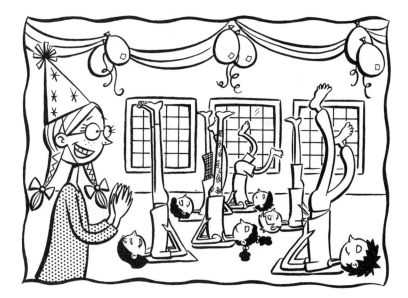

Yogini birthday candles!

And don't forget to make a wish for fish! Have each party guest make a wish, then do Fish Pose (see Chapter 17).

At the end of the journey, give every guest a present by doing a guided deep relaxation. Have all the guests lie down on their backs in Shavasana, and ask an adult to talk the group into a relaxed state (see Chapter 19 for more about getting into this pose). Then, ask the adult to speak the following words, or something similar:

Turn your attention to your breath. Feel it moving in and out of your nose. Follow the sound and the feeling of your breath. Listen to your breath. [Pause]

Now, assign your breath a color, to make it easier to follow. Notice the color moving all the way down into your belly, then back out through your nose. [Pause] Watch your colored breath. Relax and breathe. [Pause]

Imagine the color slowly leaving your breath. Return your breathing to normal. [Pause]

Imagine that today is your birthday. Think about what kind of weather you would like to have. [Pause] On your birthday, you can do what you would most like to do. Choose an activity. Maybe you will go somewhere. [Pause] Think about who you will go with. [Pause] Now try to imagine yourself doing the activity or visiting your chosen place. Look around at everything. Look slowly so that you don't miss anything. [Pause] Now listen to the sounds, both the sounds from things nearby and the faraway sounds. [Pause]

Now, you've just received the present you've dreamed of the most. Use your hands to touch it and feel it. How does it feel? [Pause] Play with it for a while. [Pause]

Now it is time to eat your cake. First inhale through your nose and smell the cake. How does it smell? Think about how it might taste. Imagine eating it (without actually eating anything). [Pause]

Spend some more time celebrating your birthday. Enjoy. Be peaceful. Have fun! [Pause]

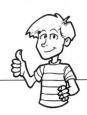

For Kids Only

A yoga party can be a great first step to a yoga club. If you and your friends have an awesome time doing yoga together, why not make it a regular thing? Who says you have to have an official holiday to have a yoga party, or just an informal yoga get-to-gether? With yoga, every day is a cause for a celebration!

Now, slowly deepen your breath as you prepare to awaken your body. [Pause] *Then, slowly begin to move your toes.* [Pause] *Now your fingers.* [Pause] *Gently move your ankles and wrists.* [Pause]

Stretch your body as if you were a cat waking from a nap. [Pause] *Bring your knees in to your chest and gently roll over to your side, making a pillow with your hands. Keep your eyes closed.* [Pause]

Slowly open your eyes half way as you use your hands to come up, sitting in Pretzel Pose.

Parents might place kids' party favors on their bellies right before they open their eyes or get up. This makes a great incentive for kids to lie down and chill for awhile!

We hope you had a great party! The best thing about a yoga party is that you can have lots of them, and every one of them can be completely different. All yoga parties have something in common, however: They make lasting memories!

The Least You Need to Know

➤ Yoga makes a great party theme for a child's birthday party or other celebration.

➤ Keep kids safe by holding the party in a secure and age-appropriate location with good supervision.

➤ Invitations, decorations, food, and favors needn't be expensive. You can make everything you need out of stuff you probably already have at home.

➤ Organize a series of active, fun, theme-related yoga poses and games.

➤ Parental or adult involvement at a level that engages and pleases kids makes a yoga kid's party ultimately successful.

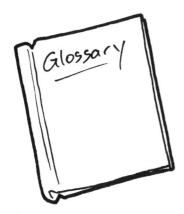

Glossary

Adho Mukha Shavasana   The Sanskrit term for Downward Facing Dog Pose.

Adho Mukha Vrikshaasana   The Sanskrit term for Handstand.

allopathic medicine   Standard, conventional Western medicine as taught in most medical schools and as practiced by most medical doctors in the West.

altar   A spiritual space to keep personally meaningful objects and symbolic representations as well as tools associated with yoga and/or meditation. An altar can be a tribute to selfhood as well as a focus for meditation and contemplation.

alveoli   The grape-like clusters at the ends of the bronchioles and covered with capillaries, where oxygen and carbon dioxide are exchanged.

ashram   A spiritual retreat, originally associated with Hinduism but now commonly used to describe a place where yoga is taught and/or practiced.

attention deficit disorder (ADD)   *See* attention deficit hyperactivity disorder (ADHD).

attention deficit hyperactivity disorder (ADHD)   Sometimes called attention deficit disorder (ADD), this condition is characterized by the child's inability to sustain attention for a length of time considered appropriate for age, excessive talking and interrupting, a tendency to shift from one uncompleted activity to another, difficulty in remaining seated, listening to directions, following instructions, and waiting for his or her turn.

Baddha Konasana   The Sanskrit term for Butterfly Pose.

Bakasana   The Sanskrit term for Crow Pose.

bandhas   Yoga energy-retention techniques.

Bhujangaasana   The Sanskrit term for Snake or Cobra Pose.

Bidalasana   The Sanskrit term for Cat Pose.

bronchial tubes   The section of airway leading from the larynx to the lungs.

bronchioles   Branches of the bronchial tubes that terminate in alveoli.

capillaries   Tiny blood vessels in which oxygen and carbon dioxide are exchanged.

cardiopulmonary   Referring to the joint workings of the heart and lungs.

cardiovascular   Referring to the heart and blood vessels.

chakras   Energy centers in the body thought to be concentrated centers of prana or life-force energy, connected by energy channels. The seven primary chakras are located along the spinal column, at the base of the spine, behind the abdomen, behind the navel, behind the solar plexus, behind the heart, in the throat, on the forehead, and at the crown of the head.

complementary medicine   A holistic approach to healthcare using natural medicine techniques.

developmental arithmetic disorder (DAD)   A condition related to dyslexia and characterized by an inability to correctly process graphic symbols, resulting in difficulty with arithmetic.

developmental reading disorder (DRD)   *See* dyslexia.

developmental writing disorder (DWD)   A condition related to dyslexia and characterized by an inability to correctly process graphic symbols, resulting in difficulty writing.

Dhanurasana   The Sanskrit term for Bow Pose.

diaphragm   A muscular membrane that separates the chest and abdominal cavities. It is roughly disk shaped and expands downward when the lungs expand with an inhalation, then moves upward to help push air out of the lungs with each exhalation.

dyslexia   Also called developmental reading disorder (DRD), this condition is a reading disability resulting from an inability to correctly or completely process graphic symbols.

Eightfold Path   The path of yoga as described by Patanjali in his Yoga Sutras, including values (yamas), expressions of values (niyamas), exercises (asanas), breathing techniques (pranayama), sense withdrawal (pratyahama), concentration (dharana), meditation (dhyana), and interaction with divinity (samadhi).

flow   Also called flow series, this term refers to a yoga vinyasa, or a combination of yoga poses synchronized with breathing and strung together into a flowing motion.

Garudaasana   The Sanskrit term for Eagle Pose.

Halaasana   The Sanskrit term for Plow Pose.

hatha yoga   A branch of yoga on which most modern yoga is based. *Ha* means sun and *tha* means moon, symbolizing the balancing and joining of opposites.

insomnia   The chronic inability to fall asleep or to stay asleep long enough or well enough to feel alert during the day.

integrative medicine   A combination approach to healthcare using both allopathic and natural or complementary medicine, depending on the need.

lacto vegetarian   Someone who doesn't eat any animal products except for milk.

lacto-ovo vegetarian   Someone who doesn't eat meat, fish, or fowl, or other products that involved the killing of an animal, but who eats dairy products and eggs.

larynx   Following the pharynx, the larynx contains the vocal chords or voice box and leads to the trachea.

ligaments   Bands of tissue that connect bone to bone and support the joints.

lochia   The fluid and blood a woman passes for several weeks after giving birth as the body rids itself of excess fluid.

Makaraasana   The Sanskrit term for Crocodile Pose.

mandala   A picture of a circular pattern that draws the eye to its center, to help the mind focus on a single point.

mandala meditation   A form of meditation in which the meditator gazes at a mandala while meditating.

mantra yoga   A form of yoga that uses the chanting of mantras.

mantras   Words or groups of words meant to invoke certain beneficial vibrations, personal associations, and focus when chanted.

Marichiasana   The Sanskrit term for Deer Pose.

Matsynasana   The Sanskrit term for Fish Pose.

meditation   A technique for relaxing and disciplining the mind by teaching it to become very still and aware of the moment, not jumping around to what happened before or what might happen next. Meditation can be practiced by sitting still, walking slowly, or lying down. Yoga exercises help to control the body so it isn't distracting during meditation, one of the original purposes of yoga.

mindfulness   A state of awareness in which a person is consciously present in each moment as it happens rather than dwelling in the past or the future, or automatically performing behaviors.

mudra   The Sanskrit word for "seal," mudra refers to positions and movements other than asanas (yoga exercises) specifically designed to seal energy or prana in the body. The word commonly refers to certain hand positions used during meditation and breathing exercises in which fingers and thumb touch in various positions to form a circuit.

namaste   A Sanskrit word that means "I recognize and honor the divine light within you." It is a nice way to greet or say good-bye to someone, and an especially nice way to end a yoga practice when more than one yogini is involved.

natural medicine   Sometimes called holistic or alternative medicine, natural medicine seeks to adjust the body's own energy to bring about greater self-healing power.

niyamas   Productive habits to cultivate that will help the yogini honor his or her own spirit by maximizing physical, emotional, and spiritual potential, including shauca (purity), santosha (contentment), tapas (discipline), svadhyaya (self-study), and ishvara-pranidhana (devotion to the divine).

Om   A word meant to imitate the original sound of the universe at creation and the vibration that connects all beings in the world. It is a mantra repeated to help focus the mind during meditation, symbolizing unity with all things. It also makes a great vibration when spoken by a group, connecting everyone to each other.

Padmaasana   The Sanskrit term for Lotus Pose.

Patanjali   A man who lived in India, probably sometime around the second century C.E., although no one is sure of the exact date. He systematized centuries of yoga thought and practice into a collection of aphorisms called the Yoga Sutras.

pharynx   The passageway that connects the nasal passages to the vocal chords.

prana   The Hindu word for the life-force energy in the body and the environment that can be taken in and transformed within the body through special breathing techniques called pranayama, and energy retention techniques called bandhas.

pranayama   Yoga breathing techniques designed to infuse the body with prana.

Purva Uttanasana   The Sanskrit term for what we call Slide Pose.

rajasic   The Sanskrit word used to describe a food (or any other influence) that has an effect of agitation, movement, and increased activity on the body and mind.

samyama   A state of being resulting from the complete and thorough investigation of a subject. It is the point when that subject (which could be anything, from yoga to playing the piano) is completely understood. According to yoga philosophy, samyama results from extended contemplation of, focus on, concentration about, meditation on, and study of a subject.

Sarvangaasana   The Sanskrit term for Candle Pose, also called shoulder stand.

sattvic   The Sanskrit word used to describe a food (or any other influence) that has an effect of balance, lightness, and clarity on the body and mind.

Setu Bandha Sarvangaasana   The Sanskrit term for Bridge Pose.

Shavasana   Sanskrit for "corpse pose" or "dead pose," this deep relaxation pose, which we prefer to call "peaceful pose," is meant to bring the body into complete and total deep relaxation by lying flat on the floor, face up, and centering the mind while relinquishing control of the body.

sprain   An injury to a joint resulting from stretched or torn ligaments.

strain   A tearing of muscles or tendons.

Supta Parivartanasana   The Sanskrit term for what we call Twister Pose.

Surya Namaskar   The Sanskrit term for Yoga Sun Dance, often called Sun Salutation.

Tadasana   The Sanskrit term for Mountain Pose.

tamasic   The Sanskrit word used to describe a food (or any other influence) that has an effect of laziness, heaviness, and inactivity on the body and mind.

tendons   Bands of tissue that connect muscle to bone.

trachea   The section of airway leading from the larynx to the bronchial tubes.

Urdhva Dhanursana   The Sanskrit term for Wheel Pose.

Ushtraasana   The Sanskrit term for Camel Pose.

Vasisthasana   The Sanskrit term for Rainbow Pose.

vegan   Someone who doesn't consume any animal products, including dairy products and eggs.

vegetarian   Someone who limits his or her consumption of animal products in a specific way.

vinyasa   A Sanskrit word used to refer to multiple yoga poses synchronized with breathing and strung together into a flowing motion. In contemporary Western yoga classes, vinyasa is often referred to as "flow" or "flow series."

Virabhadraasana   The Sanskrit term for Warrior Pose, used in this book to refer to Warrior Poses I, II, and III.

Vrikshasana   The Sanskrit term for Tree Pose.

yamas   Yoga guidelines for personal thought, behavior, and reaction to one's environment and other people, including ahimsa (non-violence), satya (truthfulness), asteya (not stealing), brahmacharya (chastity), and aparigraha (avoidance of greed).

yoga   Literally "union," yoga is a system of physical and mental exercises meant to synchronize body and mind for a healthier and more aware whole self.

Yoga Sutras   A collection of aphorisms by the ancient Indian sage Patanjali, in which is detailed, among other things, yoga's Eightfold Path, consisting of a list of five values called yamas, a list of five habits of expressions of values called niyamas, and discussions of the importance of yoga exercises (asanas), breathing techniques (pranayama), sense withdrawal (pratyahara), concentration (dharana), meditation (dhyana), and interaction with divinity (samadhi).

yogi   Anyone who practices yoga. Traditionally, the term referred to a man who practices yoga, but today it commonly refers to any adult practicing yoga.

yogini   A child (from infant to teenager) who practices yoga. Traditionally, the term referred to a female yoga practitioner, but because "yogi" is generally used for all adult yoga practitioners, we have chosen "yogini" as our term to represent the child who practices yoga.

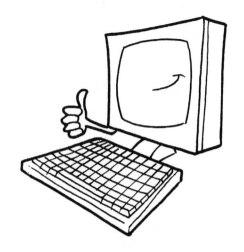

Resources

The world is full of great resources for yoginis. This list includes many of the picture books, yoga and other related books, videos, Web sites, and other resources we have found helpful. We hope you find them helpful, too.

Picture Books

So many excellent and delightful picture books exist for children that we can only begin to scratch the surface, but following are a few of our favorites.

Barner, Bob. *Dem Bones*. San Francisco, California: Chronicle Books, 1996.

Cherry, Lynne. *The Great Kapok Tree: A Tale of the Amazon Rain Forest*. San Diego, California, New York and London: Gulliver Green Books, 1990.

Curtis, Chara M. *All I See Is Part of Me*. Bellvue, Washington: Illumination Arts, 1989.

Hoose, Philip, and Hannah Hoose. *Hey, Little Ant*. Berkeley, California: Tricycle Press, 1998.

Marozollo, Jean. *Pretend You're a Cat*. New York: Penguin Books, 1990.

Most, Bernard. *The Cow That Went OINK*. California, New York, and London: Red Wagon Books, 1990.

Perry, Sarah. *If*. Venice, California: Children's Library Press, 1995.

Wood, Douglas. *Old Turtle*. Duluth, Minnesota: Pfeifer-Hamilton Publishers, 1992.

Yoga and Related Books

Reading is a fantastic way to learn about yoga, your own body, how to improve your health, or anything at all! The following books have all proved helpful to us in our yoga and related pursuits. We think you will enjoy them, too.

Balestrino, Philip. *The Skeleton Inside You*. New York: Junior Books, 1989.

Bowen, Connie. *I Believe in Me: A Book of Affirmations*. Unity Village, Missouri: Unity Books, 1997.

Budilovsky, Joan, and Eve Adamson. *The Complete Idiot's Guide to Yoga*. New York: Alpha Books, 1998.

Chanchani, Swati, and Rajiv Chanchani. *Yoga for Children: A Complete Illustrated Guide to Yoga Including a Manual for Parents and Teachers*. New Delhi: UBSPD, 1995.

Childre, Doc Lew. *Teaching Children to Love: 80 Games and Fun Activities for Raising Balanced Children in Unbalanced Times*. Boulder Creek, California: Planetary Publications, 1996.

Children of Yogaville. *Hatha Yoga for Kids!* Buckingham, Virginia: Integral Yoga Publications, 1990.

Cohen, Kenneth K. *Imagine That: A Child's Guide to Yoga*. Buckingham, Virginia: Integral Yoga Publications, 1983.

Cook, Deanna F. *The Kid's Multicultural Cookbook: Food and Fun Around the World*. Charlotte, Vermont: Williamson Publishing Co., 1995.

Curtis, Sandra R. *The Joy of Movement in Early Childhood*. New York and London: Teachers College Press, 1982.

Das, Baba Ram. *Be Here Now*. New York: Crown Publishers, Inc., 1978.

Dass, Baba Hari. *A Child's Garden of Yoga*. Santa Cruz, California: Sri Rama, 1980.

Dennison, Paul E. and Gail E. Dennison. *Brain Gym: Simple Activities for Whole Brain Learning*. Ventura, California: Edu Kinesthetics, 1992.

Gardner, Howard. *Frames of the Mind*. New York: HarperCollins Publishers, 1983.

Garth, Maureen. *Earthlight: New Meditations for Children.* New York: HarperCollins Publishers, 1997.

——. *Moonbeam: A Book of Meditations for Children.* New York: HarperCollins Publishers, 1992.

——. *Starbright: Meditations for Children.* New York: HarperCollins Publishers, 1991.

Hirschi, Gertrud. *Basic Yoga for Everybody.* York Beach, Maine: Samuel Weiser, Inc., 1998.

Khalsa, Shakta Kaur. *Fly Like a Butterfly: Yoga for Children.* Portland, Oregon: Rudra Press, 1998.

Koch, Isabelle. *Like a Fish in Water: Yoga for Children.* Rochester, Vermont: Inner Traditions, 1999.

Luby, Thia. *Children's Book of Yoga: Games and Exercises Mimic Plants and Animals and Objects.* Santa Fe, New Mexico: Clear Light Publishers, 1998.

——. *Yoga for Teens.* Santa Fe, New Mexico: Clear Light Publishers, 2000.

Mainland, Pauline. *A Yoga Parade of Animals.* Boston, Massachusetts: Element Books, 1998.

Murdock, Maureen. *Spinning Inward: Using Guided Imagery with Children for Learning, Creativity and Relaxation.* Boston, Massachusetts and London: Shambhala, 1987.

Payne, Lauren Murphy. *Just Because I Am: A Child's Book of Affirmation.* Minneapolis, Minnesota: Free Spirit Publishing, Inc., 1994.

Roxman, Deborah. *Meditating with Children: The Art of Concentration and Centering.* Boulder Creek, California: Planetary Publications, 1994.

Schiffman, Erich. *Yoga: The Spirit and Practice of Moving into Stillness.* New York: Pocket Books, 1996.

Stark, Freddy. *Gray's Anatomy: A Fact Filled Coloring Book.* Philadelphia, Pennsylvania and London: Running Press, 1991.

Stewart, Mary, and Kathy Phillips. *Yoga for Children.* London: Webster's International Publishers, 1992.

Sumar, Sonia. *Yoga for the Special Child: A Therapeutic Approach for Infants and Children with Down Syndrome, Cerebral Palsy, and Learning Disabilities.* Buckingham, Virginia: Special Yoga Publications, 1998.

Trivell, Lisa. *I Can't Believe It's Yoga for Kids!* New York: Hatherleigh Press, 2000.

Weiss, Stefanie Iris. *Everything You Need to Know about Yoga: An Introduction for Teens.* New York: The Rosen Publishing Group, Inc., 1999.

Weller, Stella. *Yoga for Children.* San Francisco, California: HarperCollins Publishers, 1996.

Williams, Mary L. *Cool Cats Calm Kids.* Atascadero, California: Impact Publishers, 1996.

Williams, Mary Sue, and Sherry Shellenberger. *How Does Your Engine Run? A Leaders Guide to the Alert Program for Self-Regulation.* Albuquerque, New Mexico: Therapy Works, Inc., 1996.

Magazines

Yoga Journal

Yoga International

Videos, Games, and Activity Sets

Empowerment Activity Book: Discover the Rainbow in You, Imaginazium.

The Human Body: Discover the Wonders of the Human Body: The Skeleton, the Primary Organs, the Body Systems, and How They All Work Together! Nick Graham, M.D.

The Yoga Garden Game: A Cooperative Game for Ages 4 and Up, Jennifer Durand.

Yoga Kit Instruction Book: Fun and Fitness, Imaginazium.

YogaKids: An Easy, Fun-Filled Adventure for Children Ages 3–10 (video), Marsha Wenig, Living Arts.

Music

Africa Fete '98, Island Records.

The Classical Child Volume 1, Ernie Mavrides, Sophia Sounds.

Cloud Fantasy, Eco-Voyage Natures Relaxing Sounds with Music, Madacy Music Group, Inc.

Deep Forest, Celine Music.

Disney's Sebastian: from The Little Mermaid, Worler's Music, Inc.

Don't Worry, Be Happy, words and music by Bobby McFerrin.

A Gift of Love, Deepak and Friends, Rasa.

Jeremiah Was a Bullfrog (Joy to the World), Hoyt Axton, Youngheart.

The Lion King, Walt Disney Records.

More Classical Music for People Who Hate Classical Music, Maxiplay.

The Mozart Effect: Music for Children, Volume 1, Don Campbell, HNH International, Ltd. and Spring Hill Music, Inc.

Mozart for Meditation: Quiet Music for Quiet Times, Polygram.

Music from YogaKids, Chris Bennett and Marsha Wenig, Living Arts.

Ocean Moods, Natural Wonders, World Disc Productions.

Raffi in Concert with the Rise and Shine Band, Troubadour Records, Ltd.

Romantica, Putumayo World Music.

Sacred Earth Drums, David and Steve Gordon, Sequoia Records.

Silly Favorites, Music for Little People.

Songs My Children Taught Me, Mark Isham, Windham Hill Productions Inc.

Songs of Healing, On Wings of Song and Robert Gass, Spring Hill Music.

The Vanishing Rain Forest, Eco-Voyage Nature's Relaxing Sounds with Music, Madacy Music Group, Inc.

Voices of the Rainforest: A Day in the Life of the Kaluli People, Bosavi, Papua New Guinea.

Wee Sing Silly Songs, Pamela Conn Beall and Susan Hagen Nipp, Price Stern Sloan.

Yoga Zone: Music for Meditation, Windham Hill Records.

Props

Herbal Animal Eye Pillows
Herbal Animals, Inc.
P.O. Box 556
Bethesda, MD 20827
Phone: 301-469-7800
Web site: www.herbal-animals.com

Relaxation Blankets
Kozē by Komitor
512 7th Avenue
New York, NY 10018
Phone: 212-921-2524
Web site: www.komitor.com

Thera-Ball
Thera-Band
1245 Home Avenue
Akron, OH 44310
Phone: 1-800-321-2135
Web site: www.thera-band.com

Total Well Being Props, Clothing, and Gifts
Living Arts
P.O. Box 2908
Venice, CA 90291-2939
Phone: 1-800-254-8464
Web site: www.livingarts.com

Toys and Props
Oriental Trading Company, Inc.
P.O. Box 2676
Omaha, NE 68103-2676
Phone: 1-800-228-2269
Web site: www.oriental.com

Yoga Props
Tools for Yoga
2 Green Village Road, Suite 202
Madison, NJ 07928
Phone: 973-966-5311

Web Sites

American Eagle Foundation
www.eagles.org/moreabout.html

Crocodilian Biology Database
www.flmnh.ufl.edu/natsci/herpetology/brittoncrocs/cbd-faq-q2.htm

Crocodilians Web page
crocodilian.com/

Herbal Animals
www.herbal-animals.com

Kozē by Komitor
www.komitor.com

Living Arts
www.livingarts.com

Next Generation Yoga
www.nextgenerationyoga.com

Oriental Trading Company, Inc. (catalog)
www.oriental.com

Thera-Band
www.thera-band.com

Useless Facts Library
www.southhouse.com/useless/factlib1.htm

When Johnny Comes Marching Home Again (hear the song)
members.tripod.com/~Randy_T/johnny.html

Yoga for the Special Child
www.specialyoga.com

The Yoga Garden Game
www.theyogagarden.com

YogaKids
www.yogakids.com

Certified Children's Yoga Teachers

See the following Web sites for updated certified children's yoga instructors:

www.nextgenerationyoga.com

www.specialyoga.com

www.yogakids.com

Index

A

acupuncture, 320
ADD (attention deficit disorder), 121
ADHD (attention deficit hyperactivity disorder), 333-334
Adho Mukha Vrikshasana (Handstand Pose), 223-224
adulthood, 341
All I See Is Part of Me, 363
Alligator Pose, 194-195
allopathic medicine, 320-321
altars, 92
Alternate Nostril Breathing, 141, 272
alveoli, 129
American-style eating habits, 310-312
    families, 311-312
    kids, 310-311
anatomy, 78-79
anger management, 70-73
animals
    poses, 162, 185
        Alligator, 194-195
        Antelope Dash, 190
        Baby Cobra, 176
        Bear Walk, 191-192
        Birds, 166
        Bucking Bronco, 186
        Cactus, 183-184
        Camel, 181-182
        Cat, 162
        Cow, 163-164
        Crocodile, 193-194
        Deer, 187
        Dog, 164-165
        Father Snake, 178-179
        Giraffe Walk, 189-190
        Mother Snake, 177-178
        Mouse, 166
        Owl, 179-180
        Roadrunner, 182
        Shark, 192
        T. rex, 195
        Unicorn, 187-189
    exploring own animal natures, 160-161
    games, 160-161, 253
    observing behaviors, 161-162
Antelope Dash Pose, 190
"Ants Go Marching" March, 209-210
arms, exercises, 26, 285
asanas (exercises), 47, 57. *See also* exercises; poses
ashram, 92
Assist Me exercise, 250-251
associative play, 290
asthma, 322-323
athletics, effects of yoga on, 118
    balanced exercise programs, 118
    maximizing potentials, 120
attention deficit disorder. *See* ADD
attire, 93, 157

B

Baby Breathing, 272, 283
Baby Cobra Pose, 176
Baby Lift Pose, 279
back pain, 324
backpacks, 324
balance, 24
balanced exercise programs, 118
Balloon Breathing, 138, 276
Barner, Bob, 363
Bear Walk Pose, 191-192, 273
Belly Breathing, 137, 271
benefits of yoga
    developmental, 30
        enhancement of natural development, 34
        grade-schoolers, 33
        infants, 31-33
        preschoolers, 32
        special-needs children, 34
        teens, 33
        toddlers, 32
    health
        flexibility, 23
        internal, 16-22
        joint strengthening, 24
        motor coordination, 22
        sleep habits, 28
        spinal, 25-27
        stability and balance, 24
        stamina, 24
Bicycle Pose, 238-239
Bird Poses, 166
    Crow, 173-174
    Eagle, 168
    Flamingo, 167
    Pigeon, 169
    Seagull, 172
    Swan, 171
Boat Poses, 212
    Rowboat, 212-214

body
cross-training, 8
mind-body relationship, 4, 9
    stress management, 67-68
    self-love, 76-77
strengthening physical skills, 7
bonding, parent/child experience, 74, 281
books (resources), 109, 364
boosting self-esteem, 9
Bow Pose, 227
boys. *See* male yoginis
Breath of Fire breathing exercise, 140
breathing, 130
    calm breathing exercises
        Alternate Nostril, 141
        Breathing Staircase, 142-143
        Fly Like a Bird, 141
    chakras, 135-136
    energizing breathing exercises
        Breath of Fire, 140
        Bunny Breathing, 139
        Lion's Breath, 139-140
        Reach for the Sun, 139
        Wood Chopper, 139
    heart's functions, 130
    lung's functions, 129
    postpartum moms, 271-272
    pranas, 127-129
Bridge Pose, 230
bronchioles, 129
Bucking Bronco Pose, 186
Bunny Breathing, 139
Butterfly Pose, 152-153, 276

C

Cactus Pose, 183-184
cake recipes, 352-353

calm breathing exercises
    Alternate Nostril, 141
    Breathing Staircase, 142-143
    Fly Like a Bird, 141
calming of senses (pratyahara), 47, 58
Camel Pose, 181-182, 273, 278
Candle Pose, 241-242
capillaries, 129
cardiopulmonary system, 18-20
cardiovascular system, 18-22
Cat Pose, 162, 273
cerebral palsy, 336
certified yoga teachers, Web sites, 369
chakras, 135-136
challenging poses, 239
    Candle, 241-242
    Fish, 243-244
    Headstand, 244-245
    Lotus, 240-241
    Plow, 242-243
    Pretzel, 239
Chant 'n' Clap chanting game, 133
chanting, 131
    games, 133
    mantras, 132
    songs, 134
Cherry, Lynne, 363
Chi Kung, 250
childhood development
    enhancement of natural development, 34
    milestones, 30
        grade-schoolers, 33
        infants, 31-33
        preschoolers, 32
        teens, 33
        toddlers, 32
    special-needs children, 34
chiropractic care, 321
circulatory system, 16
classes, 112
    finding local classes, 112-113

resources, 112-113
teachers
    meeting, 113
    qualifications, 114-115
trial class, 113
cleanliness (niyama guidelines), 53, 300
clothes. *See* attire
Cloud Floating relaxation exercise, 261
Club Sandwich Pose, 304-305
clubs, 115
    organizational steps, 116
    sample plan, 117
Cobra Family Pose, 303
colic, 284, 322
colors, association with chakras, 135-136
committing to a higher power (niyama guidelines), 56-57
Complete Idiot's Guide to Yoga, The, 364
concentration poses, 326
conflict resolutions
    parents, 73
    stress management, 72
constipation, 18, 323-324
contentment (niyama guidelines), 53
controlling sexual urges (yama guidelines), 51-52
cooperative play, 290
coordination poses, 22, 233
    Bicycle, 238-239
    Crossovers, 237-238
    eye exercises, 234-235
    Toe-Ups, 235-236
    Windmill, 236
Cow Pose, 163-164, 273
creating yoga spaces
    at home, 88-90
    permanent spaces, 92-93
    requirements, 91
    uncluttered environments, 91
    versus playrooms, 90
Crocodile Pose, 193-194

Crocodilian Biology Database Web site, 368
cross-training, 8
Crossovers, 237-238
Crow Pose, 173-174
Curtis, Chara, 363

D

DAD, 333-335
dad poses, 277-279
Dancing Poses, 203-205
de-cluttering yoga spaces, 91
decorations for parties, 350-351
deep relaxation, infants, 288-289
Deer Pose, 187
Dem Bones, 363
depression, postpartum, 274
desert creature poses, 176
  Baby Cobra, 176
  Cactus, 183-184
  Camel, 181-182
  Father Snake, 178-179
  Mother Snake, 177-178
  Owl, 179-180
  Roadrunner, 182
developmental milestones, 30
  enhancement of natural development, 34
  grade-schoolers, 33
  infants, 31-33
  preschoolers, 32
  teens, 33
  toddlers, 32
Dhanurasana (Bow Pose), 227
dharana (focusing techniques), 48, 58-59
dhyana (meditation), 48, 59
diarrhea, 323-324
digestive system, 16-18
Dog Pose, 164-165
Down's Syndrome, 335-336
Downward Facing Dog Pose, 38

Driving My Car Pose, 210
DWD, 333-335
dyslexia, 333

E

Eagle Pose, 168
eating disorders, 52
eating habits
  American-style, 310-312
  developing healthy habits, 315-316
  family meals, 316
  mindful eating, 316
  snacks, 317-318
  yoga-style, 312-315
  vegetarianism, 314-315
Eightfold Path, 47
  asanas (exercises), 57
  dharana (focusing techniques), 58-59
  dhyana (meditation), 59
  family involvement, 60
  niyamas (healthy habits), 48, 53
    ishvar-pranidhana (committing to a higher power), 56-57
    santosha (contentment), 53
    saucha (cleanliness), 53
    svadhyaya (self-study), 55-56
    tapas (self-discipline), 54
  pranayama (breathing exercises), 58
  pratyahara (calming of senses), 58
  samadhi (spiritual communion), 60
  yamas (values), 48-49
    ahimsa (live in peace), 49-50
    aparigraha (greediness), 52
    asteya (refusing to steal), 50-51

brahmacarya (controlling sexual urges), 51-52
  satya (truth), 50
emotions, expressing through yoga, 65
endocrine system, 16
energizing breathing exercises
  Breath of Fire, 140
  Bunny Breathing, 139
  Lion's Breath, 139-140
  Reach for the Sun, 139
  Wood Chopper, 139
energy forces, pranas, 127-129
environmental stresses, 64
equilibrium of motions, 200
execretory system, 16
exercise programs
  balancing with yoga, 118
  coaxing children to exercise, 119-120
exercises. *See also* poses
  breathing, 58
    Alternate Nostril, 141
    Balloon, 138
    Breath of Fire, 140
    Breathing Staircase, 142-143
    Bunny Breathing, 139
    Fly Like a Bird, 141
    Lion's Breath, 139-141
    postpartum moms, 271-272
    Reach for the Sun, 139
    Wood Chopper, 139
  Crossovers, 237-238
  eyes, 234-235
  infants, 34
    arms, 36, 285
    Baby Breather, 283
    feet, 35
    footsies, 283-284
    hips, 284-285
    inversions, 287-288
    knees, 284
    leg lifts and knee bends, 36
    Sleep Pose, 285
    tummy poses, 286

partner yoga
  Assist Me, 250-251
  Mirror Me, 249-250
  Partner Straddle
    Stretching, 248
  relaxation, visual imagery,
    260-264, 274
  toddlers
    toddler's-choice trips,
      293
    trip to the park, 292-293
    trip to the zoo, 291
  Toe-Ups, 235-236
eye exercises, 234-235

F

families
  commitment to a yoga
    routine, 95
  eating habits, 311-312
  family meal traditions, 316
  group yoga, 13-14
  sibling harmony, 306
  walking the yoga path, 60
Family Picnic Pose, 303
Father Snake Pose, 178-179
favors, parties, 353-354
feet
  infant exercises, 35
  footsie exercise, 283-284
  massages, 305
female yoginis, 80, 343-345
  menstruation, 344
  womanhood, 344
fierce animal poses
  Alligator, 194-195
  Bear Walk, 191-192
  Crocodile, 193-194
  Shark, 192
  T. rex, 195
finger foods, 351-352
Fish Pose, 243-244
Flamingo Pose, 167
flexibility poses, 23, 225
  Bow, 227
  Bridge, 230

Sandwich, 228-229
Twister, 226-227
Untying Knots, 225
Wheel, 230
X, 231-232
Flopping Rag Doll Pose, 206
Flower Pose, 153-154
Fly Like a Bird breathing
  exercise, 140, 272
focusing techniques
  (dharana), 48, 58-59
Follow That Mantra chanting
  game, 133
foods
  American-style eating,
    310-311
  parties, 351
    cakes, 352-353
    finger foods, 351-352
  snacks, 317-318
  yoga-style eating, 312
    rajasic, 313
    sattvic, 313
    tamasic foods, 313
    vegetarianism, 314-315
footsie exercise, 283-284
footwear, 93
Frog Pose, 152

G

games
  animals, 160-161
  "Ants Go Marching"
    March, 209-210
  chanting, 133
  group yoga, 252
    Animal Enigma, 253
    inventing games, 255
    Synchronized Yoga,
      254-255
    Whisper in My Ear, 252
    Yogini's Choice, 252
  parties, 354-356
  resources, 366

gas, 323-324
Giraffe Walk Pose, 189-190
girls. *See* female yoginis
gland massages, 20-22
grade-schoolers
  developmental milestones,
    33
  poses, 38-39
  yoginis, 12
*Great Kapok Tree: A Tale of the
  Amazon Rain Forest*, 363
greediness (yama guidelines),
  52
group yoga
  families, 13-14
  games, 252
    Animal Enigma, 253
    inventing, 255
    Synchronized Yoga,
      254-255
    Whisper in My Ear, 252
    Yogini's Choice, 252
  Group Flower Pose, 40
  practices, 108

H

Halaasana (Plow Pose),
  242-243
Half Bow Pose, 37
hand positions (mudras),
  134-135
Handstand Pose, 223-224, 278
Hari Om (mantra), 133
harmony between siblings,
  306
Headstand Pose, 244-245
healing techniques, 320
  acupuncture, 320
  chiropractic care, 321
  homeopathy, 320
  massage therapy, 320
  naturopathy, 321
  reiki, 321
health benefits
  flexibility, 23

internal, 16-17
   digestive and elimination, 18
   heart and lungs, 18-20
   massages, 20-22
joint strengthening, 24
motor coordination, 22
natural remedies, 322
   asthma, 322-323
   back pain, 324
   colic, 322
   sprains, 325
   upset stomachs, 323-324
sleep habits, 28
spinal, 25
   nervous system, 27
   postures, 26-27
stability and balance, 24
stamina, 24
niyamas (healthy habits), 47-48
   ishvar-pranidhana (committing to a higher power), 56-57
   santosha (contentment), 53
   saucha (cleanliness), 53
   svadhyaya (self-study), 55-56
   tapas (self-discipline), 54
heart
   resting heartrate, 19-20
   role in breathing process, 130
Helicopter Pose, 24
herbal animal eye pillows, 367
Herbal Animals Web site, 368
Hero Pose, 216
Hey, Little Ant, 363
higher powers (niyama guidelines), 56-57
hip exercises, 284-285
holding poses, 215
home yoga spaces, 88-90
homeopathy, 320
honoring yoga spaces, 94

Hoose, Hannah, 363
Hoose, Philip, 363
hypermobility, 335-336
hypocerebratonicity, 337

I

I Believe in Me: A Book of Affirmations, 364
If, 363
imaginative exploration, 146
immobility, 336-337
independence of teen yoginis, 340-341
indoor yoga practices, 106-107
infants
   developmental milestones, 31-33
   exercises
      arms, 285
      Baby Breather, 283
      footsies, 283-284
      hips, 284-285
      inversions, 287-288
      knees, 284
   parent/child bonding experience, 281
   poses, 34-36
      Sleep Pose, 285
      tummy poses, 286
   relaxation, 288-289
   siblings' reactions, 295-297
   yoginis, 12
insomnia, 28
integumentary system, 16
integrative medicine, 321
intelligences
   interpersonal, 105
   intrapersonal, 106
   kinesthetic, 105
   linguistics, 103
   logical, 104
   musical, 104
   visual, 104

internal health, 16-17
   digestive and elimination, 18
   heart and lungs, 18-20
   massages, 20, 22
interpersonal intelligence (learning style), 105
intrapersonal intelligence (learning style), 106
inventing
   games, 255
   poses, 82-83
inversions, 242, 287-288
invitations for parties, 350

J-L

Japanese Sitting Pose, 276
joints, strengthening, 24

karma, 51
kinesthetic intelligence (learning style), 105
knee exercises, 284
Kozē by Komitor Web site, 368

lacto vegetarians, 314
lacto-ovo vegetarians, 314
larynx, 129
learning-challenged children, 121, 332
   ADHD, 333-334
   DAD, 333-335
   DWD, 333-335
   dyslexia, 333
learning styles, personality quiz, 99-102
   communicators, 103
   interpersonal, 105
   intrapersonal, 106
   master of logic, 104
   musical intelligence, 104
   touch-oriented, 105
   visual intelligence, 104
leg exercises, 36
Lion's Breath breathing exercise, 139-140

live in peace (yama guidelines), 49-50, 299
liver massages, 21-22
Living Arts Web site, 369
location of chakras, 135-136
lochia, 273
logical intelligence, 104
Lotus Pose, 240-241, 273
lungs, breathing process, 129

M

magazines (resources), 366
Makaraasana (Crocodile Pose),
193-194
male yoginis, 80, 341-343
strength-building, 342
transition to manhood,
342
mandala meditation, 104
manhood, 342
mantra yoga, 104
mantras, 132-134
chanting games, 133
songs, 134
Marichyasana (Deer Pose),
187
Marozollo, Jean, 363
massage therapy, 320
massages
feet, 305
glands, 20, 22
internal organs, 20, 22
liver, 21-22
master of logic (learning
style), 104
mats, 93
Matsynasan (Fish Pose),
243-244
meditation, 9
dharana, 59
dhyana, 48
mandala meditation, 104
meetings, yoga clubs, 116-117
menstruation, 344

milestones of childhood
development, 30
grade-schoolers, 33
infants, 31-33
preschoolers, 32
teens, 33
toddlers, 32
mind
building a strong mind, 8
meditation, 9
mind-body relationship,
4, 9
self-love, 76-77
stress management,
67-68
mindfulness, 65-66
Mirror Me exercise, 249-250
moms (postpartum)
breathing exercises,
271-272
depression, 274
poses, 270-275
Bear Walk, 273
Butterfly, 276
Camel, 273
Cat, 273
Cow, 273
Japanese Sitting Pose,
276
Mountain, 274
Mouse, 273
Shavasana relaxation,
274
Snake, 273
Tree, 274
Warrior II, 277
Yoga Sun Dance, 274
"monkey mind," 67-68
Most, Bernard, 363
Mother Snake Pose, 177-178
motor coordination, 22
Mountain Pose, 149, 274
Mouse Pose, 166, 273
movement, 199
poses
Boat, 212-214
Driving My Car, 210
Flopping Rag Doll, 206

Rock and Roll, 211-212
Roller Coaster Spin,
205-206
Volcano Blast, 207-208
Yoga Dancing, 203-205
equilibrium, 200-201
rhythm, 200
mudras (hand positions),
134-135
muscular system, 16
music (resources), 366-367
musical intelligence (learning
style), 104

N

Namaste, 264
naming yoga clubs, 116
natural medicine, 320
healing techniques, 320
acupuncture, 320
chiropractic care, 321
homeopathy, 320
massage therapy, 320
naturopathy, 321
reiki, 321
remedies, 322
asthma, 322-323
back pain, 324
colic, 322
sprains, 325
upset stomachs, 323-324
versus allopathic medicine,
321
nature
imaginative exploration,
146
observation, 5-6
poses, 149
Butterfly, 152-153
Flower, 153-154
Frog, 152
Mountain, 149
Rainbow, 155
Star, 154
Tree, 150-152
respecting, 147-148

walks, 157
   attire, 157
   observations, 157-158
naturopathy, 321
nervous system, 16, 27
Next Generation Yoga Web
   site, 369
next generation yoginis, 345
niyamas (healthy habits), 47,
   53
   ishvar-pranidhana (com-
      mitting to a higher
      power), 56-57
   santosha (contentment),
      53
   saucha (cleanliness), 53
   svadhyaya (self-study),
      55-56
   tapas (self-discipline), 54

O

Old Turtle, 363
Om (mantra), 46, 133
Om Jothi (mantra), 133
Om Shanti (mantra), 133
onlooker play, 290
optional props, 93-94
organization of yoga clubs,
   116-117
Oriental Trading Company
   Web site, 369
outdoor yoga practices,
   106-107
Owl Pose, 179-180

P

Padmaasana (Lotus Pose),
   240-241
parallel play, 290
paralysis, 336-337
parenting
   cultivating contentment,
      54
   encouraging child, 109-110

model behaviors, 73
parent/child bonding experience, 74, 281
self-discipline, 54
parties, 348
   decorations, 350-351
   favors, 353-354
   foods, 351
      cakes, 352-353
      finger foods, 351-352
   invitations, 350
   necessities, 348
   poses, 354-356
   safety, 349
   themes, 349
Partner Straddle Stretching
   exercise, 248
partner yoga exercises, 247
   Assist Me, 250-251
   Mirror Me, 249-250
   Partner Straddle Stretching,
      248
Parvatasana (Hero Pose), 216
Paschima Uttanasana
   (Sandwich Pose), 228-229
Patanjali, 47
PDD (pervasive develop-
   mental delay), 121
permanent yoga spaces, 92-93
Perry, Sarah, 363
personality quiz (learning
   styles), 99-102
   communicators, 103
   interpersonal, 105
   intrapersonal, 106
   master of logic, 104
   musical intelligence, 104
   touch-oriented, 105
   visual intelligence, 104
pervasive developmental
   delay. *See* PDD
pharynx, 129
physical skills
   cross-training, 8
   strengthening, 7
physically challenged children, 122, 335
   cerebral palsy, 336

Down's Syndrome, 335-336
hypocerebratonicity, 337
immobility, 336-337
paralysis, 336-337
picture books (resources), 363
Pigeon Pose, 169
playrooms versus yoga spaces,
   90
Plow Pose, 242-243
poses. *See also* exercises
   birds
      Crow, 173-174
      Eagle, 168
      Flamingo, 167
      Pigeon, 169
      Seagull, 172
      Swan, 171
   challenging, 239
      Candle, 241-242
      Fish, 243-244
      Headstand, 244-245
      Lotus, 240-241
      Plow, 242-243
      Pretzel, 239
   concentration, 326
   coordination, 233
      Bicycle, 238-239
      Crossovers, 237-238
      eye exercises, 234-235
      Toe-Ups, 235-236
      Windmill, 236
   dads, 277-279
   desert creatures, 176
      Baby Cobra, 176
      Cactus, 183-184
      Camel, 181-182
      Father Snake, 178-179
      Mother Snake, 177-178
      Owl, 179-180
      Roadrunner, 182
   Downward Facing Dog
      Pose, 38
   farm animals, 162
      Bird, 166
      Cat, 162
      Cow, 163-164
      Dog, 164-165
      Mouse, 166

fierce animals
  Alligator, 194-195
  Bear Walk, 191-192
  Crocodile, 193-194
  Shark, 192
  T. rex, 195
flexibility, 225
  Bow, 227
  Bridge, 230
  Sandwich, 228-229
  Twister, 226-227
  Untying Knots, 225
  Wheel, 230
  X, 231-232
grade-schoolers, 38-39
Group Flower Pose, 40
group yoga, 252-255
Half Bow, 37
Helicopter Pose, 24
holding, 215
infants, 34-36
inventing, 82-83
movement
  Boat, 212-214
  Driving My Car, 210
  Flopping Rag Doll, 206
  Rock and Roll, 211-212
  Roller Coaster Spin,
    205-206
  Volcano Blast, 207-208
  Yoga Dancing, 203-205
nature, 149
  Butterfly, 152-153
  Flower, 153-154
  Frog, 152
  Mountain, 149
  Rainbow, 155
  Star, 154
  Tree, 150, 152
parties, 354-356
postpartum moms. *See*
  postpartum moms
preschoolers, 38
Shavasana relaxation
  before bedtime, 264
  ending practice, 264
  establishing right envi-
    ronment, 258

practice times, 265
  visual imagery, 260-264
siblings, 302
  Club Sandwich, 304-305
  Cobra Family, 303
  Family Picnic, 303
  foot massages, 305
  Puppy Play with
    Downward Facing
    Dog, 302
Sleep Pose, 285
strength, 216
  Handstand, 223-224
  Hero Pose, 216
  Slide, 222
  Superperson, 217
  Table, 221-222
  Warrior I, 218-220
  Warrior II, 220
  Warrior III, 221
teens, 39-40
toddlers, 36-37
tummy poses, 286
wild animals, 185
  Antelope Dash, 190
  Bucking Bronco, 186
  Deer, 187
  Giraffe Walk, 189-190
  Unicorn, 187-189
Yoga Sun Dance, 201-203
postpartum moms
  breathing exercises,
    271-272
  depression, 274
  poses, 270-275
    Bear Walk, 273
    Butterfly, 276
    Camel, 273
    Cat, 273
    Cow, 273
    Japanese Sitting, 276
    Mountain, 274
    Mouse, 273
    Shavasana relaxation,
      274
    Snake, 273
    Tree, 274
    Warrior II, 277
    Yoga Sun Dance, 274

postures, 26-27
practices
  learning styles, 99-106
  routines, 109
  special-needs children, 330
  structure guidelines, 98
  types, 106
    group, 108
    indoors, 106-107
    outdoors, 106-107
    solo, 108
    supervised, 108
    unsupervised, 108
pranas, 127-129
pranayama (breathing exercises), 47, 58
pratyahara (calming of
  senses), 47, 58
preschoolers
  developmental milestones,
    32
  poses, 38
  yoginis, 12
Pretend You're a Cat, 363
Pretzel Pose, 239, 273
progressive stages of yoga, 79
props, 93
  herbal animal eye pillows,
    367
  mats, 93
  optional props, 93-94
  relaxation blankets, 368
  thera-ball, 368
Puppy Play with Downward
  Facing Dog Pose, 302
Purvottanasana (Slide Pose),
  222

Q-R

qualifications of teachers,
  114-115

Rainbow Pose, 155
Rainbow relaxation exercise,
  260
Rainforest relaxation exercise,
  262-264
rajasic foods, 313

Reach for the Sun breathing exercise, 139
refusing to steal (yama guidelines), 50-51
reiki, 321
relaxation
    blankets, 368
    infants, 288-289
    Shavasana, 258
        before bedtime, 264
        ending practice, 264
        establishing right environment, 258
        postpartum moms, 274
        practice times, 265
        visual imagery, 260-264
    visual imagery exercises, 260
        Cloud Floating, 261
        ending practice, 264
        Rainbow relaxation, 260
        Rainforest relaxation, 262-264
religions, spirituality of yoga, 46-47
remedies (natural), 322
    asthma, 322-323
    back pain, 324
    colic, 322
    sprains, 325
    upset stomachs, 323-324
reproductive system, 17
resources
    books, 109, 364
    classes, 112-113
    games, 366
    magazines, 366
    music, 366-367
    picture books, 363
    videos, 109, 366
respect
    sibling synchronicity, 299
    nature, 147-148
respiratory system, 17-20
Return to Love, A, 82
rhythm, 200
Roadrunner Pose, 182
Rock and Roll Pose, 211-212

Roller Coaster Spins, 205-206
routines
    family commitments, 95
    practices, 109
    sample, 98
Rowboat Pose, 212-214

S

safety at yoga parties, 349
Sailboat Pose, 212
samadhi (spiritual communion), 48, 60
samples
    club plans, 117
    routines, 98
samyama (concept of yoga), 122-123
Sandwich Pose, 228-229
Sarvangaasana (Candle Pose), 241-242
sattvic foods, 313
Seagull Pose, 172
self-discipline (niyama guidelines), 54, 299-300
self-esteem, 9, 81-82
self-knowledge (anatomy), 77-79
self-love, teaching, 76,
    mind-body union, 76-77
    trust, 77
self-study (niyama guidelines), 55-56
senses, calming, 58
Setu Bandha Sarvangaasana (Bridge Pose), 230
sexual urges (yama guidelines), 51-52
Shark Pose, 192
Shavasana relaxation, 258, 277-279
    before bedtime, 264
    ending practice, 264
    establishing right environment, 258
    postpartum moms, 274
    practice times, 265
    visual imagery, 260-264

siblings
    bonding with yoga, 298
    dealing with new baby, 295-297
    harmony, 306
    poses, 302
        Club Sandwich, 304-305
        Cobra Family, 303
        Family Picnic, 303
        foot massages, 305
        Puppy Play with Downward Facing Dog, 302
    synchronicity steps
        cleanliness, 300
        live in peace, 299
        respect, 299
        self-control, 299
        self-discipline, 300
        sharing, 299
        spiritual journeys, 301
        studying together, 301
        truthfulness, 299
        worries, 300
skeletal system, 17
Skeleton Inside You, 364
sleep habits
    improving, 28
    insomnia, 28
    Shavasana relaxation, 264
Sleep Pose, 37, 285
Slide Pose, 222
snacks, 317-318
Snake poses, 176, 273
    Baby Cobra Pose, 176
    Father Snake Pose, 178-179
    Mother Snake Pose, 177-178
socializer (learning style), 105-106
solitary play, 290
solo practices, 108
songs, mantra songs, 134
spaces for yoga
    at home
        creating, 88
        surveying qualities, 88-90

honoring, 94
permanent spaces, 92-93
requirements, 91
uncluttered environments, 91
versus playrooms, 90
special-needs children, 34, 121, 330
designing practice schedules, 330
learning-challenged, 121, 332
ADHD, 333-334
DAD, 333-335
DWD, 333-335
dyslexia, 333
physically challenged, 122, 335
cerebral palsy, 336
Down's Syndrome, 335-336
hypocerebratonicity, 337
immobility, 336-337
paralysis, 336-337
spinal health benefits of yoga, 25
nervous system, 27
postures, 26-27
spiritual communion (samadhi), 48, 60
spirituality
embracing of all religions, 46-47
finding spiritual identity, 46
yoga without spiritual aspects, 46
sibling synchronicity, 301
sports, effects of yoga on, 118
balanced exercise programs, 118
maximizing potentials, 120
sprains, 325
stability, 24
Staircase breathing exercises, 142-143

stamina, 24
Star Pose, 154
stealing (yama guidelines), 50-51
sticky mats, 93
stillness, 258
strains, 325
strength poses, 216
Handstand, 223-224
Hero, 216
Slide, 222
Superperson, 217
Table, 221-222
Warrior I, 218, 220
Warrior II, 220
Warrior III, 221
strength-building
joints, 24
male yoginis, 342
mental capacities, 8
physical skills, 7-8
stress management, 64
anger, 70
competition, 71
conflict resolutions, 72
environmental stressors, 64
expressing emotions, 65
internal stressors, 64
mind-body relationship, 67-68
mindfulness, 65-66
modeling parent behaviors, 73
positive behaviors, 64
structure of practices, 98
Sun Salutation, 201-203, 274
Superperson Pose, 217
supervised practices, 108
Supta Parivartanasana (Twister Pose), 226-227
Surya Namaskar (Yoga Sun Dance), 201-203
Swan pose, 171
synchroncity of siblings, steps
cleanliness, 300
live in peace, 299
respect, 299

self-control, 299
self-discipline, 300
sharing, 299
spiritual journeys, 301
studying together, 301
truthfulness, 299
worries, 300
Synchronized Yoga game, 254-255

T

Table Pose, 221-222
tamasic foods, 313
Tarzan Holler exercise, 195-196, 278
teachers
meeting, 113
qualifications, 114-115
teen yoginis, 12
adulthood, 341
developmental milestones, 33
independence, 340-341
poses, 39-40
themes for parties, 349
Thera-Ball, 368
Thera-Band Web site, 369
thyroid gland, 21
toddler yoginis, 12
developmental milestones, 32
exercises
toddler's-choice trip, 293
trip to the park, 292-293
trip to the zoo, 291
learning through play, 289
poses, 36-37
Toe-Up exercises, 235-236
touch-oriented
learning styles, 105
trachea, 129
tradition of yoga, 5-6
Tree Pose, 150-152, 274
trip to the park exercise, 292-293

trip to the zoo exercise, 291
trust, teaching self-love, 77
truthfulness, sibling synchronicity, 299
truths (yama guidelines), 50
tummy poses, 286
Twister Pose, 226-227
T. rex Pose, 195

U

uncluttered environments (yoga spaces), 91
Unicorn Pose, 187-189
union, mind-body relationship, 4, 9
    stress management, 67-68
    self-love, 76-77
unoccupied play, 290
unsupervised practices, 108
Untying Knots Pose, 225
upset stomachs, 323-324
Urdhva Dhanurasana (Wheel Pose), 230
Useless Facts Library Web site, 369

V

values (yamas), 47-49
    ahimsa (live in peace), 49-50
    aparigraha (greediness), 52
    asteya (refusing to steal), 50-51
    brahmacarya (controlling sexual urges), 51-52
    satya (truth), 50
vegetarianism, 314-315
videos (resources), 109, 366
vinyasa (multiple poses), 200-203
Virabhadrasana I (Warrior I Pose), 218-220
Virabhadrasana II (Warrior II Pose), 220

Virabhadrasana III (Warrior III Pose), 221
visual imagery exercises
    postpartum moms, 274, 277
    relaxation, 260
        Cloud Floating, 261
        ending practice, 264
        Rainbow, 260
        Rainforest, 262-264
visual intelligence (learning styles), 104
vital signs, 19-20
Volcano Blast Pose, 207-208

W

walks, nature walks, 157
    attire, 157
    observations, 157-158
Warrior I Pose, 218-220
Warrior II Pose, 220
Warrior III Pose, 221
Web sites
    Crocodilian Biology Database, 368
    Crocodilians, 368
    Herbal Animals, 368
    Kozē by Komitor, 368
    Living Arts, 369
    Next Generation Yoga, 369
    Oriental Trading Company, 369
    Thera-Band, 369
    Useless Facts Library, 369
    Yoga Garden Game, 369
    YogaKids, 369
Wheel Pose, 230
Whisper in My Ear game, 252
wild animal poses, 185
    Antelope Dash, 190
    Bucking Bronco Pose, 186
    Deer Pose, 187
    Giraffe Walk, 189-190
    Unicorn, 187-189
Williamson, Marianne, 82

Windmill Pose, 236
Wise Owl Pose, 179-180
womanhood, 344
Wood Chopper breathing, 139
Wood, Douglas, 363
worries, sibling synchronicity, 300

X-Z

X Pose, 231-232

yamas (values), guidelines 47-49
    ahimsa (live in peace), 49-50
    aparigraha (greediness), 52
    asteya (refusing to steal), 50-51
    brahmacarya (controlling sexual urges), 51-52
    satya (truth), 50
yoga
    description of, 4
        traditions, 5-6
        union between body and mind, 4
    developmental benefits, 30
        enhancement of natural development, 34
        grade-schoolers, 33
        infants, 31-33
        preschoolers, 32
        special-needs children, 34
        teens, 33
        toddlers, 32
    health benefits
        flexibility, 23
        internal, 16-20, 22
        joint strengthening, 24
        motor coordination, 22
        sleep habits, 28
        spinal, 25-27
        stability and balance, 24
        stamina, 24

without spirituality, 46
yoginis, 11
    grade-schoolers, 12
    infants, 12
    preschoolers, 12
    teens, 12
    toddlers, 12
Yoga Dancing, 203-205
Yoga for the Special Child, 34,
    282
Yoga Garden Game Web site,
    369
Yoga Sun Dance, 201-203, 274
yoga-style eating habits, 312
    rajasic foods, 313
    sattvic foods, 313
    tamasic foods, 313
    vegetarianism, 314-315
YogaKids Web site, 369
Yogini's Choice game, 252
yoginis, 11
    females, 343-345
    grade-schoolers, 12, 38-39
    infants, 12, 34-36
    learning styles, 99-106
    males, 341-343
    next generation, 345
    preschoolers, 12, 38
    special-needs children, 121
        learning challenges, 121
        physical challenges, 122
    teens, 12
        adulthood, 341
        independence, 340-341
        poses, 39-40
    toddlers, 12
        exercises, 291-293
        learning through play,
            289
        poses, 36

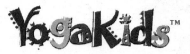

Adventures in Health, Harmony, and Education

"Bringing peace and understanding through yoga ... one child at a time."

Are you interested in teaching yoga to children?

Share the gifts of yoga with children!

Become a Certified YogaKids™ Facilitator.

Marsha Wenig's YogaKids™ Facilitator Certification Program provides you with a unique set of teaching skills that work magic with children. YogaKids is the only program that uses yoga as a springboard into other areas of learning. It integrates reading, storytelling, games, music, and other arts into a complete curriculum to engage the "whole child" in the multiple intelligences theory of learning—employing ecology, anatomy, earth care, and life lessons that echo the yogic principles of interdependence, oneness and FUN!

> *"Marsha Wenig manages to enchant while she teaches and give the essence and spirit of yoga while making it a whole lot of fun. Would that the rest of education could be this profound and exciting ..."*

—*Dr. Jean Houston, author, educator, and visionary*

Marsha Wenig is the creator of the internationally acclaimed video *YogaKids*™. She is a recipient of both the Parent's Choice Award and honors from The Coalition for Quality Children's Media. Her Certification Program is currently training hundreds of educators, parents, and health care professionals around the world to share yogic wisdom with children.

YogaKids™ video, audio tape, and T-shirts are available to order. The video and audio tape are sold together for $15. T-shirts are $15. A special package of the *YogaKids*™ video, audio tape, and T-shirt is available for $28. (Add $5 for shipping and handling on each package.)

Become a part of the YogaKids™ Bridge of Diamonds Foundation. The Bridge of Diamonds is committed to empowering children to love themselves and one another. Its aim is to link children together through the practice and living of the YogaKids™ philosophy. Like diamonds shining brightly, children globally will join together and build a bridge that illuminates the world for us all.

For more information on the Bridge of Diamonds Foundation, YogaKids™ products, a free brochure and schedule of upcoming YogaKids™ programs, or to register for a Phase 1 YogaKids™ Training, call 1-800-968-0694, visit our Web site at www.yogakids.com, or send this coupon to:

YogaKids
2501 Oriole Trail #8
Long Beach, IN 46360

Name: _____

Address: _____

City/State/Zip: _____

Telephone/e-mail: _____

Please send me free information on: _____

_____

Please send the following items: _____

_____

_____ A check or money order is enclosed

_____ Please charge: _____ American Express   _____ Visa   _____ MasterCard

Account number: _____

Expiration date: _____

Signature: _____

Indiana residents add 5% sales tax.

Payment to be made in U.S. funds. Prices and availability are subject to change at any time without notice.

This coupon entitles you to take $25 off the price of the Phase 1 YogaKids Introductory Weekend.